NOVEL STRATEGIES IN THE DESIGN AND PRODUCTION OF VACCINES

ADVANCES IN EXPERIMENTAL MEDICINE AND BIOLOGY

Recent Volumes in this Series

Volume 389
INTRACELLULAR PROTEIN CATABOLISM
Edited by Koichi Suzuki and Judith S. Bond

Volume 390
ANTIMICROBIAL RESISTANCE: A Crisis in Health Care
Edited by Donald L. Jungkind, Joel E. Mortensen, Henry S. Fraimow,
and Gary B. Calandra

Volume 391
NATURAL TOXINS 2: Structure, Mechanism of Action, and Detection
Edited by Bal Ram Singh and Anthony T. Tu

Volume 392
FUMONISINS IN FOOD
Edited by Lauren S. Jackson, Jonathan W. DeVries, and Lloyd B. Bullerman

Volume 393
MODELING AND CONTROL OF VENTILATION
Edited by Stephen J. G. Semple, Lewis Adams, and Brian J. Whipp

Volume 394
ANTIVIRAL CHEMOTHERAPY 4: New Directions for Clinical Application and Research
Edited by John Mills, Paul A. Volberding, and Laurence Corey

Volume 395
OXYTOCIN: Cellular and Molecular Approaches in Medicine and Research
Edited by Richard Ivell and John A. Russell

Volume 396
RECENT ADVANCES IN CELLULAR AND MOLECULAR ASPECTS OF
ANGIOTENSIN RECEPTORS
Edited by Mohan K. Raizada, M. Ian Phillips, and Colin Sumners

Volume 397
NOVEL STRATEGIES IN THE DESIGN AND PRODUCTION OF VACCINES
Edited by Sara Cohen and Avigdor Shafferman

NOVEL STRATEGIES IN THE DESIGN AND PRODUCTION OF VACCINES

Edited by

Sara Cohen and **Avigdor Shafferman**

Israel Institute for Biological Research
Ness-Ziona, Israel

Springer Science+Business Media, LLC

Library of Congress Cataloging-in-Publication Data

On file

Proceedings of the 39th OHOLO Conference on Vaccines: Novel Strategies in Design and Production, held May 7–11, 1995, in Eilat, Israel

DOI 10.1007/978-1-4899-1382-1

© 1996 Springer Science+Business Media New York
Originally published by Plenum Press, New York in 1996
MyCopy version of the original edition 1996

10 9 8 7 6 5 4 3 2 1

www.springer.com/mycopy

39TH OHOLO CONFERENCE

Eliat, Israel, May 7-11, 1995

SCIENTIFIC ORGANIZING COMMITTEE

Avigdor Shafferman	Israel Institute for Biological Research, Ness-Ziona, Israel
Sara Cohen	Israel Institute for Biological Research, Ness-Ziona, Israel
Moshe White	Israel Institute for Biological Research, Ness-Ziona, Israel
Shaul Reuveny	Israel Institute for Biological Research, Ness-Ziona, Israel
Baruch Velan	Israel Institute for Biological Research, Ness-Ziona, Israel

SCIENTIFIC ADVISORY COMMITTEE

Ruth Arnon	Weizmann Institute, Rehovot, Israel
Jonathan Gershoni	Tel-Aviv University, Tel-Aviv, Israel
Rino Rappuoli	IRIS, Siena, Italy
Amos Panet	B.T.G., Jerusalem, Israel
Jerald Sadoff	WRAIR, Washington D.C., United States
Florian Schödel	Inserm, Lyon, France
Raymond Spier	Surrey University, Guildford, United Kingdom

ALEXANDER KOHN

1919-1994

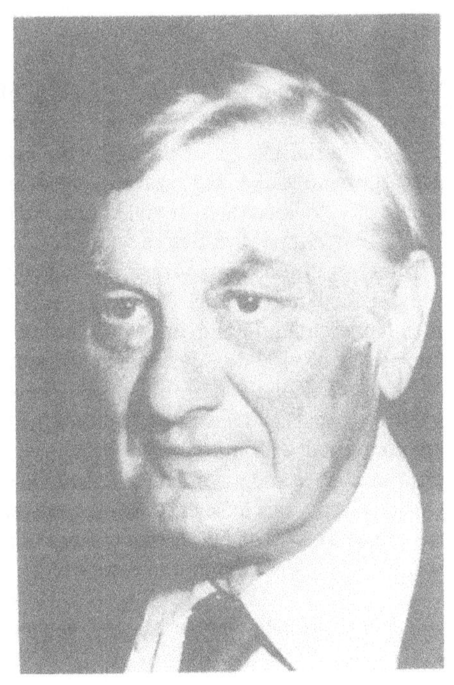

The tradition of the OHOLO Conferences was initiated 39 years ago in 1955 in Oholo on the banks of the Lake of Galilee. The aim of these was to bring together scientists from abroad and from Israel and set the grounds for ongoing scientific interactions. The founder and the driving force behind the OHOLO Conference was Professor Alexander Kohn, known to everybody by his nickname Leshek. By finding the right balance between serious scientific discussions and a very friendly atmosphere, Leshek established the specific character of the OHOLO meetings. Leshek was famous for his generous hospitality. He spared no effort in providing a warm welcome to the guests, from tours of historic sites to entertainment in the evening, the epitome of which were his productions, depicting the topic of the specific conference in a humoristic way. He pursued this task until his retirement from the Israel Institute for Biological Research, IIBR Ness Ziona in 1984.

Professor Alexander Kohn was born on March 8, 1919, in Poland. At the age of 18 he emigrated to Israel where he studied microbiology at the Hebrew University in Jerusalem from 1937-1940. Being aware of the fate of the Jewish people during the Second World War, he joined the Jewish Brigade (8th Army) and fought in North Africa and Italy through 1946. After an absence of 6 years, he resumed his studies in the Hebrew University, and received his M.Sc. degree in bacteriology in 1947. His Ph.D. thesis, dealing with the behavior of microorganisms in the air under normal and artificial conditions, was awarded to him in 1952.

Leshek joined IIBR in 1952 and very soon became one of the leading faculty members of the institute. In 1956 he was appointed Head of the Department of Biophysics, in 1960 he became Deputy Director for Research, and in 1970 he was appointed the position of Director of IIBR. His activity at IIBR was interspersed with sabbatical leaves at the Institute of Microbiology, Rutgers University, where he collaborated with Prof. W. Szybalski, at the Molecular Biology and Virus Laboratory, University of California at Berkeley, at the Imperial Cancer Research Foundation, London, and at the Virus Oncology Laboratory, University of Chicago.

Prof. Kohn acted as Vice President of the Israel Association for the Advancement of Science, as well as president of the Israel Society for Microbiology, and served as member of the editorial boards of the *Israel Journal of Medical Science*, the *Journal of Medical Virology*, and *Gene*. He was appointed as Professor for Microbiology at the Tel-Aviv University, Medical School and later acted as senate member.

Prof. Kohn's main research activity revolved around viruses and development of viral vaccines, for human and veterinary diseases. In addition, he was fascinated by the process of virus-cell interactions (budding), which eventually led him to numerous studies of membrane structure and function. During the last period of his life, he applied his vast knowledge of viral diseases to development of methods for rapid viral diagnostics.

Prof. Kohn's scientific publications totaled more than two hundred papers in reviewed journals and meetings. He was an editor and author of six books. His two last books are connected with moral issues related to research. *False Prophets* deals with fraud and error in science and medicine, and *Fortune and Failure* deals with missed opportunities and chance discoveries in science. Humor played a central part in Prof. Kohn's life. He was the founder and editor of the *Journal of Irreproducible Research* (J.I.R.), a satirical journal where scientists laugh at science and themselves.

Leshek died on November 29, 1994, after a short illness. His wife Chana, his son Yoram and his daughter Ruth, and four grandchildren at his bedside.

PREFACE

Vaccination is one of the most efficient and cost effective methods of promoting human health and has been in clinical use for at least 200 years. Nevertheless, infectious diseases continue to constitute a constant threat to the well being of humanity. Common pathogens, once believed to be under control, acquire increased virulence and resistance to drugs, while exotic microorganisms emerged from hidden reservoirs to cause yet incurable diseases in humans. These changes, together with epidemic outbreaks related to political and socio-economic instabilities, increase the needs for the development of new, advanced vaccines. In this volume, devoted to the proceedings of the 39th OHOLO Conference, we present some of the recent strategies for the design and production of novel vaccines.

The advent of recombinant DNA technology has stimulated the production of several subunit vaccines. In spite of the obvious advantages to this approach, the limited immunogenicity of many subunit candidates has hindered their development. Strategies to enhance the immunogenicity of subunit vaccines is therefore critical. Several approaches toward this goal, including design of novel adjuvants and delivery systems as well as design of advantageous carriers, are presented here. Among the carriers evaluated here are polypeptides (flagellin, HBV core antigen, β-galactosidase), attenuated virions (Vaccinia, Sindbis), and nonpathogenic licensed bacteria (*Salmonella*).

The developments in molecular biology have also provided the tools for design of a new generation of live vaccines. Live attenuated vaccines and native detoxified toxins, derived in the past by empirical methods, can now be engineered by precise molecular tailoring to offer a greater level of safety. This approach is exemplified in this volume by the generation of genetically modified pertusis and cholera toxin vaccines, hybrid SFV/Sindbis alphavirus, and attenuated bacterial vaccines for anthrax and cholera.

An additional development in the field of bacterial vaccines is related to the recent large-scale application of subcellular fractions as demonstrated here for staphylcocci polysaccharide vaccine and meningococcal outer membrane protein. This was brought about by improving immunogenicity of these fractions by appropriate formulation.

The recent most revolutionary development in vaccination is related to nucleic acid vaccines. Such vaccines are of particular interest not only for novelty of the concept but also for practical advantages, as well as their capacity to generate both cellular and humoral responses. The power of this approach is exhibited in this volume by evaluation of DNA-based vaccines to influenza, HIV and *Mycobacterium tuberculosis*.

The development of novel vaccines relies very much on the availability of effective procedures for their production and evaluation in humans. Advances in vaccine production in recent years include development of well characterized, validated manufacturing processes with appropriate in-process controls as exemplified here in production of hepatitis and influenza vaccines and formulation of various combination vaccines. Determination of efficacy in preclinical and specifically in clinical trials is the ultimate step in vaccine development. The complexity of such evaluation is demonstrated for HIV, and an example for efficacy assessment in humans under field conditions is presented for a live *Shigella* vaccine.

These proceedings cannot, obviously, encompass all the advances made in vaccine development during the recent years. Nevertheless, the directions and strategies presented here offer reasons for hope that many novel vaccines for prevention, control, and possibly eradication of diseases will be available for use in the near future.

We are obliged to all the contributors to this volume and to our colleagues: Ruth Arnon, Jonathan Gershoni, Amos Panet, Rino Rappuoli, Shaul Reuveny, Jerald Sadoff, Florian Schödel, Raymond Spier, Baruch Velan, and Moshe White.

ACKNOWLEDGMENTS

The organizing committee of the 39th OHOLO Conference gratefully acknowledges the generous support of the following organizations:

- Amgen Inc., Thousand Oaks, California
- Behringwerke AG, Marburg, Germany
- Biocine SpA, Siena, Italy
- BioTechnology General Ltd., Rehovot, Israel
- Interpharm Laboratories Ltd., Ness-Ziona, Israel
- Joseph Meyerhoff Fund Inc., Baltimore, Maryland
- Lederle-Praxis Biologicals, Pearl River, New York
- Merck & Co., Inc.-Merck Research Laboratories, Rahway, New Jersey
- Ministry of Science and the Arts, Jerusalem, Israel
- Ministry of Tourism, Jerusalem, Israel
- SmithKline Beecham Biologicals, Rixensart, Belgium
- The British Council, Tel-Aviv, Israel
- The Israel Academy of Sciences and Humanities, Jerusalem, Israel

CONTENTS

Recombinant Antigens and Presentation Vectors

1. Synthetic Vaccines for Infectious and Autoimmune Diseases 1
   Michael Sela

2. Host Range Restricted, Non-Replicating Vaccinia Virus Vectors as Vaccine
   Candidates 7
   Bernard Moss, Miles W. Carroll, Linda S. Wyatt, Jack R. Bennink,
   Vanessa M. Hirsch, Simoy Goldstein, William R. Elkins,
   Thomas R. Fuerst, Jeffrey D. Lifson, M. Piatak, Nicholas P. Restifo,
   Willem Overwijk, Ronald Chamberlain, Steven A. Rosenberg, and
   Gerd Sutter

3. Hybrid Hepatitis B Virus Core Antigen as a Vaccine Carrier Moiety:
   II. Expression in Avirulent *Salmonella spp.* for Mucosal Immunization ... 15
   F. Schödel, S. Kelly, S, Tinge, S. Hopkins, D. Peterson, D. Milich, and
   R. Curtiss III

4. Synthetic Recombinant Vaccine Induces Anti-Influenza Long-Term Immunity
   and Cross-Strain Protection 23
   Ruth Arnon and Raphael Levi

5. Alphavirus-Based Expression Systems 31
   Charles M. Rice

6. Alphavirus Hybrid Virion Vaccines 41
   A. Shafferman, S. Lustig, Y. Inbar, M. Halevy, P. Schneider, T. Bino,
   M. Leitner, H. Grosfeld, B. Velan, F. Schödel, and S. Cohen

7. DNA Vaccines for Bacteria and Viruses 49
   J. B. Ulmer, R. R. Deck, A. Yawman, A. Friedman, C. Dewitt, D. Martinez,
   D. L. Montgomery, J. J. Donnelly, and M. A. Liu

Bacterial Vaccines – Novel Approaches

8. New Vaccines against Bacterial Toxins 55
    Rino Rappuoli, Mariagrazia Pizza, Gill Douce, and Gordon Dougan

9. Parameters for the Rational Design of Genetic Toxoid Vaccines 61
    W. Neal Burnette

10. Protective Immunity Induced by *Bacillus anthracis* Toxin Mutant Strains 69
    C. Pezard., J-C. Sirard, and M. Mock

11. Bacterial Outer Membrane Protein Vaccines: The Meningococcal Example 73
    Jan T. Poolman

Strategies for HIV Vaccine

12. Changing Paradigms for an HIV Vaccine 79
    Alan M. Schultz

13. Complexed HIV Envelope as a Target for an AIDS Vaccine 91
    J. M. Gershoni, G. F. Denisova, D. Raviv, B. Stern, and J. Zwickel

14. HIV–Peplotion Vaccine: A Novel Approach to Vaccination against AIDS by
    Transepithelial Transport of Viral Peptides and Antigens to Langerhans
    Cells for Induction of Cytolytic T Cells by HLA Class I and CD1
    Molecules for Long Term Protection 97
    Yechiel Becker

Adjuvants and Delivery Systems

15. The Role of Adjuvants and Delivery Systems in Modulation of Immune
    Response to Vaccines 105
    Rajesh K. Gupta, Paul Griffin, Jr., An-Cheng Chang, Rachel Rivera,
        Roger Anderson, Bradford Rost, Douglas Cecchini, Mary Nicholson, and
        George R. Siber

16. Unique Immunomodulating Properties of Dimethyl Dioctadecyl Ammonium
    Bromide (DDA) in Experimental Viral Vaccines 115
    D. Katz, S. Lehrer, O. Galan, B. Lachmi, S. Cohen, I. Inbar, I. Samina,
        B. Peleg, D. Heller, H. Yadin, D. Chai, E. Freeman, H. Schupper, and
        P. Fuchs

Production Processes and Clinical Evaluation

17. Challenges in the Development of Combination Vaccines 127
    Ronald W. Ellis

18. Polysaccharide Conjugate Vaccines for the Prevention of Gram-Positive
    Bacterial Infections 133
    Robert Naso and Ali Fattom

19. Production of Influenza Virus in Cell Cultures for Vaccine Preparation 141
     O.-W. Merten, C. Hannoun, J.-C. Manuguerra, F. Ventre, and S. Petres

20. Analysis of *Bordetella pertussis* Suspensions by ELISA and Flow Cytometry ... 153
     W. Jiskoot, J. Westdijk, C. H. K. Reubsaet, and E. C. Beuvery

21. Clinical Trials of *Shigella* Vaccines in Israel 159
     D. Cohen, S. Ashkenazi, M. Green, M. Gdalevich, M. Yavzori, N. Orr,
     G. Robin, R. Slepon, Y. Lerman, C. Block, I. Ashkenazi, D. Taylor,
     L. Hale, J. Sadoff, R. Schneerson, J. Robbins, M. Wiener, and J. Shemer

Vaccine Development - General Consideration

22. Hypothesis: How Licensed Vaccines Confer Protective Immunity 169
     John B. Robbins, Rachel Schneerson, and Shousun C. Szu

23. Therapeutic Vaccines: A Pandoric Prospect 183
     R. E. Spier

Index 191

1

SYNTHETIC VACCINES FOR INFECTIOUS AND AUTOIMMUNE DISEASES

Michael Sela

Department of Chemical Immunology
The Weizmann Institute of Science
Rehovot, Israel 76100

The ideal vaccine is one that is stable, safe, administered orally in a single dose at birth, 100% effective, reasonably priced, and protective for a lifetime. Unfortunately, there is no such vaccine (Dowdle and Orenstein, 1995). The development of vaccines has been one of the most important achievements in immunology and medicine. The existing vaccines, which consist mostly of killed or live attenuated microbial agents or their isolated components, have led to the eradication of smallpox and have diminished the incidence, morbidity and mortality in a large number of infectious diseases, including polio, measles and diphtheria. The current procedures of vaccines preparation present, nevertheless, problems such as whether a particular viral vaccine preparation is completely killed or sufficiently attenuated, the difficulty in preparing enough material for vaccine production, and the genetic variation in viruses.

1. VACCINES AGAINST INFECTIOUS DISEASES

For all the above reasons, considerable effort is now exerted towards development of synthetic vaccines (Arnon, 1986; Sela and Arnon, 1992). Our own work on the development of synthetic antigens (Sela, 1969) led us to the concept of synthetic vaccines (Sela, 1974: Arnon, 1972).

Following a clear distinction between sequential and conformation-dependent antigenic determinants (epitopes), we showed that the attachment of the synthetic 'loop' peptide of lysozyme to a multichain poly-DL-alanine carrier, results in a conjugate provoking antibodies reacting with the intact lysozyme (Arnon *et al.*, 1971). The reaction occurs with a unique region within the native protein (the 'loop' region) and it is conformation-dependent. The inevitable conclusion of these studies was that a new approach to vaccination is possible, for the simple reason that if this holds for one protein, it may hold for others, including viral coat proteins and bacterial toxins.

The concept of synthetic vaccines must include, not only the ability to produce immunogenic molecules capable of provoking antibodies and specifically sensitized cells of the appropriate specificity that can induce protection, but also several other 'ingredients',

Novel Strategies in Design and Production of Vaccines
Edited by S. Cohen and A. Shafferman, Plenum Press, New York, 1996

1

crucial to any strategy of development of new vaccines. These should include attempts towards built-in adjuvanticity, consideration of genetic background of the species immunized, concern about the possibility of antigenic competition, and efforts to obtain prolonged immunity.

The synthesis of the epitopes desired for the vaccines may be either chemical or by genetic engineering. Most of the studies in our laboratory were devoted to the chemical approach. In early studies we showed that it is possible to prepare synthetic antigens provoking antibodies capable of neutralizing a virus, namely, MS2 bacteriophage (Langbeheim *et al.*, 1976), thus demonstrating for the first time the feasibility of the approach. Actually, an antiviral response induced by a peptide was reported as early as 1963. Using a natural hexapeptide obtained from an enzymatic digest of tobacco mosaic virus protein, conjugated to bovine serum albumin, Anderer (Anderer, 1963), succeeded in eliciting antibodies with a limited inhibitory capacity towards the infectivity of the virus. Ruth Arnon and her colleagues have shown that such a response can be elicited by synthetic peptides and their conjugates, such as influenza (Muller *et al.*, 1982), and this is the topic of her presentation at this Conference.

In the last fifteen years synthetic antigens have been prepared, capable of provoking antibodies neutralizing bacterial toxins as well, such as diphtheria (Audibert *et al.*, 1981) and cholera (Jacob *et al.*, 1983). Furthermore, using these systems as experimental models, we also showed that it is possible to prepare conjugates in which the appropriate synthetic epitope related to the biological system investigated, and a synthetic adjuvant, MDP (N-acetylmuramyl-D-alanyl-L-isoglutamine), are attached covalently to the same polymeric carrier, and that the resulting conjugate, when administered in aqueous solution, leads to neutralizing antibodies (Arnon *et al.*, 1980; Audibert *et al.*, 1982; Jacob *et al.*, 1986). These findings demonstrate that it is possible to design synthetic peptide vaccines with built-in adjuvanticity.

2. TOWARDS VACCINES AGAINST AUTOIMMUNE DISEASES

In a typical vaccine against an infectious disease, one increases the immune response against an antigen, or a mosaic of epitopes on an antigen, in a specific manner, without otherwise affecting the immune system. Similarly, one would like in the case of autoimmune diseases, to decrease the response to epitopes causing the disease (or aggravating it), without otherwise interfering with the immune system of the individual. A necessary condition for this approach is at least a guess concerning the nature of the responsible antigen. Another difference between the two approaches is that vaccines against infectious diseases are prophylactic, whereas in the case of autoimmune diseases the vaccines would be of a therapeutic nature.

Autoimmune diseases may be the result of the action of specific T cells and/or antibodies. Therefore, preventing their formation by either elimination or suppression should be of therapeutic value. In the case of T cells, this may occur at the level of class II antigens on the antigen-presenting cells (APC), where the immunomodulating 'vaccine' might successfully compete with the self antigen responsible for the autoimmune phenomenon, or at the level of the T cell receptor, where an immune response to the variable segments of its specific α and β chains might abolish the autoimmune reaction.

In our previous studies on experimental allergic encephalomyelitis and multiple sclerosis, we showed that a synthetic amino acid copolymer, denoted Cop-1, can suppress the onset of the disease in experimental animals (reverting the disease in monkeys), and is capable of reducing the number of attacks in patients with the exacerbating-remitting type of multiple sclerosis (Sela and Arnon, 1992). Cop-1 has been tested successfully in a phase

III double-blind clinical trial in 11 centers in the USA as a candidate drug for the exacerbating-remitting type of multiple sclerosis.

One possible mechanism of action of Cop-1 has been investigated, using myelin basic protein (MBP) specific T cell lines and clones with various H-2 restrictions and antigenic specificities. We have shown that, specifically, Cop-1 could competitively inhibit T cell responses to MBP (Teitelbaum *et al.*, 1988). The effect of Cop-1 on both the proliferative response and IL-2 secretion induced by MBP in all these T cell lines and clones has been investigated. All the lines and clones were affected by Cop-1. In seven of them, Cop-1 specifically inhibited the response to MBP, and in one, Cop-1 was able to induce proliferation. Inhibition of the response to MBP was shown to be specific to Cop-1, and only T cell lines responsive to MBP were affected by Cop-1. These results suggest that Cop-1 or Cop-1-derived peptides can bind to the relevant major histocompatibility complex (MHC) molecules and competitively inhibit the binding of MBP. Consequently, activation of MBP effector cells is blocked.

Cop-1 can also inhibit the response to MBP of various specific human T cell lines and clones, and similarly, MBP inhibited T cell clones specific to Cop-1, irrespective of their DR restriction (Teitelbaum *et al.*, 1992). The inhibition was demonstrated only in the presence of antigen presenting cells (APCs), indicating that the site of competition between MBP and Cop-1 is most probably the MHC class II binding site. The direct binding of Cop-1 to MHC molecules on living APCs has now been corroborated by using its biotinylated derivative (Fridkis-Hareli *et al.*, 1994). Cop-1 and MBP bound in a promiscuous manner to different types of APC of various H-2 and HLA haplotypes. The specificity of the binding was confirmed by its inhibition with either the relevant anti-MHC class II antibodies or unlabeled analogs. Cop-1 exhibited the most extensive and rapid binding to the APC. It is our belief that the successful competition of Cop-1 with MBP for the groove on MHC class II molecule, serves as the first stage in the mechanism of action of Cop-1 in the exacerbating-remitting stages of multiple sclerosis.

More recently, we have described a similar approach to another autoimmne disease, myasthenia gravis (MG). This disease is a well-characterized autoimmune disorder, the symptoms of which are caused by an antibody-mediated autoimmune response to the nicotinic acetylcholine receptor (AChr) (Lindstrom *et al.*, 1988). Although the presence of pathogenic autoantibodies was once considered to be crucial to the development of MG, several lines of experimental evidence indicate that T cells play an important role in mediating this disease. This is not surprising, since helper T cells are necessary for an efficient antibody response in the case of all antigens except those few which are thymus independent. Nevertheless, it is still unclear what initiates and regulates autoimmune reactivity in MG, and there is no definitive cure for this disease.

Previous studies showed that two peptides, p195-212 and p259-271, representing amino acids 195-212 and 257-271 of the human AChR α subunit significantly stimulated peripheral blood lymphocytes of MG patients in comparison to healthy controls. In addition, a correlation was demonstrated between the capacity of peripheral blood lymphocytes of MG patients to proliferate in response to p195-212 and p259-271 and to HLA-PB5 and HLA-DR3 respectively (Brocke *et al.*, 1988). Extension of this research using inbred mouse strains revealed that p195-212 and p259-271 are immunodominant T cell epitopes for SJL and BALB/c mice, respectively, and are cryptic epitopes for C3H.SW mice (Brocke *et al.*, 1990).

It has been proposed that T cell responses may be inhibited by peptides that bind to MHC class II restriction elements but do not activate specific T cells. Such inhibitory peptides may be used to specifically treat autoimmune diseases by inhibiting the pathogenic T cell responses (Teitelbaum *et al.*, 1988; Sakai *et al.*, 1989). We have designed and synthesized a number of analogs of p195-212 and p259-271 containing single amino acid substitutions. These analogs were screened for their ability to inhibit T cell responses to p195-212 and p259-271 both *in vitro* and *in vivo*.

Two analogs, the p195-212 analog, #455, containing a $Met_{207} \rightarrow$ Ala substitution, and the p259-271 analog, #306, containing a $Glu_{262} \rightarrow$ Lys substitution, were capable of inhibiting T cell responses triggered by the myasthenogenic T cell epitopes. Cells of the p195-212 specific murine T cell line, TCSJL195-212, proliferated in the presence of p195-212 (stimulation index SI = 632) but not in response to the analog #455 (SI = 2.1). Moreover, the proliferative responses of the TCSJL195-212 line to p195-212 were inhibited up to 100% in the presence of the analog #455 at a stimulator/inhibitor ratio of 1:10. Similarly, the p259-271 specific murine T cell line, TCBALB/c259-271, did not proliferate in the presence of the analog #306 (SI = 1), as compared to SI = 289 for p259-271. The proliferative responses of the TCBALB/c259-271 line were inhibited up to 93% in the presence of #306 (stimulator:inhibitor = 1:200) (Katz-Levy *et al.*, 1993).

It was of interest to determine whether the analogs were capable of inhibiting a T cell population more heterogeneous than the long-term cultures. To this end analog #306 was used to inhibit p259-271 primed lymph node (LN) cells in an *in vitro* proliferation assay. It was found that the proliferative response of the LN cells was inhibited by 66% at a stimulator:inhibitor ratio of 1:100. Since the analogs could inhibit T cell proliferative responses in vitro , we tested their ability to inhibit in vivo priming of LN cells. Hence, mice were primed with the myasthenogenic peptides in complete Freund's adjuvant concomitant with administration of the analogs (either i.v. or i.p.) in aqueous solution. Therefore, the proliferative capacity of the LN cells in response to the parent peptides was tested ex vivo. Administration of analog #455 led to decreased proliferative responses of up to 70% by LN cells from peptide-primed SJL mice. Similarly, administration of analog #306 led to decreased proliferative responses of up to 85% by p259-271 primed LN cells from BALAB/c mice. Similar results were obtained whether the analogs were administered i.v. or i.p. (Katz-Levy *et al.*, 1993).

The main goal of this research has been to identify analogs that can be used for immunomodulatory therapy in myasthenic patients. Preliminary studies have shown that analogs #455 and #306 could inhibit up to 100% of p195-212 and p259-271 specific proliferative responses in these patients. The ability of analogs #455 and #306 to inhibit T cell responses, both *in vitro* and *in vivo*, indicates that they are good candidates for immunomodulatory therapy for MG patients.

In conclusion, synthetic approaches bring hope both for improvements in vaccination against infectious diseases, and for new treatment of autoimmune diseases, based on antagonists to epitopes provoking such diseases.

REFERENCES

Anderer, F.A., 1963, Preparation and properties of an artificial antigen immunologically related to tobacco mosaic virus. *Biochim. Biophys. Acta* 71:246-248.

Arnon, R., 1972, Synthetic vaccines - dream or reality. In "Immunity and viral and rickettsial diseases," eds. A. Kohn and A.M. Klingberg, Plenum Press, New York, pp. 209-222.

Arnon, R., 1986, Synthetic peptides as the basis for future vaccines. *TIBS* 11:521-524.

Arnon, R., Maron, E., Sela, M., and Anfinsen, C.B., 1971, Antibodies reactive with native lysozyme elicited by a completely synthetic antigen. *Proc. Natl. Acad. Sci. USA* 68:1450-1454.

Arnon, R., Sela, M., Parant, M., and Chedid, L., 1980, Antiviral response elicited by a completely synthetic antigen with built-in adjuvanticity. *Proc. Natl. Acad. Sci. USA* 77:6769-6772.

Audibert, F., Jolivet, M., Chedid, L., Alouf, J.E., Bouquet, P., Rivaille, P., and Siffret, O., 1981, Active antitoxic immunization by a diphtheria toxin synthetic oligopeptide. *Nature* 289:593-595.

Audibert, F., Jolivet, M., Chedid, L., Arnon, R., and Sela, M. 1982, Successful immunization with a totally synthetic diphtheria vaccine. *Proc. Natl. Acad. Sci. USA* 79:5042-5046.

Brocke, S., Brautbar, C., Steinman, L., Abramsky, O., Rothbard, J., Neumann, D., Fuchs, S., and Mozes, E., 1988, *In vitro* proliferative responses and antibody titers specific to human acetylcholine receptor synthetic peptides in patients with myasthenia grais and relation to HLA class II genes. *J. Clin. Invest.* 82:1894-1900 .

Brocke, S., Dayan, M., Rothbard, J., Fuchs, S., and Mozes, E., 1990, The autoimmune response of different mouse strains to T-cell epitopes of the human acetylcholine receptor alpha subunit. *Immunology* 69:495-500.

Dowdle, W.R., and Orenstein, W.A., 1995, Quest for life-long protection by vaccination. In "Infectious diseases in an age of change", ed B. Roizman, National Academy of Sciences, Washington, D.C., pp. 235-247.

Fridkis-Hareli, M., Teitelbaum,D., Gurevich, E., Pecht, I., Brautbar, C., Kwon, O.J. Brenner, T., Arnon, R., and Sela, M., 1994, Direct binding of myelin basic protein and synthetic copolymer 1 to class II major histocompatibility complex molecules on living antigen-presenting cells - specificity and promiscuity. *Proc. Natl. Acad. Sci. USA* 91:4872-4876.

Jacob, C.O., Arnon, R., and Sela, M., 1986, Anti-cholera response elicited by a completely synthetic antigen with built-in adjuvanticity administered in aqueous solution. *Immunol. Lett.* 14:43-48.

Jacob, C.O., Sela, M., and Arnon, R., 1983, Antibodies against synthetic peptides of the B subunit of cholera toxin: cross-reaction and neutralization of the toxin. *Proc. Natl. Acad. Sci. USA* 80, 7611-7615.

Katz-Levy, Y., Kirshner, S.L., Sela, M., and Mozes, E., 1993, Inhibition of T cell reactivity to myasthenogenic epitopes of the human acetylcholine receptor by synthetic analogs. *Proc. Natl. Acad. Sci. USA* 90:7000-7004.

Langbeheim, H., Arnon, R., and Sela, M., 1976, Antiviral effect on MS-2 coliphage obtained with a synthetic antigen. *Proc. Natl. Acad. Sci. USA* 73:4636-4670.

Lindstrom, J., Shelton, D., and Fuji, Y., 1988, Myasthenia gravis. *Adv. Immunol.* 42:233-284.

Muller, G.M., Shapira, M., and Arnon, R., 1982, Anti-influenza response achieved by immunization with a synthetic conjugate. *Proc. Natl. Acad. Sci. USA* : 79:569-573.

Sakai, K., Zamwil, S.S., Mitchell, D.J., Hodgkinson, S., Rothbard, J.B., and Steinman, L., 1989, Prevention of experimental encephalomyelitis with peptides that block interaction of T cells with major histocompatibility complex antigens. *Proc. Natl. Acad. Sci. USA* 86:9470-9474.

Sela, M., 1974, Vaccins synthetiques - un reve ou une realite? *Bull. Inst. Pasteur* 72:73-86.

Sela, M., and Arnon, R., 1992, Synthetic approaches to vaccines for infectious and autoimmune diseases. *Vaccine* 10:991-999.

Teitelbaum, D., Aharoni, R., Arnon, R., and Sela, M., 1988, Specific inhibition of the T cell response to myelin basic protein by the suppressive copolymer COP 1. *Proc. Natl. Acad. Sci. USA* 85:9724-9728.

Teitelbaum, D., Milo, R., Arnon, R., and Sela, M., 1992, Synthetic copolymer 1 inhibits human T-cell lines specific for myelin basic protein. *Proc. Natl. Acad. Sci. USA* 89:137-141.

2

HOST RANGE RESTRICTED, NON-REPLICATING VACCINIA VIRUS VECTORS AS VACCINE CANDIDATES

Bernard Moss,[1] Miles W. Carroll,[1] Linda S. Wyatt,[1] Jack R. Bennink,[1]
Vanessa M. Hirsch,[2] Simoy Goldstein,[2] William R. Elkins,[2]
Thomas R. Fuerst,[3] Jeffrey D. Lifson,[3] M. Piatak,[3] Nicholas P. Restifo,[4]
Willem Overwijk,[4] Ronald Chamberlain,[4] Steven A. Rosenberg,[4] and
Gerd Sutter[1]

[1] Laboratory of Viral Diseases, National Institute of Allergy and Infectious
     Diseases
   National Institutes of Health, Bethesda, Maryland 20892
[2] Laboratory of Infectious Diseases, National Institute of Allergy and
     Infectious Diseases
   National Institutes of Health, Rockville, Maryland 20852
[3] GeneLabs Technologies
   Redwood City, California 94063
[4] Surgery Branch, National Cancer Institute
   National Institutes of Health, Bethesda, Maryland 20892

1. INTRODUCTION

The use of a recombinant virus containing a heterologous gene of another microorganism as a live vaccine was suggested more than 10 years ago (Mackett et al., 1982; Panicali and Paoletti, 1982). Vaccinia virus was considered for such a purpose because of its success as a smallpox vaccine and ease and economy of production, distribution and administration (Fenner et al., 1988). The extensive experimental use of recombinant vaccinia viruses was facilitated by the construction of plasmid transfer vectors containing a vaccinia virus promoter, one or more convenient restriction endonuclease sites for inserting a foreign gene, flanking DNA sequences for homologous recombination into a non-essential site of the vaccinia virus genome and for selection and/or screening of recombinant viruses (Chakrabarti et al., 1985; Mackett et al., 1984). Humoral and cell mediated immune responses to an expressed foreign protein and protection of experimental animals against challenge with the corresponding pathogen were demonstated in a variety of animal model systems (Cox et al., 1992; Moss, 1991).

Initial testing of recombinant vaccinia viruses in humans has been reported. A first generation recombinant vaccinia virus AIDS vaccine was considered to be immunogenic and safe (Cooney et al., 1991). Nevertheless, the occurrence of rare adverse reactions to smallpox

Novel Strategies in Design and Production of Vaccines
Edited by S. Cohen and A. Shafferman, Plenum Press, New York, 1996

vaccination and the increased susceptibility of immunodeficient individuals has made further attenuation and improved safety a priority for new human vaccines based on vaccinia virus. Attenuation can be achieved by deleting genes that contribute to virulence but are non-essential for replication in tissue culture (Buller et al., 1988; Buller et al., 1985; Tartaglia et al., 1992) or by insertion of lymphokine genes (Flexner et al., 1987; Ramshaw et al., 1987). An alternative approach is to use one of several highly attenuated strains of vaccinia virus that were developed but not extensively used during the smallpox eradication campaign. One of these, known as modified vaccinia virus Ankara (MVA), is avirulent in normal or immunosuppressed animals and elicited no adverse reactions in 120,000 humans, many of whom were at risk for the conventional smallpox vaccine (Hochstein-Mintzel et al., 1972; Mayr and Danner, 1979; Mayr et al., 1975; Mayr et al., 1978; Stickl et al., 1974; Werner et al., 1980).

MVA was generated by over 500 passages of the parental strain in chicken embryo fibroblasts, during which it became severely host restricted and unable to propagate efficiently in mammalian cells. In this respect, MVA resembles Avipoxviruses which are also being developed as safe vaccines (Taylor et al., 1992). Compared to the parental vaccinia virus, MVA contains six major deletions of genomic DNA resulting in the loss of 30,000 base pairs (bp) or 15% of its genetic information (Meyer et al., 1991). The block in replication of MVA in human and other mammalian cells occurs at a step in virion assembly, allowing unimpaired expression of early and late viral or recombinant genes (Sutter & Moss, 1992). Thus, MVA is an efficient as well as a safe vector system. Here, we review examples of the use of recombinant MVA to protectively immunize against influenza virus, simian immunodeficiency virus (SIV), and neoplastic cells in animal model systems.

2. IMMUNIZATION WITH MVA

2.1. Immunization against Influenza Virus

Influenza virus infection of mice provides an experimental model for vaccination against a respiratory disease. Previous studies demonstrated that recombinant vaccinia viruses expressing the influenza virus hemagglutinin gene (*ha*) induced type-specific humoral and cell mediated immune responses and protectively immunized mice against a lethal influenza virus challenge (Andrew et al., 1986; Bennink et al., 1984). Recombinant vaccinia viruses expressing the influenza virus nucleoprotein gene (*np*) induced a less protective but cross-reactive CTL response (Andrew et al., 1986; Yewdell et al., 1985). To evaluate MVA as a candidate vaccine, both the *ha* and *np* regulated by vaccinia virus synthetic strong early/late promoters were inserted into the MVA genome to form MVA-INF$_{ha/np}$ (Sutter et al., 1994). Preliminary experiments verified that the genes were expressed and that the recombinant virus did not cause a spreading infection or discernible cytopathathology in monolayers of mouse L929 cells. Mice inoculated intramuscularly with MVA-INF$_{ha/np}$ developed humoral and CTL immune responses to influenza virus proteins in a dose-dependent manner. A single vaccination with 10^4 or more infectious units of MVA-INF$_{ha/np}$ protected mice against a challenge with 100 times the lethal dose of influenza virus (Table 1; Sutter et al., 1994). Surprisingly, all parameters of immunity including protection were similar or better than those induced by standard intradermal vaccination with equivalent doses of replication competent vaccinia virus strain WR expressing influenza *ha* and *np*. (The lower dose of recombinant virus required for protection than for detectable hemagglutinin inhibition probably reflects different sensitivities of the *in vivo* and *in vitro* assays). Protection was also achieved by nasal vaccination, although higher vaccine doses were required (Table 1).

Table 1. Protection against lethal challenge with influenza virus[1]

Inoculation site	Vaccine	Dose[2]	Increased HI titer[3]	Survivors[4]
Intramuscular	MVA	8	0/8	0/8
	WR	6	0/8	0/8
	WR-INF$_{ha/np}$	4	0/8	5/8
		5	1/8	8/8
		6	4/8	8/8
	MVA-INF$_{ha/np}$	4	0/16	14/16
		5	3/16	16/16
		6	7/8	8/8
Intranasal	MVA	6	0/8	0/8
	MVA-INF$_{ha/np}$	4	0/8	0/8
		5	0/8	0/8
		6	0/8	6/8

[1]data from Sutter et al. (1994) with permission.
[2]log tissue culture infectious dose$_{50}$ or plaque forming unit/animal.
[3]Number of animals with >4 fold increase in hemagglutinin (HI) titer / total animals for each group.
[4]Surviving animals/ total animals challenged for each group; 100 LD$_{50}$ Influenza A/PR/8 challenge delivered to 10-week-old-mice, 4 weeks post vaccination.

2.2. Immunization against SIV

SIV and human immunodeficiency virus (HIV) are closely related viruses with similar genome organizations and CD4 lymphocyte/macrophage tropism. Moreover, SIV causes an immunodeficiency disease in macaques that has many of the features of AIDS. For these reasons, SIV has been used as an HIV surrogate for vaccine studies. Good protection has been obtained by vaccination with live attenuated SIV (Daniel et al., 1992). Varying degrees of protection, perhaps partly due to differences in challenge strains, were observed with recombinant vaccinia viruses alone or combined with other immunogens (Giavedoni et al., 1993; Hu et al., 1992; Israel et al., 1994). MVA could provide a safer alternative to conventional vaccinia virus-based vaccines particularly in populations in which AIDS is prevalent.

A recombinant MVA (MVA-SIV$_{env/gag/pol}$) virus containing the complete envelope and gag-polymerase coding regions of HIV-1 regulated by a strong synthetic vaccinia virus early/late promoter and a moderate natural vaccinia virus early/late promoter, respectively, was constructed (Hirsch et al., 1995). For comparative purposes, the same SIV genes were inserted into the Wyeth (WY) vaccine strain of vaccinia virus to generate WY-SIV$_{env/gag/pol}$. We verified that the SIV genes were expressed by both recombinant viruses in monkey BS-C-1 cells. Twelve juvenile rhesus macaques, divided into four groups, were immunized four times over a period of 28 weeks with MVA-SIV$_{env/gag/pol}$ (n = 4), WY-SIV$_{env/gag/pol}$ (n = 4), MVA control virus (n = 2) or WY control virus (n = 2). After 44 weeks, animals receiving either recombinant virus were also vaccinated with 250 µg of whole SIV, inactivated with psoralen and ultraviolet light (Johnson et al., 1992), in saline. No visible lesions were formed after the intramuscular inoculations of 5 X 10^8 infectius units of MVA or MVA-SIV$_{env/gag/pol}$, whereas typical cutaneous lesions occured after the first intradermal injection of 10^8 infectious units of WY viruses. MVA-SIV$_{env/gag/pol}$ induced a sustained antibody response to both env and gag proteins whereas WY-SIV$_{env/gag/pol}$ induced detectable antibody only to the

Table 2. Responses of vaccinated macaques to SIV challenge

Parameter	MVA or WY controls	MVA-SIVenv/gag/pol	WY-SIVenv/gag/pol
Anamnestic antibody	No	Yes	Yes
PBMC viremia	Persistent in 3 of 4	Transient in 3 of 4	Persistent in 4 of 4
Acute phase			
Antigenemia	3 of 4	None	1 of 4
Plasma viral RNA	High	Severely reduced	Reduced
PBMC viral copies	High	Reduced	Reduced
Lymph nodes			
Morphology	Hyperplastic	Normal	Hyperplastic
In situ	Numerous positive	Negative (3 of 4)	Positive
Virus load	High	Low	Moderate
CD4 lymphocytes	Low (3 of 4)	Low (1 of 4)	Low (4 of 4)
Survivors	1 of 4	4 of 4	1 of 4

envelope protein. *In vitro* neutralizing activity to SIV was transient, peaking after the second recombinant virus administration, and was not enhanced by the inactivated whole SIV.

Four weeks after the final boost, all macaques were challenged by intravenous injection with 50 monkey infectious doses of cell-free, uncloned, homologous SIV (sm/E660) that had been generated in macaque peripheral blood lymphocyte cultures (Goldstein et al., 1994). The results of the SIV challenge are summarized (Table 2; Hirsch et al., 1995). All of the control animals, immunized with non-recombinant MVA or WY strains of vaccinia virus, were infected and three had severe disease requiring them to be sacrificed at 14, 22, and 54 weeks post challenge; the fourth appears healthy with a low virus load and a normal CD4 count. In contrast to the control animals, the macaques that had been vaccinated with recombinant viruses all displayed a rapid anamnestic antibody response to SIV. Although the vaccinated macaques were infected with SIV, virus replication was restricted particularly in three of the four that received MVA-SIV$_{env/gag/pol}$. In the latter, plasma viremia was absent, the viral load in peripheral blood mononuclear cells was reduced, lymph nodes contained 1% or less of the virus from control animals and the architecture was normal, the CD4 counts were maintained, and the animals are still healthy after 62 weeks. The fourth MVA-SIV$_{env/gag/pol}$ immunized macaque has lymphadenopathy and a low CD4 count. The group vaccinated with WY-SIV$_{env/gag/pol}$ was less well protected than the group vaccinated with MVA-SIV$_{env/gag/pol}$: three of the four macaques had to be sacrificed between 51 and 58 weeks because of secondary infections and the fourth has lymphadenopathy and a low CD4 count. At this time, we cannot determine whether inherent genetic differences between the vectors accounted for the better immunity induced by recombinant MVA compared to recombinant WY or whether differences in the dose or route of inoculation were important. Further vaccine trials with MVA-SIV$_{env/gag/pol}$ are in progress.

2.3. Immunization against Neoplastic Cells

Tumor-associated antigens, that are recognized by CD8[+] CTL, are potential targets for cancer immunotherapy. To evaluate MVA as a vector for tumor antigens, we used a murine model system that was previously tested with recombinant vaccinia and fowlpox viruses (Bronte et al., 1995; Wang et al., 1995). The BALB/c colon carcinoma cell line CT26.WT was stably transfected with the *Escherichia coli lacZ* gene, which encodes β-galactosidase, to generate CT26.CL25. BALB/c mice, immunized intramuscularly with MVA expressing

Table 3. Protection against neoplastic cells

Vaccination intramuscular	Dose[1]	CT26.WT number of metastases[2]	CT26.CL25 number of metastases[2]
None		411	>500
MVA	10^8	>500	>500
MVA-βgal	10^8	>500	0
MVA-βgal	10^6	>500	2

[1]Infectious units.
[2]Pulmonary nodules per lung, average of 5 animals.

the *lacZ* model tumor antigen (MVA-βgal), were protected against intravenous challenge with a lethal number of CT26.CL25 cells (Table 3). Pulmonary metastases and death occurred in control animals vaccinated with MVA-βgal and challenged with CT26.WT or vaccinated with parental MVA and challenged with CT26.CL25 (Table 3). Therefore, protection was specific for virus and cell-lines expressing the model tumor antigen. In treatment experiments using mice bearing 3-day established pulmonary tumors, either prolonged survival or a reduction in the number of metastases was obtained by immunization with MVA-βgal or by adoptive transfer of *in vitro* stimulated splenocytes from normal mice vaccinated with MVA-βgal. Comparative studies suggested that MVA-βgal might be more effective than WR-βgal (a replication-competent vaccinia virus expressing β-galactosdiase) when used for treatment of established tumors.

3. SUMMARY

Three model sytems were used to demonstrate the immunogenicity of highly attenuated and replication-defective recombinant MVA. (1) Intramuscular inoculation of MVA-IN-$F_{ha/np}$ induced humoral and cell-mediated immune responses in mice and protectively immunized them against a lethal respiratory challenge with influenza virus. Intranasal vaccination was also protective, although higher doses were needed. (2) In rhesus macaques, an immunization scheme involving intramuscular injections of MVA-SIV$_{env/gag/pol}$ greatly reduced the severity of disease caused by an SIV challenge. (3) In a murine cancer model, immunization with MVA-βgal prevented the establishment of tumor metastases and even prolonged life in animals with established tumors. These results, together with previous data on the safety of MVA in humans, suggest the potential usefulness of recombinant MVA for prophylactic vaccination and therapeutic treatment of infectious diseases and cancer.

REFERENCES

Andrew, M. E., Coupar, B. E. H., Ada, G. L. and Boyle, D. B., 1986, Cell-mediated immune response to influenza virus antigens expressed by vaccinia virus recombinants, *Microb. Path.* 1:443-452.

Bennink, J. R., Yewdell, J. W., Smith, J. W., Moller, C. and Moss, B., 1984, Recombinant vaccinia virus primes and stimulates influenza virus HA-specific CTL, *Nature* 311:578-579.

Bronte, V., Tsung, K., Rao, J. B., Chen, P. W., Wang, M., Rosenberg, S. A. and Restifo, N. P., 1995, IL-2 enhances the function of recombinant poxvirus-based vaccines in the treatment of established pulmonary metastases, *J. Immunol.* 154:5282-5292.

Buller, R. M., Chakrabarti, S., Cooper, J. A., Twardzik, D. R. and Moss, B., 1988, Deletion of the vaccinia virus growth factor gene reduces virus virulence, *J. Virol.* 62:866-877.

Buller, R. M. L., Smith, G. L., Cremer, K., Notkins, A. L. and Moss, B., 1985, Decreased virulence of recombinant vaccinia virus expression vectors is associated with a thymidine kinase-negative phenotype, *Nature* 317:813-815.

Chakrabarti, S., Brechling, K. and Moss, B., 1985, Vaccinia virus expression vector: Coexpression of β-galactosidase provides visual screening of recombinant virus plaques, *Mol. Cell. Biol.* 5:3403-3409.

Cooney, E. L., Collier, A. C., Greenberg, P. D., Coombs, R. W., Zarling, J., Arditti, D. E., Hoffman, M. C., Hu, S. L. and Corey, L., 1991, Safety of and immunological response to a recombinant vaccinia virus vaccine expressing HIV envelope glycoprotein, *Lancet* 337: 567-572.

Cox, W. I., Tartaglia, J. and Paoletti, E., 1992, Poxvirus recombinants as live vaccines, *Recombinant poxviruses*. (Binns, M. M. and Smith, G. L., eds.), 123-162. CRC Press, Boca Raton.

Daniel, M. D., Kirchhoff, F., Czajak, S. C., Sehgal, P. K. and Desrosiers, R. C., 1992, Protective effects of a live attenuated SIV vaccine with a deletion in the nef gene, *Science* 258:1938-1941.

Fenner, F., Henderson, D. A., Arita, I., Jezek, Z. and Ladnyi, I. D., 1988, *Smallpox and its eradication*, World Health Organization, Geneva.

Flexner, C., Hugin, A. and Moss, B., 1987, Prevention of vaccinia virus infection in immunodeficient nude mice by vector-directed IL-2 expression, *Nature* 330:259-262.

Giavedoni, L. D., Planelles, V., Haigwood, N. L., Ahmad, S., Kluge, J. D., Marthas, M. L., Gardner, M. B., Luciw, P. A. and Yilma, T. D., 1993, Immune response of rhesus macaques to recombinant simian immunodeficiency virus-gp130 does not protect from challenge infection, *J. Virol.* 67:577-583.

Goldstein, S., Elkins, W. R., London, W. T., Hahn, A., Goeken, R., Martin, J. E. and Hirsch, V. M., 1994, Immunization with whole inactivated vaccine protects from infection by SIV grown in human but not macaque cells, *J. Med. Primatol.* 23: 75-82.

Hirsch, V. M., Goldstein, S., Chanock, R., Elkins, W. R., Sutter, G., Moss, B., Sisler, J., Lifson, J. and Fuerst, T., 1995, Limited virus replication following SIV challenge of macaques immunized with attenuated MVA vaccinia expressing SIVsm *env* and *gag-pol*, *Vaccines* 95:195-200.

Hochstein-Mintzel, V., Huber, H. C. and Stickl, H., 1972, Virulenz und immunogenität eines modifizierten vaccinia-virus (Stamm MVA), *Z. Immun.-Forsch.* 144:140-145.

Hu, S.-L., Abrams, K., Barber, G. N., Moran, P., Zarling, J. M., Langlois, A. J., Kuller, L., Morton, W. R. and Beneviste, R. E., 1992, Protection of macaques against SIV infection by subunit vaccines of SIV envelope glycoprotein gp160. *Science* 255:456-459.

Israel, Z. R., Edmonson, P. F., Maul, D. H., O'Neill, S. P., Mossman, S. P., Thiriart, C., Fabry, L., Van Opstal, O., Bruck, C., Bex, F., Burny, A., Fultz, P. N., Mullins, J. I. and Hoover, E. A., 1994, Incomplete protection, but suppression of virus burden, elicited by subunit simian immunodeficiency virus vaccines, *J. Virol.* 68:1843-1853.

Johnson, P. R., Montefiori, D. C., Goldstein, S., Hamm, T. E., Zhou, J. Y., Kitov, S., Haigwood, N. L., Misher, L., London, W. T., Gerin, J. L., Allison, A., Purcell, R. H., Chanock, R. M. and Hirsch, V. M., 1992, Inactivated whole SIV vaccine in Macaques - evaluation of protective efficacy against challenge with cell-free virus or infected cells, *AIDS Res. Human Retroviruses*, 8:1501-1505.

Mackett, M., Smith, G. L. and Moss, B., 1982, Vaccinia virus: a selectable eukaryotic cloning and expression vector, *Proc. Natl. Acad. Sci. USA*, 79:7415-7419.

Mackett, M., Smith, G. L. and Moss, B., 1984, General method for production and selection of infectious vaccinia virus recombinants expressing foreign genes, *J. Virol.* 49:857-864.

Mayr, A. and Danner, K., 1979, Bedeutung von tierpocken für den menschen nach aufhebung der pflichtimpfung gegen pocken, *Berl. Münch. Tierärztl. Wochenschr.* 92:251-256.

Mayr, A., Hochstein-Mintzel, V. and Stickl, H., 1975, Abstammung, eigenschaften und verwendung des attenuierten vaccinia-stammes MVA, *Infection* 3:6-14.

Mayr, A., Stickl, H., Müller, H. K., Danner, K. and Singer, H., 1978, Pockenimpfstamm MVA: marker, genetische struktur, erfahrungen mit der parenteralen schutzimpfung und verhalten im abwehrgeschwächten organismus, *Zbl. Bakt. Hyg. I.Abt. Orig. B* 167:375-390.

Meyer, H., Sutter, G. and Mayr, A., 1991, Mapping of deletions in the genome of the highly attenuated vaccinia virus MVA and their influence on virulence, *J. Gen. Virol.* 72:1031-1038.

Moss, B., 1991, Vaccinia virus: a tool for research and vaccine development. *Science* 252:1662-1667.

Panicali, D. and Paoletti, E., 1982, Construction of poxviruses as cloning vectors: insertion of the thymidine kinase gene from herpes simplex virus into the DNA of infectious vaccinia virus, *Proc. Natl. Acad. Sci. USA* 79:4927-4931.

Ramshaw, A., Andrew, M. E., Phillips, S. M., Boyle, D. B. and Coupar, B. E. H., 1987, Recovery of immunodeficient mice from a vaccinia virus/IL-2 recombinant infection, *Nature* 329:545-546.

Stickl, H., Hochstein-Mintzel, V., Mayr, A., Huber, H. C., Schäfer, H. and Holzner, A., 1974, MVA-stufenimpfung gegen pocken. Kleinische erprobung des attenuierten pocken-lebendimpfstoffes, stamm MVA. *Dtsch. Med. Wschr.* 99:2386-2392.

Sutter, G. and Moss, B., 1992, Nonreplicating vaccinia vector efficiently expresses recombinant genes, *Proc. Natl. Acad. Sci. USA* 89:10847-10851.

Sutter, G., Wyatt, L. S., Foley, P. L., Bennink, J. R. and Moss, B., 1994, A recombinant vector derived from the host range-restricted and highly attenuated MVA strain of vaccinia virus stimulates protective immunity in mice to influenza virus, *Vaccine* 12:1032-1040.

Tartaglia, J., Perkus, M. E., Taylor, J., Norton, E. K., Audonnet, J. C., Cox, W. I., Davis, S. W., Vanderhoeven, J., Meignier, B., Riviere, M., Languet, B. and Paoletti, E., 1992, NYVAC - A highly attenuated strain of vaccinia virus, *Virology* 188:217-232.

Taylor, J., Weinberg, R., Tartaglia, J., Richardson, C., Alkhatib, G., Breidis, D., Appel, M., Norton, E. and Paoletti, E., 1992, Nonreplicating viral vectors as potential vaccines: recombinant canarypox virus expressing measles virus fusion (F) and hemagglutinin (HA) glycoproteins, *Virology* 187:321-328.

Wang, M., Bronte, V., Chen, P. W., Gritz, L., Panicali, D., Rosenberg, S. A. and Restifo, N. P., 1995, Active immunotherapy of cancer with a non-replicating recombinant fowlpox virus encoding a model tumor-associated antigen. *J. Immunol.* 154:4685-4692.

Werner, G. T., Jentsch, U., Metzger, E. and Simon, J., 1980, Studies on poxvirus infection in irradiated animals, *Arch. Virol.* 64:247-256.

Yewdell, J. W., Bennink, J. R., Smith, G. L. and Moss, B., 1985, Influenza A virus nucleoprotein is a major target for cross-reactive anti-influenza virus cytotoxic T lymphocytes, *Proc. Natl. Acad. Sci. USA* 82:1785-1789.

3

HYBRID HEPATITIS B VIRUS CORE ANTIGEN AS A VACCINE CARRIER MOIETY

II. Expression in Avirulent *Salmonella spp.* for Mucosal Immunization

F. Schödel,[1]* S. Kelly,[2] S, Tinge,[2] S. Hopkins,[3] D. Peterson,[4] D. Milich,[5] and R. Curtiss III[6]

[1] INSERM U 80, Pavillon P, Hôpital Edouard Herriot
69437 Lyon Cedex 03, France
[2] Megan Animal Health
St. Louis, Missouri 63110
[3] Department of Biochemistry, ISREC, University of Lausanne
Epalinges, Switzerland
[4] Department of Biochemistry, Virginia Commonwealth University
Richmond, Virginia, 23298
[5] Department of Molecular Biology, The Scripps Research Institute
La Jolla, California, 92037
[6] Department of Biology, Washington University
St. Louis, Missouri 63130

1. ABSTRACT

Hepatitis B virus (HBV) core antigen (HBcAg) is a highly immunogenic subviral particle. We and others have defined insertion sites for heterologous epitopes and successfully used hybrid particles to generate B and T cell immunity (reviewed in: Schödel et al. 1994a, 1995). Here we shall review recent progress in constructing avirulent *Salmonella spp.* expressing hybrid HBcAg particles carrying different epitopes. Hybrid HBcAg particles carrying virus neutralizing epitopes of the hepatitis B virus pre-S region or repeat epitopes of plasmodial circumsporozoite antigens were previously described (Schödel et al. 1992, 1994b). *Salmonella spp.* can be attenuated by defined genetic means so that they become avirulent, yet preserve invasiveness after oral uptake.

Hybrid HBcAg-pre-S particles were expressed in *Salmonella typhimurium* and *S. typhi* vaccine strains. A single oral immunization of mice with such live recombinant *S. typhimurium* strains elicited a high titered serum anti-pre-S1 IgG response. Similarly, circumsporozoite repeat epitopes of three different malaria parasites were expressed as

HBcAg-CS hybrids in recombinant *S. spp.* and were found to be highly immunogenic after oral immunization.

To analyze mucosal immune responses, BALB/c mice were immunized with recombinant *phoP^c S.typhimurium* expressing HBcAg by various mucosal routes (Hopkins et al., 1995). All routes of immunization resulted in high titered serum and local antibodies against HBcAg and *S. typhimurium* LPS. However, nasal immunization was most efficient in generating pulmonary IgA and rectal immunization in eliciting rectal IgA, suggesting some compartmentalization of the mucosal immune response.

2. INTRODUCTION

Salmonella spp. can be rendered avirulent by defined genetic manipulations while retaining invasiveness across the intestinal epithelium after oral uptake (for reviews see Curtiss, 1990; Schödel, 1992). Antigenic determinants of other pathogens can be synthesized in avirulent *Salmonella* strains by recombinant techniques. Such live recombinant *Salmonella* strains have been shown to stimulate immune responses when delivered orally or when applied to mucosal surfaces. However, many genes encoding viral envelope or capsid antigens cannot be expressed in an immunogenic form in prokaryotes because their expression is toxic and/or the recombinant antigens are not correctly processed and/or do not fold correctly. HBsAg for example, which is the major component of current HBV vaccines cannot be expressed in an immunogenic form in prokaryotes. If one plans to use *Salmonella spp.* as carriers for vaccination against viral diseases, especially when the goal is to elicit virus neutralizing antibodies, the challenge is to identify forms of the critical viral epitopes which can be expressed in *Salmonella spp.* in a stable and immunogenic manner.

We have previously shown that in mice only a minority of *Salmonella* proteins elicit high titered serum antibodies after a single oral immunization with live avirulent *Salmonella typhimurium* vaccine strains (Schödel et al, 1994c). It is therefore necessary to identify carrier proteins which convey their enhanced immunogenicity to carried epitopes.

We have concentrated our efforts on the use of hepatitis B virus (HBV) core antigen (HBcAg) as a carrier moiety for HBV and non-HBV epitopes in recombinant *Salmonella spp.*

HBcAg is a 183 amino acid, 21kDa protein that spontaneously assembles to form particles, even when the core gene alone is expressed in prokaryotes (for reviews see Schödel et al., 1994a; 1995). We have used HBcAg primarily as a carrier for virus-neutralizing epitopes of the HBV pre-S region (Schödel et al. 1990; 1992), HIV V3 loop epitopes (von Brunn et al., 1993) and dominant antibody binding sites on the circumsporozoite antigen repeat sequences of three different malaria parasites (Schödel et al. 1994b).

3. EXPERIMENTAL AND DISCUSSION

3.1. HBcAg-pre-S Particles Expressed in *Salmonella*

Candidate oral HBV vaccines were constructed based on the expression of hybrid HBcAg -pre-S particles in recombinant *Salmonella* strains. The pre-S1 and pre-S2 region of the HBV surface antigens harbour protective peptidic epitopes, that unlike the major SAg epitopes are not dependent on the assembly of a lipid membrane containing particle for their conformation (Milich, 1988). We intended to exploit the intrinsic protective (probably T-cell mediated) characteristics of HBcAg (see: Schödel et al., 1993b) and endow it with the ability to raise virus neutralizing antibodies. Such hybrid HBc/pre-S particles could be stably expressed in various *aroA* or *cya crp S. typhimurium* and *S. dublin* vaccine strains (kindly provided by Bruce Stocker and Roy Curtiss) (Schödel et al., 1990, 1994d and unpublished data). At first we analyzed the oral immunogenicity of live recombinant *S. typhimurium* strains synthesizing a hybrid truncated HBcAg in which two overlapping antibody binding sites of the pre-S2 region were fused to the C-terminus (Schödel et al., 1990). A single oral immunization of BALB/c mice with the live recombinant *Salmonellae* elicited high titered serum IgG antibody responses against HBcAg, with an IgG2a dominated broad IgG subclass distribution similar to that found after parenteral immunization with HBcAg (Schödel et al., 1990). Due to the less immunogenic position of the pre-S2 epitopes at the C-terminus of HBcAg (Schödel et al., 1992) only a low titered antibody response to pre-S2 could be observed. Anti-HBcAg seroconversion required only a single oral dose of approximately 5 x 10^6 CFU of the Δcya Δcrp *S. typhimurium* strain χ 4064(pFS14PS2) in B10.S (Schödel et al., 1993a) and the recombinant *S. typhimurium* χ 4064(pFS14PS2) elicited serum anti HBc antibodies in all 6 of 6 mouse strains with different MHC haplotypes tested (M. Battegay, R. Zinkernagel, D. Milich and F. Schödel, unpublished data). However, a single oral immunization of BALB/c mice with a *S. typhimurium cya crp* strain χ 4064(pNS27-53PS2) synthesizing a hybrid HBc/preS particle in which the pre-S1 sequence is internally inserted gave rise to substantial anti-pre-S serum antibody titres (Schödel et al., 1994d).

3.2. Non-Antibiotic Resistant Expression

For potential clinical use of such multivalent *salmonellae* based vaccine strains, the absence of antibiotic resistant markers is required. We have therefore developed non antibiotic resistant plasmids expressing HBc/preS hybrid genes in avirulent *S. typhimurium* and *S. typhi* strains (Schödel et al., 1994 and unpublished data). These plasmids are based on a balanced-lethal host-vector combination adopted for this purpose by the Curtiss group (Nakayama, 198; Galan et al., 1990). The carrier strains have a deletion in the gene coding for aspartate ß-semialdehyde dehydrogenase (*asd*), an enzyme required in the cell wall synthesis of gram negatives. The wild-type *asd* gene is provided *in trans* from the plasmids. In the absence of diaminopimelic acid, which is not available in mammalian tissues, the cells losing the plasmid lyse. With such *asd* complementing plasmids we have been able to construct *S. typhimurium* and *S. typhi* strains stably expressing hybrid HBc/pre-S and other hybrid HBc genes. These recombinant *S. typhimurium* are immunogenic after a single oral dose in mice (Schödel et al., 1994d).

The first recombinant *cya crp cdt S. typhi* expressing hybrid HBcAg-pre-S particles which were tested in phase I clinical trials by the oral and rectal routes of administration were clinically safe but insufficiently immunogenic for the carried antigen and not highly immunogenic for *S. typhi* antigens (in collaboration with the Center for Vaccine Development, Maryland University and the Dept. of Gynecology, Univers. of Lausanne, C. Tackett, M. Levine, G. Losonsky, S. Kelly, S. Tinge, F. Schödel, D. Nardelli, J-P. Krähenbühl, S. Hopkins, J. Le Grandi and R. Curtiss, unpublished results). It remains an important task to identify suitably attenuated *Salmonella spp.* which combine safety with sufficient immunogenicity for carried antigens in humans.

3.3. *Salmonella* Expressing Hybrid HBcAg Malarial Genes

Apart from the potential as a carrier of HBV virus neutralizing epitopes in recombinant live oral vaccine strains, HBcAg could have potential as a carrier of other pathogen epitopes in oral vaccine strains. We have therefore expressed hybrid genes containing *Plasmodium falciparum*, *P. yoelii* and *Plasmodium berghei* circumsporozoite (CS) gene repeat regions as internal fusions with the core gene in *S. typhimurium* or *S. typhi*. Again,

Table I. Serum antibodies in BALB/c 6 weeks after a single oral immunization with
χ 4064(pC75CS2)[a]

Antigen	Immunoglobulin Titre (1/)						
	IgA	IgM	IgG	IgG1	IgG2a	IgG2b	IgG3
LPS	100	0	12,800	800	6,400	3,200	6,400
(NANP)$_n$	800	6,400	102,400	12,800	102,400	25,600	204,800

a Groups of ten female BALB/c mice were immunized orally with a single dose of 2.2×10^9 CFU *S. typhimurium* χ 4064 (pC75CS2) in 20 µl PBS as previously described (Schödel et al. 1994d). Sere were collected before immunization and at regular intervals after immunization. Pooled sera were analyzed by solid phase ELISA with *S. typhimurium* LPS (1.0 µg/well) and the *P. falciparum* CS repeat synthetic peptide [NANP]$_4$ (200 ng/well) as the solid-phase ligands. Titers are indicated as the highest serum dilution yielding an OD492>3 times above preimmune serum.

the recombinant genes can be stably expressed to high levels (Schödel et al. 1994b). A single oral immunization of BALB/c mice with *cya crp S. typhimurium* χ 4064 synthesizing hybrid HBcAg/CS particles elicits high titered serum CS specific antibody responses (Table I). Even when delivered by recombinant *S. typhimurium*, hybrid HBcAg-CS particles elicit a broad IgG isotype response. The Ig isotype distribution against the CS repeat amino acid sequence NANP$_4$ in the experiment shown is remarkably similar to the primary anti-[DP$_4$NPN]$_2$ (*P. berghei* CS repeat sequence) observed in BALB/c mice immunized with hybrid HBcAg-CS2 particles in complete Freund's adjuvant (Schödel et al., 1995) despite the differences in epitope and, more significantly, delivery of the immunogen. BALB/c mice immunized with the *P. berghei* CS repeat particles were protected between a 100% and 90% in repeat experiments from *P. berghei* challenge (Schödel et al., 1994b). The serum antibody titres reached after a single oral immunization with recombinant *S. typhimurium* expressing the same hybrid HBcAg -CS - while impressive - do not reach the same highly protective level (data not shown).

In collaboration with Roy Curtiss and colleagues we have again constructed avirulent, non antibiotic resistant *S. typhi* strains expressing high levels of hybrid HBcAg-CS (*P. falciparum*) using the same balanced-lethal host vector combination. To date, one of these strains, χ 4632(pYBC75CS2), was tested for immunogenicity in mice. When given i.p. to CD1 mice in hog gastric mucin high titered anti-NANP IgG serum responses were elicited (Sandra Kelly, Steve Tinge, Roy Curtiss and F. Schödel, unpublished data).

3.4. Gene Dosage Effects

It is so far unknown which level of foreign gene expression is critical for immunogenicity of a carried antigen in live recombinant *Salmonella spp*. In one experimental system it has been demonstrated that the immunogenicity after oral feeding of the *Escherichia coli* heat-labile enterotoxin subunit B expressed by avirulent *S. typhimurium* correlates with the level of *in vitro* , but not *in vivo* expression (Cardenas et al. 1994). We employed the *asd* expression system for hybrid HBcAg particles to study the impact of gene dosage on *S. typhimurium in vitro* growth characteristics, plasmid stability and *in vivo* immunogenicity. Maintaining the same *S. typhimurium asd* gene and hybrid HBcAg-pre-S expression cassette under *trc* promoter control on the plasmid as described (Schödel et al, 1994d) we exchanged the p15a origin of replication with two variants of a ColE1 origin of replication situated on AccI-Xba I fragments derived from pUC19 to yield plasmid pYA3168 or pBR322 to yield pYA3167 (Steve Tinge, unpublished data). Exchange of the p15 a with a ColE1 origin of replication resulted in a higher *in vitro* level of expression of the hybrid HBcAg-preS gene as expected. The *in vitro* stability of the expression plasmid decreased, with the pUC19

Table II. Serum anti-pre-S1 and anti-LPS IgG (1/) in BALB/c, 5 weeks after oral immunization with χ 4550[a]

| | | Antibody titre (1/) | |
| | | Antigen | |
Plasmid	Animal	LPS	pre-S1/2
pYNS27-53PS2	1	102,400	3200
	2	3200	1600
	3	12,800	0
	4	200	3200
	5	6400	0
	6	3200	0
	7	6400	12,800
	8	1600	3200
	9	400	204,800
pYA3167	10	1600	0
	11	51,200	51,200
	12	800	25,600
	13	25,600	3200
	14	0	51,200
	15	3200	51,200
	16	0	1600
	17	1600	1600
	18	100	1600
pYA3168	19	3200	0
	20	400	0
	21	1600	0
	22	6400	0
	23	400	0
	24	0	0
	25	0	0
	26	400	0
	27	6400	0

[a] Groups of ten female BALB/c mice were immunized orally with a single dose of approximately 10^9 CFU S. typhimurium χ 4550 harbouring one of three indicated plasmids pYNS27-53PS2, pYA3167 or pYA3168. Sera were collected before immunization and at regular intervals after immunization. Individual sera were analyzed by solid phase ELISA with *S. typhimurium* LPS (1.0 μg/well) (Sigma) and a recombinant hepatitis B virus pre-S antigen (200 ng/well) (Delos et al. 1991) as the solid-phase ligands as described (Schödel et al. 1994d). Titers are indicated as the highest serum dilution yielding an OD492>3 times above preimmune serum.

derived ColE1 yielding the lowest level of stability. This may in part explain why both the constitutive level of expression of the hybrid HBcAg-pre-S particles and the apparent plasmid DNA content in overnight cultures of transformed Δcya Δcrp Δasd χ 4550 did not significantly differ between the pBR322 (= pYA3167) and the pUC19 (=pYA3168) derivatives. To compare the immunogenicity of recombinant *S. typhimurium* expressing hybrid HBcAg-pre-S particles from different plasmid backbones, BALB/c mice were immunized with χ 4550(pYNS27-53PS2) (low copy number), χ 4550(pYA3167) (intermediate copy number) or χ 4550(pYA3167) (high copy number). When sera were analyzed for antibodies against pre-S and against *S. typhimurium* LPS, the antibody titres were similar at 5 weeks after one oral immunization with recombinants carrying the low copy number and intermediate copy number plasmid (Table II). Using the high copy number origin of replication from pUC19 produced a sharp decline in immunogenicity both for *Salmonella* and carried antigens. *S. typhimurium* χ 4550(pYA3167) grew slowly in rich media compared to the pBR322 or p15a based vectors and colonized gut or visceral tissues of mice less efficiently after oral immunization. Toxicity of the expression product(s) at high levels, not limited to the hybrid HBcAg gene, may contribute to these phenomena and to the instability of the plasmid. Note also that throughout antibody titres against *Salmonella typhimurium* LPS did not correlate well with antibody titres against a carried antigen.

3.5 Mucosal Immunogenicity

To analyze the mucosal immunogenicity and compare various routes of immunization, BALB/c mice were immunized with avirulent *phoP^c Salmonella typhimurium* expressing HBcAg by the oral, intranasal, rectal and vaginal routes (Hopkins et al., 1995). Serum and various secretions were collected and analyzed for IgA and IgG antibodies against LPS as well as HBcAg. All routes of immunization elicited high titered serum IgG antibodies against *S. typhimurium* LPS and against the carried HBc. Nasal immunization, which amounted to a mixed nasal and oral immunization, oral immunization and rectal immunization elicited gastrointestinal anti-HBc IgA. Nasal immunization was most efficient at generating HBcAg specific IgA in the lungs and rectal immunization was most efficient at generating rectal HBcAg specific IgA. The efficiency of vaginal immunization was dependent on the estrus state of the mice. Where it was efficient, saliva as well as vaginal anti-LPS IgA were elicited. Nasal immunization also elicited specific intravaginal IgA responses. It is therefore conceivable to target specific mucosal sites by varying the route of immunization with avirulent *Salmonella spp.* The safety and acceptability of these various routes will have to be established.

4. ACKNOWLEDGMENT

Parts of this research was supported by National Institute of Health grants AI20720 and AI33562 (DRM, DP, FS) and by the World Health Organisation Transdisease Vaccinology Program and the Association Française de Lutte contre la Mucoviscidose (FS).

5. REFERENCES

Cardenas, L., Dasgupta, U. and Clements, J.D. 1994. Influence of strain viability and antigen dose on the use of attenuated mutants of *Salmonella* as vaccine carriers *Vaccine* 12: 833-840

Crowther, R. A., Kiselev, N. A., Böttcher, B., Berriman, J. A., Borisova, G. P., Ose, V. and Pumpens, P. 1994. Three-dimensional structure of hepatitis B virus core particles determined by electron microscopy. *Cell,* 77: 943-950.

Curtiss, R III. Attenuated *Salmonella* strains as live vectors for the expression of foreign antigens, *In* G. C Woodrow and M. M. Levine (eds.), New Generation Vaccines. Marcel Dekker, Inc., New York, 1990, pp. 161-188.

Galan J.E., Nakayama K., and Curtiss R. III.1990. Cloning and characterization of the *asd* gene of *Salmonella typhimurium:* use in stable maintenance of recombinant plasmids in *Salmonella typhimurium. Gene* 94: 29-35.

Hopkins, S., Kraehenbuhl, J.P., Schödel, F., Potts, A., Peterson, D., De Grandi, P. and Nardelli, D. 1995. A recombinant *Salmonella typhimurium* vaccine induces local immunity by four different routes of immunization. *Infect. Immun.*63:3279-3286.

Milich, D. R. 1988 T and B cell recognition of hepatitis B viral antigens. *Immunol. Today* 9:380-386.

Nakayama K., Kelly S.M., and Curtiss R. III. 1988. Construction of an *Asd*+ expression-cloning vector: Stable maintenance and high level expression of cloned genes in a *Salmonella* vaccine strain. *Biotechnol.* 6:693-697.

Schödel, F. 1992. Prospects for oral vaccination using recombinant bacteria expressing viral epitopes. *Adv. Virus. Res.* 41:409-446.

Schödel F., Milich D.R., Will H. 1990. Hepatitis B virus nucleocapsid/pre-S2 fusion proteins expressed in attenuated *Salmonella* for oral immunization. *J. Immunol.* 145: 4317-4321.

Schödel, F., Moriarty, A.M., Peterson, D.L., Zheng, J., Hughes, J.L., Will, H., Leturcq, D.J., McGee, J.S. and Milich, D.R. 1992. The position of heterologous epitopes inserted in hepatitis B virus core particles determines their immunogenicity. *J. Virol.* 66: 106-114.

Schödel F., Peterson D., Hughes J.L., Milich D.R. 1993a. Hybrid hepatitis B virus core/pre-S particles: position effects on immunogenicity of heterologous epitopes and expression in avirulent *salmonellae* for oral vaccination.*In:* NATO ASI: Series A: Life Sciences Vol. 245: The Biology of *Salmonella*, F. Cabello, C. Hormaeche, P. Mastroeni, L. Bonina (eds.). Plenum Publishing Corp., New York, NY pp. 347-353.

Schödel F., Neckermann G., Peterson D., Fuchs K., Fuller S., Will H. and Roggendorf M. 1993b: Immunization with recombinant woodchuck hepatitis virus nucleocapsid antigen or hepatitis B virus nucleocapsid antigen protects woodchucks from woodchuck hepatitis virus infection. *Vaccine* 11: 624-628.

Schödel, F., Peterson, D., Hughes, J. and Milich, D.R. 1994a. Hepatitis B virus core particles as a vaccine carrier moiety. *Int. Rev. Immunol.* 11: 153-164.

Schödel, F., Wirtz, R., Peterson, D., Hughes, J., Warren, R., Sadoff, J. and Milich, D. 1994b. Immunity to malaria elicited by hybrid hepatitis B virus core particles carrying circumsporozoite protein epitopes. *J. Exp. Med.* 180: 1037-1046.

Schödel, F., Kelly S.M., Peterson D., Milich D., Hughes J., Tinge S., Wirtz R., and Curtiss R. 1994c. Development of recombinant *Salmonellae* expressing hybrid hepatitis B virus core particles as candidate oral vaccines. *Dev. Biol. Stand.* 82: 151-158.

Schödel, F., Kelly S.M., Peterson D.L., Milich D.R. and Curtiss R. III. 1994d. Hybrid hepatitis B virus core/pre-S proteins synthesized in avirulent *Salmonella typhimurium* and *Salmonella typhi* for oral vaccination. *Infect. Immun.* 62: 1669-1676.

Schödel, F., Peterson D., Hughes J., Wirtz R. and Milich D. 1995. Hybrid hepatitis B virus core antigen as a vaccine carrier moiety. I. Presentation of foreign epitopes. *J. Biotech.* in press.

von Brunn, A., Brand M., Reichhuber C., Morys-Wortmann C., Deinhardt F., and Schödel F. 1993. The principal neutralizing domain of HIV-1 is highly immunogenic when expressed on the surface of hepatitis B core particles. *Vaccine* 11:817-824.

4

SYNTHETIC RECOMBINANT VACCINE INDUCES ANTI-INFLUENZA LONG-TERM IMMUNITY AND CROSS-STRAIN PROTECTION

Ruth Arnon and Raphael Levi

Department of Chemical Immunology
The Weizmann Institute of Science
Rehovot, Israel

1. INTRODUCTION

The influenza viruses are responsible for many millions of infected individuals world wide and tens of thousands of deaths annually, as well as for causing considerable economic burden. The currently available influenza vaccines consist of either attenuated or inactivated viral particles. Their effectivity is limited, mainly due to the frequent antigenic variations of the external glycoproteins of the virus (*Laver and Air, 1979*), each new strain presenting a new challenge to the host immune system. Among the new strategies for vaccination, contemplated to overcome such shortcomings, are synthetic vaccines, which are based on short epitopes that should elicit protective immunity.

The influenza virus provides a very suitable model for studying the synthetic approach to vaccination, for several reasons: a) detailed information is available on the sequence, structure and function of the viral proteins, as well as on its serological specificities and genetic variations; b) various reliable assays of the virus are available for evaluating the effect of the immune response on the different viral functions; c) an established animal model in mice is available, for studying viral infection and challenge. The virus contains several major proteins of which the surface antigen haemagglutinin (HA) and the internal nucleo-protein (NP) play the most important role in the immune response elicited by the virus. In the case of influenza infection, neutralizing antibodies directed to the HA were shown to be the major factor responsible for neutralizing the virus (*Ada and Jones 1986*), whereas cytotoxic T cells (CTLs), directed mainly towards the highly conserved NP, are the key to viral clearance and recovery (*Yap and Ada 1978*). The interaction between the various cell types of the immune system was shown to be significant for the efficiency of the overall immune response (*Ada and Jones 1986*).

In our study, we used a region of the HA, comprising residues 91-108, which is conserved in all A influenza H3 strains and two NP epitopes, corresponding to amino acid

Novel Strategies in Design and Production of Vaccines
Edited by S. Cohen and A. Shafferman, Plenum Press, New York, 1996

residues 55-69 - a T helper (Th) epitope (*Gao et al. 1989*) and the epitope at position 147-158 - a CTL epitope (*Taylor et al. 1987*). Short peptides as such are usually poor immunogens and have to be administered when coupled to an appropriate carrier. We explored the possibility of presenting the epitopes when expressed in a chimeric protein, the *Salmonella* flagellin. Our results demonstrate that the products expressing these epitopes in the flagellin of *S. dublin* , are capable of protecting mice from viral challenge infection and produce efficient long-term immunity as well as cross-strain protection.

2. SYNTHETIC PEPTIDE VACCINES

In our early studies we have shown that several synthetic peptides of the HA molecule proved immunogenic and led to both humoral and cellular immunity (*Muller et al., 1982; Shapira et al., 1985a*). The peptide with the highest efficacy consisted of 18 amino acid residues corresponding to the sequence 91-108 of the HA molecule. This region, which is common to most H3 strains, was computer-predicted to be immunologically reactive, and was deliberately chosen to be part of a conserved sequence.

Indeed, a conjugate of this peptide with tetanus toxoid elicited in both rabbits and mice antibodies that reacted in a radioimmunoassay with the synthetic peptide, as well as with the intact influenza virus of several strains of type A. These antibodies were capable of inhibiting the capacity of the HA of the relevant strains to agglutinate chicken red blood cells. They also interfered with the *in vitro* growth of the virus in tissue culture, causing up to 60% reduction in viral plaque formation. Furthermore, mice immunized with the peptide-toxoid conjugate were partially protected against further challenge infection with the virus (*Muller et al., 1982*).

The peptide 91-108 does not overlap with any of the four antigenic determinants of the native HA, proposed by Wiley et al. (1981) according to the crystallographic data. It is adjacent, however, to the antigenic site D in the three-dimensional structure of the molecule. This could provide an explanation for the partial protective effect achieved by immunization with this peptide. This region resides in the interior of the HA trimer spike and is thus probably a "hidden" epitope in the native virus. However, in the infective state of the virus particle, as a result of the "opening" of the trimer, this region is exposed. This enables the antibodies raised by the synthetic peptide to react with the virus and impair its infectivity.

3. SYNTHETIC PEPTIDE VACCINES WITH BUILT-IN ADJUVANTICITY

The results reported hitherto were achieved by immunization in complete Freund's adjuvant (CFA) for augmenting the immune reactivity. This adjuvant, which consists of a water-in-oil emulsion containing killed mycobacteria, is a very effective adjuvant evoking high-level and long-lasting immunity, but is not suitable for human use. To explore the possibility of replacing the CFA by a less harmful substance, we have employed MDP (N-Acetyl-muramyl-L-alanyl-D-isoglutamine) (*Ellouz et al, 1974*), in combination with the tetanus toxoid conjugate of the 91-108 peptide of haemagglutinin for induction of anti-influenza response. Our findings revealed that this adjuvant was capable of inducing protective immunity against a viral challenge (*Shapira et al., 1985b*). MDP was most efficient when coupled covalently to the synthetic conjugate. In that form it led to the highest protection level against *in vivo* viral challenge, even higher than that induced in the presence of CFA. It should be emphasized that this conjugate of the synthetic peptide and MDP with the tetanus toxoid is water-soluble and was administered in a physiological aqueous solution, and hence constitutes a synthetic vaccine with built-in adjuvanticity, which could be suitable for use in humans.

In a more recent study we have used instead of MDP preparations of outer membranes of meningoccoci, denoted proteosomes, for augmentation of the immune response. Immunogenic proteins and peptides can be anchored via hydrophobic interactions to these proteosomes vesicles, which then serve as both carrier and adjuvant (*Lowell, 1990*). Synthetic peptides corresponding to epitopes HA91-108, NP55-69 and NP147-158 that had the lauroyl group added to their amino termini were coupled to proteosomes (*Levi et al, 1995*). These proteosome-peptide vaccines were denoted P-91, P-55 and P-147, respectively. Proteosomes without any peptides were denoted P-control.

The synthetic peptide HA91-108 was examined for its ability to induce antibodies (IgA in lungs and IgG in serum). This peptide covalently conjugated to the lauroyl group (HA91-108-L) was administered either alone, or after anchoring to proteosomes. Mice were immunized intranasally three times with three weeks intervals between each immunization, and their response was evaluated one week after the last boost. All (5/5) of the mice immunized with P-91 elicited IgA antibodies that recognized both the synthetic peptide and the intact virus, while only 1 out of 5 mice immunized with HA91-108-L produced antibodies, and at very low levels, indicating that the proteosomes were crucial for an effective humoral response.

The ability of the proteosome-anchored T-helper peptide to mount a cellular response was monitored *in vitro* using spleen cells of mice immunized once at the base of the tail with the synthetic peptide NP55-69, either in PBS or emulsified in CFA, or with the proteosome preparation P-55 and P-control in PBS. The proliferative response to stimulation with the synthetic peptide, as manifested by thymidine uptake, was monitored. The results indicated that P-55, when injected without external adjuvant, was very effective in priming the mice and the response was comparable to that of priming with the synthetic peptide emulsified in CFA. No nonspecific response to priming with the proteosomes control was observed.

Once it was established that peptide-proteosome preparations are capable of initiating anti influenza specific humoral and cellular immune responses, the efficiency of the various preparations to protect mice from viral challenge was determined. Mice were immunized with P-91 alone, and in different combinations with the other two peptides-proteosome preparations, namely, P-55 and P-147 (carrying the Th and CTL epitopes, respectively). The mice were challenged four weeks after the last immunization and protection was evaluated. The results indicated that immunization with a P-91 alone resulted in reduction of virus titre (a difference of 1.55 Log EID_{50}). The protective effect was not improved by the combining P-91 with P-55, and slightly improved by combining with P-147. Immunization with a proteosome vaccine containing the two T cell epitopes (P-55 and P-147) without the B cell epitope (P-91) was more effective, implying that significant protection could also be mediated by stimulating only the T cell-mediated arm of the immune system.

Since comparable protection against challenge four weeks after the last immunization could be elicited by immunizing with proteosome vaccines containing either B cell or T cell epitopes, we investigated whether or not any of these vaccines induced longer lasting protection against challenge eight weeks after the last immunization. The results of these experiments demonstrated the advantage of immunizing with a combination of both B cell and T cell epitopes. Thus, immunization with the lauroyl form of the B cell epitope alone (HA91-108L) or with its proteosomes (P-91), or the combination of the two T cell epitopes (P-55 plus P-147), which protected against a challenge given four weeks after immunization, did not protect from challenge eight weeks after immunization. In contrast, protection against a challenge eight weeks after vaccination was elicited by immunizing with proteosome vaccines containing the B cell epitope (P-91) plus either the T cell helper epitope (P-55) or, to a higher extent, with the CTL epitope (P-147). The importance of priming all arms of the immune system was emphasized by the results which showed that immunization with proteosome vaccines containing the triple combination of the B cell epitope (P-91) plus both T cell epitopes (P-55 and P-147) provided the strongest protection (*Levi et al, 1995*).

4. SYNTHETIC RECOMINANT VACCINES

An alternative approach to the chemical synthesis of vaccines is the use of genetic engineering. Recombinant DNA technology can be used for the production of the relevant viral immunogenic proteins in either bacteria, yeast or animal cells, for the purpose of vaccine preparation. It can also be employed for production of live vaccines by introducing the relevant gene(s) into the genome of vaccinia virus or avirulent Salmonella mutants. We attempted to bridge the synthetic and recombinant DNA approaches with regard to the effective peptides of influenza by expressing the above mentioned epitopes in the flagellin of Salmonella vaccine strain. In earlier studies (*McEwen et al, 1992*) we described the expression of the B-cell epitope HA 91-108 in the flagellin protein, and showed that intranasal immunization with this construct led to partial protection of mice from viral challenge. More recently, we have constructed two additional recombinant bacteria expressing the Th epitope NP 55-69 and the CTL epitope NP 147-158, respectively. The flagella isolated from the three recombinant bacteria, denoted Fla-91, Fla 55 and Fla 147, respectively, were evaluated for their immunogenicity and protective capacity, when given individually or in various combinations.

4.1. Cellular Response Induced by the Recombinant Influenza Epitopes

The ability to prime for a cellular response was evaluated by injection of the hybrid flagella carrying the above three epitopes, emulsified in CFA, at the base of the tail of BALB/c mice, and monitoring the proliferation of lymphocytes from these animals in response to *in-vitro* stimulation with the three synthetic peptides. The results, monitored by thymidine incorporation, indicated that NP55-69 is indeed a strong T-helper epitope, and that NP147-158 also elicited cellular response, albeit a weaker one. These results demonstrate the ability of these recombinant preparations to effectively prime for a cellular response (*Levi et al, 1995*). The flagella expressing the HA91-108 epitope did not induce cellular response.

The local cellular immune response in the lungs was studied after intranasal immunization of BALB/c mice either with the individual hybrid flagella, or with their various combinations. The antigens were administered in PBS three times at three weeks intervals, following which, the mice were sacrificed, their lungs removed and stained for histological evaluation, one week or two months after the last boost. One week after the last boost, all the mice exhibited massive perivascular and peribroncheal lymphocytes follicular infiltration. In contrast, only mice vaccinated with the two T-cells epitopes had significant lymphocytes infiltrations also two months after the last boost.

4.2. Protective Effect against Challenge Infection

In order to evaluate the capability of the recombinant synthetic vaccines to induce long term memory and protection, groups of mice were immunized, three times at three weeks intervals, with Fla-control, or with the combinations Fla-91+Fla-147, or Fla-55+Fla-91+Fla-147 and were challenged with A/Texas/77 influenza virus, one, four or seven months, respectively, after the last booster injection. The protection was evaluated by injection of a serial dilution of the lung homogenates of each mouse into embryonated eggs, and monitoring the virus growth in the eggs, as previously described (*McEwen et al. 1992*). The results, showed that a mixture of Fla-91 + Fla 147 was quite effective, leading to a difference of 1.4 log EID_{50} from the Fla-control. However, the preparation containing all three epitopes was the most efficient one in reducing the lung virus titre (a difference of 2.2 log EID_{50}), thus indicating that the addition of the Th epitope to the other two epitopes, significantly augmented the protection. The level of infection was similar in the three groups, indicating that the protective capacity was maintained for at least seven months after the last boost (*Levi and Arnon, 1995a*). It should be noted that the isolated flagella, comprising polymerised flagellin, contain multiple copies of the influenza epitopes.

4.3. Cross-Protection Against Various A/Influenza Strains

The three epitopes used in this study were conserved ones: HA91-108 is present in all A/H3 strains, and the NP is conserved in all A strains. Hence, it was of interest to determine whether the use of these epitopes could induce cross-strain protection. BALB/c mice were immunized with Fla-control, Fla-91, Fla-91+Fla-147 or the triple combination thereof, and one month later challenged with three additional A/influenza strains: Two H3N2 subtypes (A/Aichi and A/England), and one H2N2 subtype (A/Japanese). As was expected, vaccination with epitope HA91-108 alone was effective only against H3 strains. Addition of Fla-147 (CTL epitope) to Fla-91 led to a protective effect against viruses with H2 haemagglutinin as well, probably due to CTLs activity. When the flagellin carrying the Th epitope (Fla-55) was added to the vaccine mixture, a further increase of the cross-protective capacity was observed. Hence, combined with the data of the protection from a challenge with A/Texas strain reported above, the results described herewith demonstrate that the vaccine combining all three influenza epitopes was effective against at least four different influenza strains, three H3 stains, and an H2 strain (*Levi and Arnon, 1995b*).

4.4. Protection Against Lethal Dose Infection

The results described hitherto demonstrated a protective effect manifested by reduction of viral titre. An additional parameter for evaluation was the survival of BALB/c mice from lethal viral challenge. Mice were immunized with the same preparations as above, and one month after the last boost challenged with a lethal dose of A/Texas. The results (Fig. 1A) demonstrated 100% survival in the group vaccinated with the triple combination, whereas immunization with Fla-91 and Fla-91+Fla-147 led to 10% and 67% survival, respectively, compared to a control level of 15% survival in the mice immunized with Fla-control. To further analyze the protective immunity, the weight loss (indicating disease severity) of the surviving mice was recorded. The results (Fig. 1B) showed that all three epitopes were needed for rapid regain of the weight loss. In this group already 8 days after the viral challenge the animals started gaining weight, and resumed normal weight around 20 days after the infection. In contrast, animals from all the other treatments, including the vaccination with Fla-91+Fla-147, that led to 67% survival, continued loosing weight for additional 3-4 days, and regained their weight only 40 days after the challenge.

When the lungs of mice that had survived the challenge were examined histologically (45 days after infection), those from mice immunized with Fla-91, Fla-91+Fla-147 and the control group displayed scattered inflammatory foci of granulocytes, lymphocytes and macrophages as well as abscesses, massive parenchimatic damage, exudate and cellular debris. The lungs of mice immunized with all three epitopes, on the other hand,

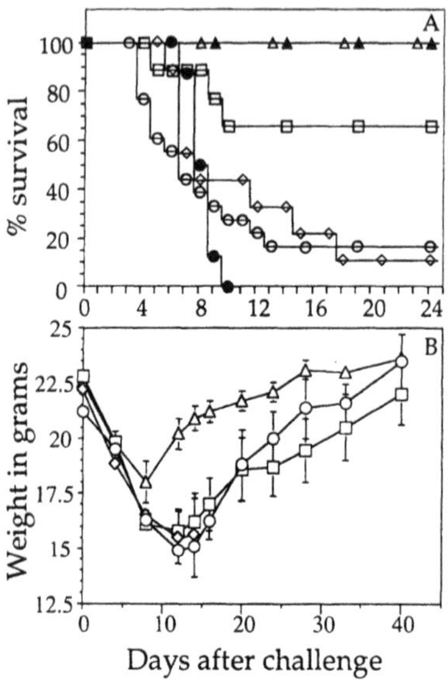

Figure 1. Protection of BALB/c mice from lethal dose challenge. Groups of 10 mice were immunized intranasally with the following combination of hybrid flagellins: Fla-91 (◇); Fla-91+Fla-147 (□) or Fla-55+Fla-91+Fla-147 (△,▲); untreated control (O,●).The schedule of administration was three times at three weeks intervals, and the challenge infection was with a lethal dose of influenza A/Texas/77 (10^{-2} HAU), given either one month (open symbols) or seven months (closed symbols) after the last boost. A- Survival rate. B- Recovery rate of the surviving mice (challenged one month after last immunization) as manifested by weight loss and regain.

appeared normal, with limited perivascular and peribroncheal foci of infiltrating lymphocytes.

In order to determine whether this protective immunity was long lasting, mice were vaccinated with the triple combination and challenged seven months after the last boost. Again, 100% of the immunized mice survived, as compared to 0% survival of the control group (Fig. 1A), indicating that the protective effect achieved by the immunization is long-term.

5. CONCLUDING REMARKS

Our results suggest that it is possible to induce anti-infleunza immune response with short peptides comprising conserved epitopes of the virus, but more than one epitope is required for the induction of efficient protection. Whereas the B-cell epitope HA 91-108 alone led only to partial protection, and each of the T-cell epitopes by itself had very limited protective effect, the combination of the HA 91-108 and the CTL epitope NP 147-158, and particularly the triple combination, including the Th epitope NP 55-69 as well, were much more effective. Protective effect was achieved with these epitopes when administered as synthetic peptides anchored to proteosomes (menigoccal outer membrane vesicles), but was even more pronounced when the epitopes were presented as recombinant constructs, within the flagellin of Salmonella vaccine strain. Both types of "vaccines" were effective after immunization by the intranasal route. Furthermore, the protection resulting from immunization with the combined recombinant epitopes persisted for up to seven months, afforded cross protection against several influenza strains and conferred resistance to lethal challenge as well as enhanced the recovery process. These findings accentuate the requirement to stimulate the various arms of the immune response - humoral, cellular, as well as cytotoxic T cells, for the induction of protective immunity, and demonstrate the potential of a synthetic recombinant vaccine, administered intranasally without external adjuvant, to induce effective broad-range, long term protection against influenza.

REFERENCES

Ada, G. L. and Jones, P. D. 1986. The immune response to influenza infection. *Curr. Top. Microbiol. Immunol.* **128**: 1.

Ellouz, F., Adam, A., Ciorbaru, R. and Lederer, E. 1974. Minimal structural requirements for adjuvant activity of bacterial peptidoglycan derivatives. *Biochim. Biophys. Res. Commun.* **53**: 1317-1325

Gao, X. M., Liew, F. Y. and Tite, J. P. 1989. Identification and characterization of T-helper epitopes in the nucleoprotein of influenza A virus *J. Immunol.* **143**: 3007

Laver, W.G., and Air, G.M. 1979. Structure and Variation in Influenza Virus. Elsevier North Holland, Amsterdam.

Levi, R., Abaud-Pirak, E., Lowell, G.H. and Arnon, R. 1995. Intranasal administration of synthetic peptides anchored to proteosomes elicits anti influenza protective immunity. *Vaccine.* (In press).

Levi R. and Arnon R. 1995a. Effective protection if mice from viral challenge by an influenza synthetic recombinant vaccine with cross-strain specificity. In: *Vaccines 1995*: Cold Spring Harbor Laboratory Press. (In press).

Levi R. and Arnon R. 1995b. Synthetic Recombinant Influenza vaccine induces efficient long-term immunity and cross-strain protection. *Vaccine.* (in press).

Lowell, G. H. 1990. Proteosomes, hydrophobic anchors, ISCOMS, and liposomes for improved presentation of peptide and protein vaccines., In: *New Generation Vaccines*. (Ed. Woodrow G.C. and Levine M.M.) Marcel Dekker, Inc., New York, pp. 141-160.

McEwen, J., Levi, R., Horwitz, R. J. and Arnon, R. 1992. Synthetic recombinant vaccine expressing influenza haemagglutinin epitope in Salmonella flagellin leads to partial protection in mice *Vaccine* **10**: 405

Müller, G.M., Shapira, M. and Arnon, R. 1982. Anti-influenza response achieved by immunization with a synthetic conjugate. *Proc. Nat. Acad. Sci.* **79**: 569-573.

Shapira, M., Misulovin, Z. and Arnon, R. 1985a. Specificity and cross-reactivity of synthetic peptides dervied from a major antigenic site of influenza hemagglutinin. *Mol. Immunol.* **22**: 23-28.

Shapira, M., Jolivet, M. and Arnon. R. 1985b. Synthetic vaccine against influenza with built-in adjuvanticity. *Int. J. Immunopharmac.* **7**: 719-723.

Taylor, P. M., Davey, J., Howland, K., Rothbard, J. and Askonas, B. A. 1987. Class I MHC molecules rather than other mouse genes dictate influenza epitope recognition by cytotoxic T-cells *Immunogen.* **26**: 267

Wiley, D.C., Wilson, I.A. and Skehel, J.J. 1981. Structural identificaiton of the antibody-binding sites of Hong Kong influenza haemagglutinin and their involvement in antegenic variation. *Nature* **289**: 366-373.

Yap, K. L. and Ada, G. L. 1978. Cytotoxic T-cells in the lungs of mice infected with an influenza A virus *Scand. J. Immunol.* **7**: 73

5

ALPHAVIRUS-BASED EXPRESSION SYSTEMS

Charles M. Rice

Washington University School of Medicine
Department of Molecular Microbiology
Box 8230, 660 S. Euclid Ave., St. Louis, Missouri 63110-1093

1. INTRODUCTION

Alphaviruses are enveloped positive-strand RNA viruses transmitted to verte-brate hosts via mosquito vectors (reviewed in 34). In the last several years, the alphavirus RNA replication and packaging machinery have been exploited for cytoplasmic expression of heterologous RNAs and proteins in animal cells (for reviews see 3, 24, 27). As transient expression systems, alphaviruses offer several potential advantages: 1) a broad range of susceptible host cells including those of insect, avian, and mammalian origin, 2) high levels of cytoplasmic RNA and protein expression without splicing and, 3) the facile construction and manipulation of recombinant RNA molecules using full-length cDNA clones from which infectious RNA transcripts can be generated by *in vitro* transcription. Several strategies are being explored using Sindbis virus (SIN), Semliki Forest virus (SFV), and Venezuelan equine encephalitis virus (VEE). These include i) construction of antigenic chimeras, ii) engineering recombinant viruses to express a second subgenomic RNA, and iii) replacement of the structural genes to produce self replicating RNA "replicons" which can be packaged into infectious particles using defective helper RNAs or packaging cell lines. Applications of these vector systems range from high level protein production in cell culture to the induction of protective immunity in animals.

2. THE ALPHAVIRUS LIFECYCLE

2.1. Virion Structure and Entry

The alphavirus particle contains a single genomic RNA complexed with 240 molecules of a basic capsid protein (C), surrounded by a lipid bilayer envelope containing 240 E1E2 glycoprotein heterodimers. Both the nucleocapsid and the envelope are organized with T=4 isosahedral symmetry (see 4). Alphaviruses can infect a variety of cell types and appear to be able to utilize more than one cell surface receptor for entry (34). After binding, several studies suggest that particles are taken up by recep-

Novel Strategies in Design and Production of Vaccines
Edited by S. Cohen and A. Shafferman, Plenum Press, New York, 1996

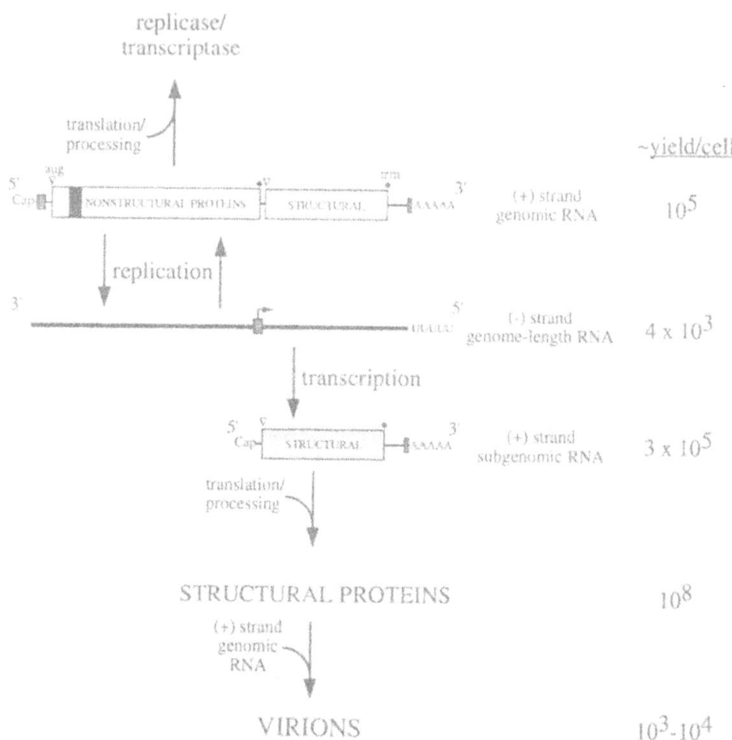

Figure 1. Alphavirus replication cycle. Translated regions of alphavirus genomic and subgenomic RNAs are shown as boxes with the nonstructural proteins and structural proteins (STRUCTURAL) indicated as open and lightly-shaded boxes, respectively. *Cis*-acting sequences important for replication and transcription are shown (small, checkered boxes) as is the sequence in the nonstructural region important for encapsidation (filled box). The start site for subgenomic mRNA transcription on the (-) strand genome-length RNA template is indicated by an arrow. Translation initiation (aug) and termination signals (trm) are indicated by open triangles and solid diamonds, respectively. See the text for further details.

tor-mediated endocytosis and that fusion of the virion envelope with the endosomal membrane is mediated by the E1 glycoprotein which undergoes a low pH-induced conformational rearrangement. The genomic RNA first serves as an mRNA for translation of viral nonstructural proteins (nsPs) required for initiation of viral RNA amplification.

2.2. RNA Replication

RNA replication occurs via synthesis of a full-length minus-strand intermediate which is used as the template for synthesis of additional genome-length RNAs and for transcription of a plus-strand subgenomic RNA from an internal promoter (Fig. 1). This subgenomic RNA, which can accumulate to levels approaching 10^6 molecules per cell, is the mRNA for translation of the structural proteins. The synthesis of minus, plus, and subgenomic RNAs appears to be temporally regulated via proteolytic processing of non-structural polyprotein replicase components by a virus encoded protease residing in the C-terminal region of nsP2 (15, 32).

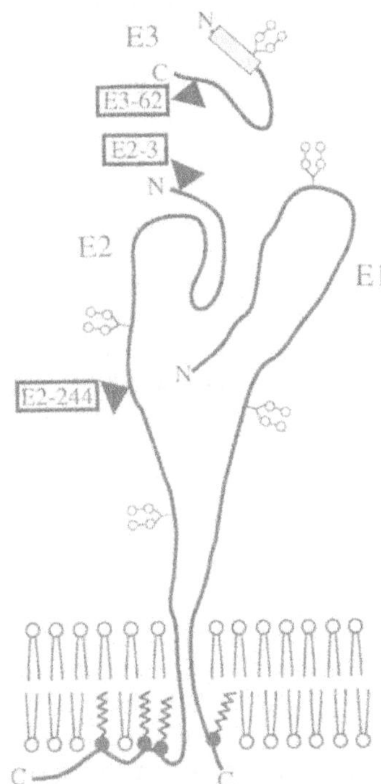

Figure 2. Permissive insertion sites for the RVFV 4D4 epitope in SIN E2. The diagram shows the SIN glycoproteins and their presumed topology with respect to a lipid bilayer. Sites of N-linked glycosylation are indicated by circles and the uncleaved PE2 signal sequence by a shaded box. Permissive sites for insertion of the 4D4 epitope are indicated by solid triangles and labeled according to their position in the respective proteins.

2.3. Translation of Structural Proteins, Virus Assembly and Release

The structural proteins are initially translated as a polyprotein (NH_2-C-E3-E2-6K-E1-COOH) which is processed co- and post-translationally to produced the mature products. Cleavage at the C/E3 site is mediated by a chymotrypsin-like protease activity residing in the C-terminal portion of the C protein. E3 and E2 are initially made as a precursor (called PE2 or P62) which is processed by a furin-like activity late during release of the virus from infected cells. The remaining processing events are mediated by host signal peptidase and give rise to the topological arrangement of the proteins shown in Fig. 2. Envelope glycoproteins E1 and PE2 form a heterdimer which migrates through the secretory pathway to the plasma membrane. In the cytoplasm, C protein subunits complex with the genome RNA to form a nucleocapsid which matures by budding through the plasma membrane, acquiring a lipid bilayer envelope with embedded viral glycoproteins.

2.4. Effects on Host Cell Biology

In permissive vertebrate cells, virus infection results in the rapid shut off of host mRNA translation and takeover of the translational machinery by viral mRNAs. The typical alphavirus growth cycle is relatively fast resulting in the release of more than 1000 virions per cell and cell death within 12-24 hours. Recent studies have shown that expression of the viral structural proteins is not required for shut off of host translation (8). In mosquito cells, the rate of virus replication is slower, often with minimal effects on the insect cell; persistent infections can be readily established.

3. INFECTIOUS ALPHAVIRUS cDNA CLONES

Studies on the use of alphaviruses as vectors have required the recovery of infectious replication competent RNA transcripts from cDNA clones. Full-length cDNA clones from which infectious RNA transcripts can be synthesized *in vitro* have been reported for SIN, SFV, VEE, and Ross River virus. These clones have proven of great value for basic studies on alphavirus replication, including the definition of RNA elements important for RNA replication, subgenomic RNA transcription and genome RNA packaging (see Fig. 1). Capped RNA transcripts, produced *in vitro* by transcription with SP6 or T7 polymerase, are used to transfect tissue culture cells, usually a continuous hamster kidney line (BHK) or secondary chicken embryo fibroblasts (CEF). Transfection is facilitated by DEAE dextran, cationic liposomes, or electroporation. In the latter method, efficiencies can approach 100% for BHK cells (19).

4. ENGINEERING ALPHAVIRUS CHIMERAS

Once the structure of poliovirus was determined, it became possible to predict surface loops in virion proteins and potential sites for insertion of heterologous peptide sequences (1). Such viable chimeric viruses have been successfully produced and can express protective epitopes from other human pathogens, providing a possible approach for creating novel vaccine strains. Along these lines, the glycoproteins of SIN have been engineered to express a heterologous protective 11 amino acid epitope (called "4D4") derived from the G2 glycoprotein of Rift Valley Fever virus (RVFV). In contrast to non-enveloped poliovirus, a high resolution structure is not available for the SIN virion or the E1E2 heterodimer. Hence, it was necessary to employ a random mutagenesis strategy to identify sites in the viral glycoproteins permissive for insertion of this and other heterologous peptides. Random insertion libraries were derived by treating plasmid DNA with DNaseI or methidiumpropyl-EDTA-Fe(II) and permissive insertion sites were mapped in the E3, E2, 6K, and E1 proteins (21; unpublished data). Permissive insertion sites in E2 are shown in Fig. 2. Several of the chimeric viruses with growth properties similar to the parental virus have been characterized (21). To examine whether these SIN chimeras might stimulate a protective immune response, mice were immunized with the panel of SIN chimeras and subsequently challenged with a lethal inoculum of RVFV. Insertions near the N terminus of the E2 glycoprotein (E2-3) or in an internal region of E2 (near amino acid #244), resulted in 4D4 epitope expression on the virion surface, and were most effective at eliciting a partially protective immune response (21).

Such full-length random insertion libraries can be used to identify permissive insertion sites for any peptide or even larger functional domains which are compatible with recovery of infectious virus. In the case of the RVFV epitope library, replacement of the 4D4-encoding oligonucleotide in the full-length random insertion library with another oligonucleotide can be accomplished in a single step and was used to identify a cluster of sites in the E3 protein permissive for insertion of an 81 residue heterologous peptide (S. London, unpublished).

These libraries are also being used to see if the surface of SIN virions can be modified to allow targeting of SIN vectors to specific cell types. Such modified viruses must be competent for assembly and release from transfected cells, but be unable to bind and enter the normally wide range of host cells that SIN infects (7). A functional heterologous ligand or binding domain must be displayed on the virion surface, and allow selective virus binding to target cells expressing the cognate binding partner. Once bound, the engineered virus must

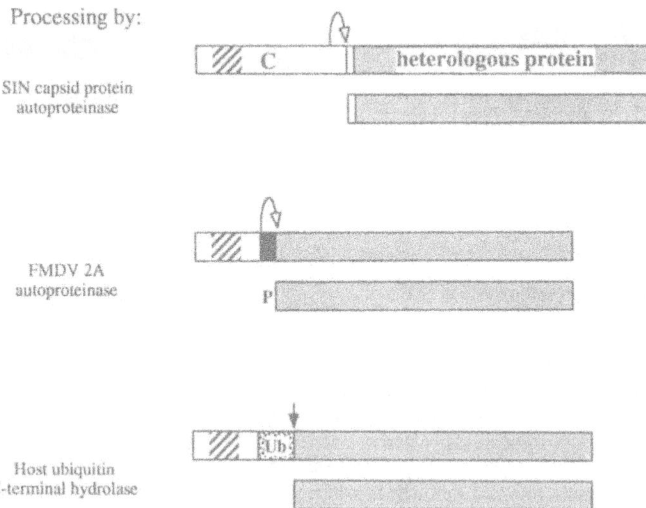

Figure 3. Double subgenomic vectors. Infectious alphavirus vectors which contain both the replication machinery and the structural proteins. Heterologous gene products are expressed by synthesis of a second subgenomic mRNA. For other symbols see Figure 1.

still be able to enter the cell and initiate replication. If successful, this technology could facilitate use of engineered alphavirus RNAs for anti-cancer and antiviral therapies.

5. REPLICATION AND PACKAGING-COMPETENT VECTORS

As mentioned earlier, several approaches have been taken for independent expression of heterologous genes using the alphavirus RNA replication machinery. The identification of the SIN subgenomic RNA promoter element allowed the construction of RNAs with additional subgenomic promoters (Fig. 3). Recombinant RNAs containing two promoters for subgenomic mRNA synthesis are referred to as double subgenomic vectors (dsSIN) (12, 29). Heterologous sequences, expressed via a second subgenomic mRNA, can be located either 3' or 5' to the structural genes. These vectors are both replication and packaging competent and allow the rapid recovery of high-titered infectious recombinant virus stocks usually in the range of 10^8-10^9 PFU/ml. In initial studies (12), dsSIN recombinants were engineered to express either bacterial chloramphenicol acetyltransferase (CAT), a truncated form of the influenza hemagglutinin (trHA), or minigenes encoding two distinct immuno-dominant cytotoxic T-cell (CTL) HA epitopes. Infection of murine cell lines with these recombinants resulted in the expression of ~10^6-10^7 CAT polypeptides/cell and efficient sensitization of target cells for lysis by appropriate MHC-restricted HA-specific CTL clones *in vitro*. In addition, priming of an influenza-specific T-cell response was observed after immunizing mice with dsSIN recombinants expressing either trHA or the immunodominant influenza CTL epitopes. Although primarily useful for short (<2 kb) heterologous sequences due to packaging constraints, this system allows the generation of high-titered recombinant virus stocks in a matter of days and has been useful for mapping and mutational analysis of class I MHC-restricted T-cell epitopes expressed via the endogenous pathway of antigen processing and presentation (13, 22).

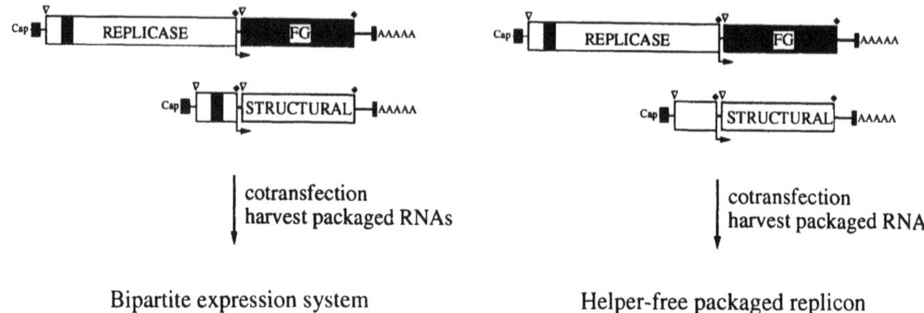

Figure 4. Replicons and DHRNAs. Shown at the top are replication and transcription competent alphavirus RNA replicons expressing a heterologous product via a subgenomic mRNA. The two RNAs shown below are packaging helpers which supply the alphavirus structural proteins after cotransfection with a replicon producing a functional replicase/transcriptase. The helper construct on the left contains the *cis*-acting signals necessary for replication and transcription as well as a packaging signal. This results in the production of infectious virus stocks with a bipartite genome structure. The helper on the right does not contain the packaging signal allowing the production of helper-free virus stocks of the packaged expression replicon.

In other studies, dsSIN recombinants have been used to map the domain of GLUT-4, the insulin-regulatable glucose transporter, which is responsible for efficient intracellular sequestration (28) and to study structure/function aspects of *rab*4 and *rab*5, two *ras*-like GTP-binding proteins which play a role in vesicular fusion and intracellular trafficking (16, 17). Another interesting application has been for gene expression studies in mosquito cells and mosquitoes (14) where engineered SIN recombinants have been used to follow virus spread in whole mosquitoes (25), to express antisense RNAs or viral proteins which are capable of specifically inhibiting replication of heterologous viruses, and for studies of normal mosquito gene function via antisense RNA-mediated inhibition.

6. ALPHAVIRUS RNA REPLICONS

The prototype replication-competent, but packaging-defective alphavirus RNA replicon was developed by replacing the SIN structural genes with the CAT gene (36)(Fig. 4, top). In cells transfected with this SIN recombinant RNA, CAT is expressed rapidly and up to 10^8 CAT polypeptides are produced per transfected cell by 16-20 hours. CAT expression could be regulated by inclusion of a *ts* mutation blocking RNA synthesis. Similar RNA replicons have also been developed for SFV (18) and VEE (R. Johnston, personal communication).

Since these RNA replicons do not express structural proteins, the level of heterologous product synthesized in transfected cells is directly related to the transfection efficiency of the recombinant RNA. Conditions for efficient RNA transfection using either cationic liposomes or electroporation have been determined for only a few cell types which limits the utility of these vectors for high level production or experiments where expression in every cell is required.

6.1. Packaging Systems

The utility of the alphavirus replicon expression systems has been markedly improved by development of a series of defective helper RNAs which allow efficient packaging of RNA replicons (2, 18). Defective helper RNAs (DHRNAs) are designed to contain the *cis*-acting sequences required for replication as well as the subgenomic RNA promoter driving expression of the structural protein genes. Packaging of SIN replicons is achieved by efficient cotransfection of BHK cells with both RNAs by electroporation (19). Replicase/transcriptase functions supplied by the vector RNA lead not only to its own amplification but also act in *trans* to allow replication and transcription of the helper RNA. This results in synthesis of structural proteins which can package the replicon with >10^8 infectious particles/ml (~ 5 x 10^9 infectious particles per electroporation) being produced after only 24 hours. Such stocks can be used, without further phenotypic selection, to infect cells for expression studies or high level protein production.

A spectrum of DHRNAs have been characterized which differ in their ability to be packaged (2, 11, 18; Fig. 4). Some DHRNAs which allow packaging of the replicon as well as themselves are useful under conditions where extensive amplification is advantageous (Fig. 4, left). Other DHRNAs allow efficient packaging of replicons, but are packaged very poorly themselves (Fig. 4, right). These helpers are useful for applications where expression of the viral structural proteins and virus spread are not desired. It is likely that the packaging capacity of alphavirus replicons for heterologous RNA will be on the order of 5 kilobases.

In addition to packaging of alphavirus RNA replicons by cotransfection with DHRNAs, continuous packaging cell lines have been developed which express a DHRNA under the control of a nuclear promoter (I. Frolov and S. Schlesinger, unpublished). Such cells can be used to rescue transfected RNA replicons and to produce large quantities of packaged replicon stocks by low multiplicity passage.

Besides reporters such as β-galatosidase and CAT, alphavirus replicons have been successfully used to express a variety of protein products (3, 24, 27). Some published examples include the neurokinin receptor (23), the HIV glycoproteins (26), and the hepatitis C virus glycoproteins (6, 20).

7. AN ALPHAVIRUS TRANSLATIONAL ENHANCER

In the course of studying the expression of proteins by alphavirus replicons, it was noticed that the level of heterologous protein expression was much lower than that observed for the authentic C protein. This observation led to the discovery of a translational enhancer in the C protein coding region (9, 33). A series of C-lacZ fusion constructs localized the element to the first ~275 bases of the subgenomic RNA (9, 33). Subsequent studies strongly suggest that an RNA element in this region of the subgenomic RNA enhances translation of the C protein in alphavirus-infected, but not uninfected cells (9, 10). SIN-lacZ replicons which lack this region express ~50 μg β-galactosidase per 10^6 cells, whereas cells infected with replicons containing the enhancer element accumulate 10-20-fold higher levels (~650 μg β-galactosidase per 10^6 cells; 9).

Such high levels of expression necessitate that the heterologous protein be expressed as a C protein fusion. Besides the incorportion of a site for specific proteolytic cleavage *in vitro*, several stratagies have been tried or are envisioned to produced high level expression of unfused product *in vivo*. One strategy employs the C protein autoproteolytic activity which cleaves at the C/PE2 junction and requires limited downstream PE2 sequences (33)(Fig. 5). A second approach involves construction of a fusion protein including the foot-and-mouth disease virus 2A autoprotease located adjacent to the N-terminal residue of the heterologous product. Self-cleavage by the 17 amino acid FMDV element should result in the production of a heterologous product with an additional N-terminal Pro residue (30). For production of proteins with authentic N termini, a ubiquitin monomer can be inserted in-frame between

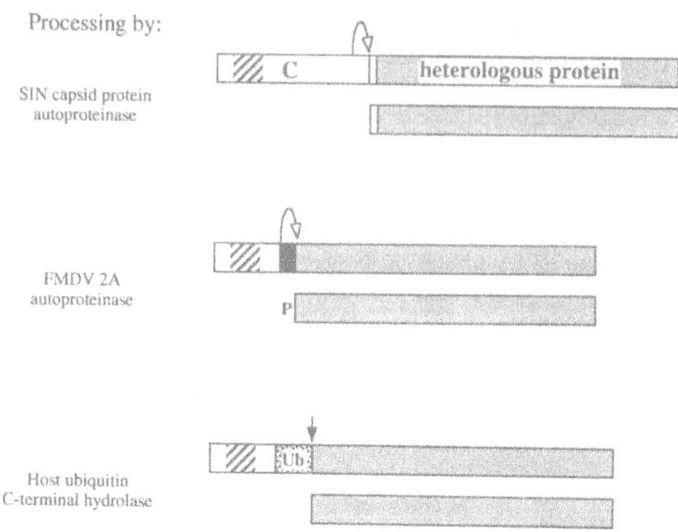

Figure 5. *In vivo* strategies for cleaving C protein fusions. See the text for explanation.

between C and the heterologous product (Fig. 5). Such constructs are cleaved efficiently *in vivo* by the host enzyme ubiquitin carboxyterminal hydrolase (see 15 and citations therein).

8. VACCINE APPLICATIONS

Given their efficient production of heterologous antigens, engineered alphavirus RNAs have significant potential for protective immunization (12, 21, 37, 38). Many strategies are just beginning to be explored. As described above, infectious particles containing either double subgenomic RNAs or packaged RNA replicons could be used. In the case of constructs expressing alphavirus structural proteins, which have the potential to spread *in vivo*, safety issues related to alphavirus pathogenicity remain a major concern. Even using the best "helper-free" packaging system, packaged replicons are likely to include low levels of packaged helper RNA or recombinant wild-type virus (35). Additional safeguards, such as mutations in the spike glycoproteins which require activation by *in vitro* proteolysis (31) or the use of packaging machinery from highly attenuated alphaviruses (5), may help to diminish the possibility of pathogenic consequences.

Alternatively, genetic immunization could be accomplished using DNA or RNA constructs lacking the structural proteins. In the case of DNA, a nuclear promoter can be used to drive expression of replication-competent SIN RNA replicons after transfection with DNA (I. Frolov and S. Schlesinger, unpublished). Although less stable than DNA, RNA vaccination should also be considered since this would result in only transient exposure to the immunizing nucleic acid minimizing the possibility of integration and undesirable mutagenic consequences. In addition, replicons can be engineered to express multiple subgenomic RNAs allowing coexpression of several protective antigens along with cytokines or other immunomodulators to enhance the generation of protective immune responses.

9. ACKNOWLEDGMENTS

The author thanks Margaret MacDonald and past and present members of the Huang, Rice and Schlesinger labs, in particular, Ilya Frolov and Sondra Schlesinger. Work on alphavirus vectors in my lab has been supported by PHS grant AI24134.

10. REFERENCES

1. Almond, J. W., and K. L. Burke. 1990. Poliovirus as a vector for the presentation of foreign antigens. Semin. Virol. **1**:11-20.
2. Bredenbeek, P. J., I. Frolov, C. M. Rice, and S. Schlesinger. 1993. Sindbis virus expression vectors: Packaging of RNA replicons by using defective helper RNAs. J. Virol. **67**:6439-6446.
3. Bredenbeek, P. J., and C. M. Rice. 1992. Animal RNA virus expression systems. Semin. Virol. **3**:297-310.
4. Cheng, R. H., R. J. Kuhn, N. H. Olson, M. G. Rossmann, H. K. Choi, T. J. Smith, and T. S. Baker. 1995. Nucleocapsid and glycoprotein organization in an enveloped virus. Cell **80**:621-630.
5. Davis, N. L., N. Powell, G. F. Greenwald, L. V. Willis, B. J. B. Johnson, J. F. Smith, and R. E. Johnston. 1991. Attenuating mutations in the E2 glycoprotein gene of Venezuelan equine encephalitis: Construction of single and multiple mutants in a full-length clone. Virology **183**:20-31.
6. Dubuisson, J., H. H. Hsu, R. C. Cheung, H. Greenberg, D. R. Russell, and C. M. Rice. 1994. Formation and intracellular localization of hepatitis C virus envelope glycoprotein complexes expressed by recombinant vaccinia and Sindbis viruses. J. Virol. **68**:6147-6160.
7. Dubuisson, J., and C. M. Rice. 1993. Sindbis virus attachment: Isolation and characterization of mutants with impaired binding to vertebrate cells. J. Virol. **67**:3363-3374.
8. Frolov, I., and S. Schlesinger. 1994. A comparison of the effects of Sindbis virus and Sindbis virus replicons on host cell protein synthesis and cytopathogenicity in BHK cells. J. Virol. **68**:1721-1727.
9. Frolov, I., and S. Schlesinger. 1994. Translation of Sindbis virus mRNA: Effects of sequences downstream of the initiating codon. J. Virol. **68**:8111-8117.
10. Frolov, I., and S. Schlesinger. 1995. Translation of Sindbis virus mRNA: analysis of sequences downstream of the initiating AUG codon that enhance translation. J. Virol. **69**: in press.
11. Geigenmuller-Gnirke, U., B. Weiss, R. Wright, and S. Schlesinger. 1991. Complementation between Sindbis viral RNAs produces infectious particles with a bipartite genome. Proc. Natl. Acad. Sci. USA **88**:3253-3257.
12. Hahn, C. S., Y. S. Hahn, T. J. Braciale, and C. M. Rice. 1992. Infectious Sindbis virus transient expression vectors for studying antigen processing and presentation. Proc. Natl. Acad. Sci. USA **89**:2679-2683.
13. Hahn, Y. S., C. S. Hahn, V. L. Braciale, T. J. Braciale, and C. M. Rice. 1992. CD8[+] T cell recognition of an endogenously processed epitope is regulated primarily by residues within the epitope. J. Exp. Med. **176**:1335-1341.
14. Higgs, S., A. M. Powers, and K. E. Olson. 1993. Alphavirus expression systems: Applications to mosquito vector studies. Parasitology Today **9**:444-452.
15. Lemm, J. A., T. Rümenapf, E. G. Strauss, J. H. Strauss, and C. M. Rice. 1994. Polypeptide requirements for assembly of functional Sindbis virus replication complexes: A model for the temporal regulation of minus and plus-strand RNA synthesis. EMBO J. **13**:2925-2934.
16. Li, G., and P. D. Stahl. 1993. Post-translational processing and membrane association of the two early endosome-associated rab GTP binding proteins (*rab*4 and *rab*5). Arch. Biochem. Biophs. **304**:471-478.
17. Li, G., and P. D. Stahl. 1993. Structure-function relationship of the small GTPase *rab*5. J. Biol. Chem. **268**:24475-24480.
18. Liljeström, P., and H. Garoff. 1991. A new generation of animal cell expression vectors based on the Semliki Forest virus replicon. BioTechnology **9**:1356-1361.
19. Liljeström, P., S. Lusa, D. Huylebroeck, and H. Garoff. 1991. *In vitro* mutagenesis of a full-length cDNA clone of Semliki Forest virus: the small 6,000-molecular-weight membrane protein modulates virus release. J. Virol. **65**:4107-4113.
20. Lin, C., B. D. Lindenbach, B. Prágai, D. W. McCourt, and C. M. Rice. 1994. Processing of the hepatitis C virus E2-NS2 region: Identification of p7 and two distinct E2-specific products with different C termini. J. Virol. **68**:5063-5073.
21. London, S. D., A. L. Schmaljohn, J. M. Dalrymple, and C. M. Rice. 1992. Infectious enveloped RNA virus antigenic chimeras. Proc. Natl. Acad. Sci. USA **89**:207-211.

22. Lovett, A. E., C. S. Hahn, C. M. Rice, T. K. Frey, and J. S. Wolinsky. 1993. Rubella virus-specific cytotoxic T-lymphocyte responses: Identification of the capsid as a target of major histocompatibility complex class I-restricted lysis and definition of two epitopes. J. Virol. **67**:5849-5858.

23. Lundstrom, K., A. Mills, G. Buell, E. Allet, N. Adami, and P. Liljeström. 1994. High-level expression of the human neurokinin-1 receptor in mammalian cell lines using the Semliki Forest virus expression system. Eur. J. Biochem. **224**:917-921.

24. Olkkonen, V. M., P. Dupree, K. Simons, O. Liljeström, and H. Garoff. 1994. Expression of exogenous protein in mammalian cells with the Semliki Forest virus vector. Meth. Cell Biol. **43**:43-53.

25. Olson, K. E., S. Higgs, C. M. Rice, J. O. Carlson, and B. J. Beaty. 1994. The expression of chloramphenicol acetyltransferase in Aedes albopictus (C6/36) cells and Aedes triseriatus mosquitoes using a double subgenomic recombinant Sindbis virus. Insect Biochem. Molec. Biol. **24**:39-48.

26. Paul, N. L., M. Marsh, J. A. McKeating, T. F. Schulz, P. Liljeström, H. Garoff, and R. A. Weiss. 1993. Expression of HIV-1 envelope glycoproteins by Semliki Forest virus vectors. AIDS Res. Human Retro. **9**:963-970.

27. Piper, R. C., J. W. Slot, G. Li, P. D. Stahl, and D. E. James. 1994. Recombinant Sindbis virus as an expression system for cell biology. Meth. Cell Biol. **43**:55-78.

28. Piper, R. C., C. Tai, J. W. Slot, C. S. Hahn, C. M. Rice, H. V. Huang, and D. E. James. 1992. The efficient intracellular sequestration of the insulin-regulatable glucose transporter (GLUT-4) is conferred by the N terminus. J. Cell Biol. **117**:729-743.

29. Raju, R., and H. V. Huang. 1991. Analysis of Sindbis virus promoter recognition *in vivo*, using novel vectors with two subgenomic mRNA promoters. J. Virol. **65**:2501-2510.

30. Ryan, M. D., and J. Drew. 1994. Foot-and-mouth disease virus 2A oligopeptide mediated cleavage of an artificial polyprotein. EMBO J. **13**:928-933.

31. Salminen, A., J. M. Wahlberg, M. Lobigs, P. Liljestrom, and H. Garoff. 1992. Membrane fusion process of Semliki Forest virus II: Cleavage dependent reorganization of the spike protein complex controls virus entry. J. Cell Biol. 349-357.

32. Shirako, Y., and J. H. Strauss. 1994. Regulation of Sindbis virus RNA replication: Uncleaved P123 and nsP4 function in minus strand RNA synthesis whereas cleaved products from P123 are required for efficient plus strand RNA synthesis. J. Virol. **185**:1874-1885.

33. Sjöberg, E. M., M. Suomalainen, and H. Garoff. 1994. A significantly improved Semliki Forest virus expression system based on translation enhancer segments from the viral capsid gene. BioTechology **12**:1127-1131.

34. Strauss, J. H., and E. G. Strauss. 1994. The alphaviruses: gene expression, replication, evolution. Microbiol. Rev. **58**:491-562.

35. Weiss, B. G., and S. Schlesinger. 1991. Recombination between Sindbis virus RNAs. J. Virol. **65**:4017-4025.

36. Xiong, C., R. Levis, P. Shen, S. Schlesinger, C. Rice, and H. V. Huang. 1989. Sindbis virus: an efficient, broad host range vector for gene expression in animal cells. Science **243**:1188-1191.

37. Zhou, X. Z., P. Berglund, G. Rhodes, S. E. Parker, M. Jondal, and P. Liljeström. 1994. Self-replicating Semliki Forest virus RNA as recombinant vaccine. Vaccine **12**:1510-1514.

38. Zhou, X. Z., P. Berglund, H. X. Zhao, P. Liljeström, and M. Jondal. 1995. Generation of cytotoxic and humoral immune responses by nonreplicative recombinant Semliki Forest virus. Proc. Natl. Acad. Sci. USA **92**:3009-3013.

6

ALPHAVIRUS HYBRID VIRION VACCINES

A. Shafferman,[1] S. Lustig,[2] Y. Inbar,[1] M. Halevy,[2] P. Schneider,[2] T. Bino,[1] M. Leitner,[1] H. Grosfeld,[1] B. Velan,[1] F. Schödel,[3] and S. Cohen[1]

[1] Department of Biochemistry and Molecular Genetics
[2] Department of Infectious Diseases
  Israel Institute for Biological Research, Ness-Ziona, Israel
[3] INSERM U 80, Pavillon P, Hôpital Edouard Herriot
  Lyon Cedex 03, France

1. INTRODUCTION

Many members of the alphavirus family are important human or veterinary pathogens. These viruses are extremely similar in molecular architecture yet differ in host range and in the pathological consequences of infection. Despite marked structural conservation, the various species are inefficient in eliciting immunological cross protection. Previously [1] we described a systematic approach for selection of epitope-cassettes of the E2 envelope of the alphavirus family that induce virus species specific protective immunity. This approach was tested and proved successful [2-5] with two viruses - Sindbis (SIN) and Semliki Forest (SF) - which are very remote phylogenetically. Vaccination was performed with recombinant peptide cassettes fused to a bacterial protein carrier (β-galactosidase) formulated with different adjuvants. In order to create a vaccine compatible with human use, we designed several live vector vaccines for presentation of the protective epitope cassette. Attenuated *salmonella* vaccine vector which can potentially allow presentation of many different cassettes and thus generation of a pan-alphavirus vaccine, proved to be inefficient. On the other hand the live attenuated viral vaccine based on a benign alphavirus such as SIN vector, appears to be promising. The principle of such vaccines is substitution of E2 epitopes of SIN virus vector with parallel protective epitopes from a different alphavirus. This system should have the advantage of presentation of specific virus epitopes in the context of the SIN alphavirus backbone which in turn could provide cross protective immunity on the basis of multiple common antigen determinants.

2. EXPERIMENTAL APPROACH

The efficiency of the different systems were evaluated for the SFV prototype representative of the family. For the study described here, the most potent protective cassette [2-4], cluster LMN (amino acids 289-352) or individual epitopes derived from it were used.

Novel Strategies in Design and Production of Vaccines
Edited by S. Cohen and A. Shafferman, Plenum Press, New York, 1996

Humoral response as well as protection from SFV challenge were followed in vaccinated mice. The efficacy of the live vaccines was compared to that of SFV-LMN-βgalactosidase (LMN-βgal) or SFV-LL-βgalactosidase (LL- βgal) fusion proteins. Vaccines based on the purified proteins were formulated in Freund's Adjuvant as described previously [3-5].

2.1 Presentation via Live *Salmonella*

Attenuated *S.typhimurium* strains were used as carriers of SFV-E2 epitopes: SL3261 (SAL) an *aro*A attenuated strain kindly provided by B. Stocker [6] and χ4072 and χ4217 *crp cya asd* strains kindly provided by R. Curtiss III [7,8]. The LPS structure of the *Salmonella* hybrids was confirmed by Urea-SDS-PAGE [9,10].

Expression of the SFV-E2 epitopes in *Salmonella* was driven by the *tac* promoter carried on two vectors: *a.* a derivative of the pTOZ plasmid [2,3] in which coding sequences of SFV-E2 protein were inserted to produce N-terminal fusion protein with βgalactosidase. *b.* a derivative of pNS14PS2 [11] which carry the modified gene of the Hepatitis B core Antigen (HBcAg) and the coding sequences of the SFV-E2-L epitope inserted within the internal loop of the HBcAg (between amino acids 74 to 81).

2.2 Presentation as Hybrid SIN Virus

The system developed by Rice et al., [12,13] for generating SIN virus libraries with random insertions of foreign epitope in the E2 envelope, was kindly provided by C. Rice and then modified to allow precise replacement of the SIN LMN cluster sequences with the parallel SFV sequences. The original restriction enzyme sites (the unique *Hind* III and *Ava*I-3161) in pMTE2 (a SIN-E2 cDNA vector) were altered and in the resulting pE2ADH15 plasmid, synthetic DNA coding for SFV LMN cluster, substituted with the SIN cDNA. The hybrid SIN/SFV-E2 cDNA was cloned into pTR2002 plasmid from which the complete 42S RNA was transcribed *in vitro* [13].

3.RESULTS AND DISCUSSION

3.1 *Salmonella* as a Carrier Vector for SFV Epitopes

Immunization with the live hybrid bacteria was compared to immunization with purified hybrid proteins emulsified with adjuvant (Table 1). Parenteral immunization with purified LMN-βgal protein (10 μg fusion protein per mouse) was much more efficient in inducing humoral response than oral immunization with live *S.typhimurium aro*A (SAL) bacteria expressing LMN-βgal (at amounts equivalent to 150μg of fused protein per mouse). This was demonstrated by: *a.* the higher levels of antibody titer (1000 fold difference) against the βgal carrier (Table 1) and *b.* immunization by live SAL/LMN-βgal did not yield detectable levels of anti-SFV antibodies while immunization with LMN-βgal with CFA induced antibodies at titers of 1:2100. To determine whether the immune system in the orally immunized mice was primed for the SFV epitopes, the mice were boosted with purified LMN-βgal. Under such conditions we were able to detect low levels of specific anti-viral antibodies (1:120, Table 1).

While the SAL/LMN-βgal proved inefficient in inducing humoral response it may nevertheless be efficient in conferring protection to mice against SFV challenge via cellular mediated immunity. It was previously shown that SAL expressing malaria antigen, induce CTL activity and protection in mice with no detectable antibody titers [15,16]. Indeed immunization with SAL/LMN-βgal conferred some protection against a low dose (1 LD$_{50}$)

Table 1. Immunization by live *Salmonella* hybrid vaccines

Immunization [a]		Antibody level - ELISA GMT[b]			
		Anti-βgal		Anti-SF	
Immunogen	Adjuvant	preboost	postboost	preboost	postboost
SAL/LMN-βgal	–	240	20,000[c]	<50	120
SAL/LL-HBcAg	–	N.D	<100	<50	460[c]
Purified LMN-βgal	+	170,000	160,000[c]	2,100	28,500[c]
Purified LL-βgal	+	150,000	170,000[c]	170	4,000[c]
Purified βgal	+	140,000	180,000[d]	N.D	<50[d]
SAL/βgal	–	450	40,000[d]	N.D	<50[d]
SAL/HBcAg	–	N.D	<100[d]	N.D	<50[d]

[a] Mice [female, 5 weeks old BALB/c (IFFA CREDO, France)] were immunized either orally with live SAL hybrid bacteria [14] or subcutaneously with purified βgal fused proteins emulsified in Freund's Adjuvant [2]. Three doses were given at two wks intervals, each dose containing either 3×10^9 bacteria or 10 µg fused protein. Ten wks post immunization, 10 µg of purified fused protein in PBS was injected intramuscularly as a booster.

[b] ELISA for anti-SFV was performed as described previously [2]. MonoQ purified βgalactosidase was used for anti-βgal ELISA. GMT - Geometric mean titer, was determined from sera collected from ten mice 10 wks post immunization (preboost) and two wks following the boost (postboost).

[c] Purified LMN-βgal boost.

[d] Purified βgal boost.

of SFV challenge (Fig. 1). Yet at higher challenge dose (250 LD_{50}) the hybrid bacterial vaccine showed no protection while the purified LMN-βgal in CFA provided full protection.

To further explore the potential of live bacterial vectors as a vaccine for presentation of viral antigens, we have tested HBcAg as a fusion carrier of SFV epitopes. Recombinant hybrid HBcAg was shown previously to be highly immunogenic either as purified core particles or when presented in *S.typhimurium* ([17] and ref. therein). In an attempt to evaluate HBV core particles as carrier for SFV epitopes, fusion genes with HBcAg were constructed by C-terminal fusion at a.a 156 of HBcAg or internal fusion between a.a 74-81. The latter configuration was found previously to be superior to other configurations of insertion ([17]). Due to limitation in the size of foreign epitopes that can be accommodated by such hybrid core, selected epitopes from the potent SFV-E2 LMN cluster were fused to HBcAg. Only one of the plasmids expressing a dimer of the L epitope of SFV-E2 (a.a 298-311) in the internal loop of HBcAg, was stable *in vitro* as well as *in vivo* . The L region was shown previously to be the minimal SFV-E2 epitope exhibiting protective efficacy when used as purified antigen in fusion with βgal [90% protection against 250 LD_{50} SFV challenge [2]].

The level of expression of the hybrid LL-HBcAg in the live SAL carrier amounted to 1% of total bacterial proteins and appeared as inclusion body aggregates rather than core particles. The humoral response of orally immunized mice with the hybrid SAL/LL-HBcAg was essentially similar to that observed for the SAL/LMN-βgal vaccine, namely, anti-SFV antibodies could be detected only after a boost with purified LMN-βgal protein. Yet the levels of the anti-SFV antibodies were significantly higher with the SAL/LL-HBcAg vaccine strain as compared with the SAL/LMN-βgal (Table 1). Furthermore the SAL/LL-HBcAg vaccine provided significant protection against infection by SFV. While all SAL/LMN-βgal immunized mice became sick with 60% recovery, in the case of SAL/LL-HBcAg 70% of the immunized mice did not develop any sign of disease (Fig 1). However, the extent of protection conferred by the SAL/LL-HBcAg live bacteria is still much lower than that provided by the same epitope (LL) when administered as purified fusion protein (compare

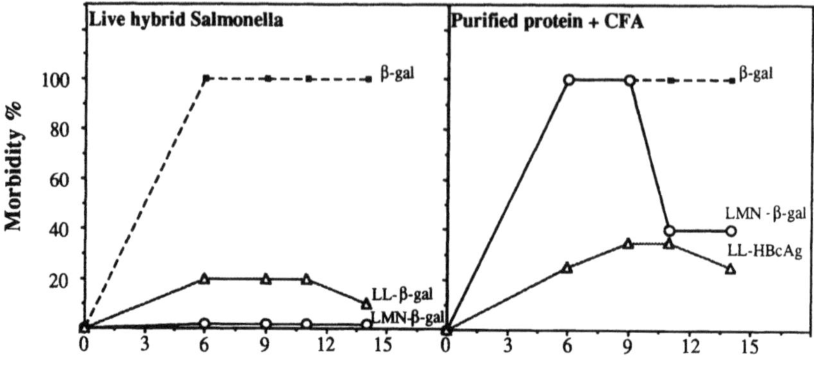

days post challenge

Figure 1. Resistance to SFV challenge, induced by hybrid *Salmonella*. Mice were immunized A. orally with live SAL expressing either βgal, or LMN-βgal, or LL-HBcAg; B. subcutaneously with the indicated purified proteins. Two wks post a booster injection with purified protein (see details in Table 1), mice were challenged with one LD_{50} of virulent SFV [2]. Mice were checked for morbidity (hind leg paralysis) and mortality for 2 wks. Mortality levels: controls βgal or SAL/βgal (50%); SAL/LMN-βgal (40%); SAL/LL-HBcAg (30%); LL-βgal (10%); LMN-βgal (0%).

LL-βgal (B) to SAL/LL-HBcAg (A) in Fig.1). These types of studies were repeated with the attenuated *S.typhimurium (cya crp asd)* strain in which the LL-HBcAg was expressed from the pYA292 plasmid (a plasmid which carry *asd* gene on which the bacteria are dependent and thus ensures survival of only plasmid bearing bacteria). Results were again disappointing with no evidence of any protection even after a boost with purified LL-βgal fused protein (data not shown).

In conclusion, in spite of the partial success in inducing some level of protection against SFV infection by one of the live *Salmonella* carrier vaccines, the system in general appears to be relatively inefficient for presentation of protective SFV epitopes.

3.2 Hybrid SIN Virus Presentation System

Initially, we prepared a hybrid SIN cDNA by replacement of the whole E2 LMN cassette coding sequences (amino acids 290-352) of SIN virus with the corresponding region from the SF virus E2 envelope glycoprotein. The resulting infectious SIN/SF RNA was able to express the hybrid E2 envelope protein in transfected BHK cells as determined by specific immunofluorescent staining, however virions could not be recovered from the cells.

Thirty four amino acids of the LMN cassette, out of the 62 amino acids which were substituted in the hybrid are unique for SFV. Assuming that the replacement of all of these amino acids may not be compatible with packaging of the hybrid virions we decided to reduce the number of substitutions to a minimum. The minimal cassette in the LMN region providing protection is confined to a 14 amino acid stretch - L cassette - in which only 8 amino acids are unique to SFV [3]. Therefore, a SIN hybrid carrying the SFV-L epitope was constructed. The SIN/SF(L) hybrid virus, unlike the SIN/SF(LMN) hybrid was successfully released from the cells and was demonstrated to be infectious although sensitive to temperature. This is best manifested by a 1000 fold reduction in PFU on BHK cells at 37°C as compared to 28°C (Table 2). For practical purposes of vaccine development it was essential to isolate temperature resistant virus. Such temperature resistant hybrid revertants, designated SIN/SFV(L)R,

Table 2. Virological and antigenic characteristics of the recombinant SIN virus vector and selected SIN/SF hybrid derivatives

Virus	L epitope type[a]			Growth properties			Virulence	
	Sequence	FA-αSF(L)		*in vitro* BHK cells[b]		*in vivo* mice viremia[c] PFU/ml	suckling mice % Survival[d]	
			HA titer	PFU/ml			IC	IP
				28°C	37°C			
SIN	SIN	–	128	10^8	10^8	3×10^5	0	20
SIN/SF(L)	SF	+	16	10^7	10^4	< 10	ND	100
SIN/SF(L)R	SF	+	16	10^7	10^7	9×10^3	100	100

[a] The nature of the L epitope of the various virions was demonstrated either by specific interaction of infected cells with anti-SFV/LMN-βgal antiserum in immunofluorescence assay [FA-αSF(L)] or by sequencing cDNA products using PCR.

[b] Virus titers of cell supernatants were determined by heamagglutination test and by plaque formation on BHK cell monolayers incubated at 28°C or 37°C.

[c] The levels of viremia were monitored 24 hrs post inoculation (Figure 2).

[d] Survival was monitored for 14 days in 1 - 2 day old suckling mice following ic or ip inoculation of 10^3 PFU of each virus .

were isolated and plaque purified at 37°C. These revertants retained the complete SFV-L sequences and were able to grow in cell cultures to relatively high titers, although both growth rate and final yield were reduced as compared to the parental SIN virus (Table 2 and data not shown). The revertants are replication competent *in vivo*, but unlike the parental SIN virus, they are non-pathogenic even to suckling mice (by the i.p. or i.c. inoculation, Table 2). Vaccination of adult mice with SIN/SF(L)R virions induced as expected, high titer of antibodies against SIN virus, similar to the levels induced by the SIN parental strain (Table 3). Similarly, these antibodies cross reacted with SFV at low levels. However, contrary to the SIN parental virus, the hybrid virions induced anti-SFV-L antibodies. Most significantly, the levels of antibodies against the L epitope of SFV induced by SIN/SF(L)R virions were comparable to those induced by infection with SF virions (Table 3).

The efficacy of the hybrid SIN/SF(L) vaccine was evaluated in a protection assay using a virulent SFV as a challenge. Mice were challenged five weeks post a single inoculation either with SIN/SF(L)R hybrid virus vaccine or with SIN parental strain or with placebo (Fig. 2). It appears that the common antigenic determinants of SIN and SFV which

Table 3. The SIN/SF(L) hybrid virus vaccine induces specific anti-SFV antibodies in infected mice

| Virus vaccine | ELISA antibody titer [a] against: | | |
	SIN virion	SF virion	SF - L peptide
SIN	30000	640	<10
SF [A7(74)][b]	1000	30000	250
SIN/SF(L)R	30000	640	80

[a] Antibody titers were determined 5 wks post immunization (Figure 2) by ELISA: anti-SIN and anti-SF virus titers were determined as described elsewhere (2) using whole virus as antigen and anti-SFV-L antibodies were determined as described previously (18) using 10μg of the L-peptide as the coating antigen. Titers are ELISA GMT.

[b] A7(74) is a nonvirulent strain of SF virus.

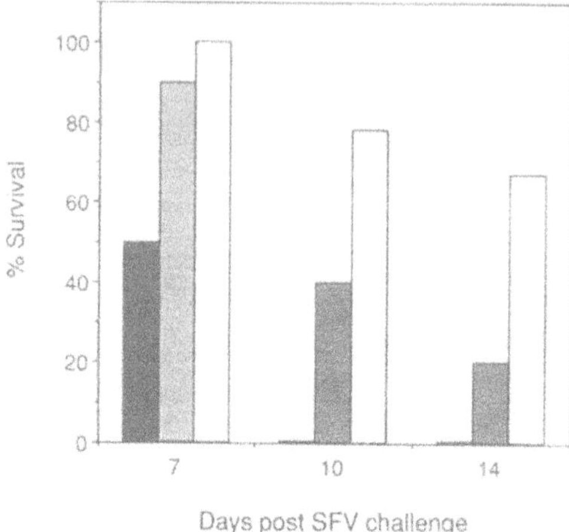

Figure 2. Protection of mice induced by hybrid SIN/SF virus against SFV challenge. Groups of weanling OF1 mice were inoculated IP with 10^5 PFU of parental SIN virus (dotted bars) or 10^9 PFU of SIN/SF(L)R hybrid virus (empty bars). Five weeks later the mice were challenged IP with 50 $IPLD_{50}$ of virulent SFV and monitored for survival (14 days). Mice of the same age and weight were inoculated with placebo (PBS) and similarly challenged (black bars).

are present on the parental vector can induce a basic level of protection (20%). Replacement of SIN amino acids with eight specific SFV amino acids (within the L epitope) was already sufficient to increase this basic level of protection - more than 70% of the animals survived the SFV challenge. All control non-inoculated mice died (Fig. 2).

The results demonstrate the feasibility of generation of live attenuated hybrid alphavirus vaccine. Furthermore, we show that cross protective immunity between distally related alphaviruses can be achieved by substitution of a very limited number of envelope amino acids. It is therefore possible to broaden the scope of protection by progressive replacements of SIN amino acids by various protective epitopes from SF virus or from any other member of the family, thereby constructing a "pan-alphavirus" live vaccine on the backbone of the benign SIN vector.

4. REFERENCES

1. Grosfeld, H., Velan, B., Olshevsky, U., Leitner, M., Lachmi, B.-E., Pinto, M. and Shafferman, A. 1988. An approach towards development of synthetic prototype model vaccine for alphaviruses. UCLA Symp. Mol. Cell. Biol. New Ser. **84:** 87-96.
2. Grosfeld, H., Velan, B., Leitner, M., Cohen, S., Lustig, S.,Lachmi, B.-E. and Shafferman, A. 1989. Semliki Forest Virus E2 envelope epitopes induce a nonneutralizing humoral response which protects mice against lethal challenge. J.Virol. **63:** 3416-3422.
3. Shafferman, A., Grosfeld, H., Leitner, M., Cohen, S., Olshevsky, U., Lachmi, B.-E., Lustig, S. and Velan, B. 1990. Selection and analysis of protective epitopes on the E2 envelope of Semliki Forest Virus. In: Vaccines 90. (Eds. Brown, F., Chanock R.M., Ginsberg, H.S. and Lerner, R.A.) Cold Spring Harbor Laboratory Press, Cold Spring Harbor, N.Y. p.p. 115-118
4. Grosfeld, H., Velan, B., Leitner, M., Lustig, S., Lachmi, B.-E., Cohen, S. and Shafferman, A. 1991. The delineation of protective epitopes on the E2- envelope glycoprotein of Semliki Forest virus.Vaccine **9:** 451-456.
5. Grosfeld, H., Lustig, S., Gozes, Y., Velan, B., Cohen, S., Leitner, M., Lachmi, B.-E., Katz, D., Olshevsky, U. and Shafferman, A. 1992. Divergent envelope E2 Alphavirus sequences spanning amino acids 297 to 352 induce in mice virus-specific protective immunity and antibodies with complement-mediated cytolytic activity. J. Virol. **66:**1084-1090.
6. Hoiseth, S.K. and Stocker, B.A.D. 1981. Aromatic-dependent *Salmonella typhimurium* are non-virulent and effective as live vaccines. Nature, **291:** 238-239.
7. Curtiss, R.III and Kelly, S.M. 1987. *Salmonella typhimurium* deletion mutants lacking adenylate cyclase and cyclic AMP receptor protein are avirulent and immunogenic. Infect. Immun., **55:** 3035-3043

8. Nakayama, K., Kelly, S.M. and Curtiss, R. III. 1988. Construction of an Asd+ expression-cloning vector: stable maintenance and high level expression of cloned genes in a *Salmonella* vaccine strain. Biotechnology, **6:** 693-797.

9. Tsai, C-M. and Frasch, C.E. 1982. A sensitive silver stain for detecting lipopolysaccharides in polyacrylamide gels. Anal. Biochem., **119:** 115- 119.

10. Hitchcock, P.J. and Brown, T.M. 1983. Morphological heterogeneity among *Salmonella* lipopolysaccharide chemotypes in silver-stained polyacrylamide gels. J. Bacteriol., **154:** 269-277.

11. Schödel, F., Milich, D.R. and Will, H. 1991. Hybrid hepatitis B virus core/pre-S particles expressed in attenuated *Salmonella* for oral immunization. In: Vaccines 91 (Eds. Brown, F., Chanock, R.M., Ginsberg, H.S and Lerner, R.A.) Cold Spring Harbor 'laboratory, Cold Spring Harbor, N.Y. p.p. 319-325.

12. Rice, C.M., Levis, R., Strauss, J.H. and Huang, H.V. 1987. Production of infectious RNA transcripts from Sindbis virus cDNA clones: mapping of lethal mutation, rescue of a temperature-sensitive marker, and *in vitro* mutagenesis to generate defined mutants. J. Virol. 3809-3819.

13. London, S.D., Schmaljohn, A.L., Dalrymple, J.M. and Rice, C.M. 1991. Infectious enveloped RNA virus antigenic chimeras. Proc. Natl. Acad. Sci. USA **89:** 207-211.

14. Cohen, S., Powell, C.J., Dubois, D.R., Hartman, A., Summers, P.L. and Eckels, K.H. 1990. Expression of the envelope antigen of dengue virus in vaccine strains of *Salmonella*. Res. Microbiol. **141:** 855-858.

15. Sadoff, J.C., Ballou, W.R., Baron, L.S., Majarian, W.R., Brey, R.N., Hockmeyer, W.T., Young, J.F., Cryz, S.J., Ou, J., Lowell, G.H. and Chulay, J.D. 1988. *Salmonella typhimurium* vaccine expressing circumsporozoite protein protects against malaria. Science (Wash. DC), **240:** 336.

16. Aggarwal, A., Kumar, S., Jaffe, R., Hone, D., Gross, M. and Sadoff, J. 1990. Oral *Salmonella*: Malaria circumsporozoite recombinants induce specific CD8[+] cytotoxic T cells. J. Exp. Med. **172:** 1083-1090.

17. Schödel, F., Kelly, S., Tinge, S., Hopkins, S., Peterson, D., Milich, D. and Curtiss, R. III. 1996. Hybrid Hepatitis B virus core antigen as a vaccine carrier moiety. In "Novel Strategies in Design and Production of Vaccines." (Eds. Cohen, S and .Shafferman, A.) Plenum Press. this volume.

18. Ariel, N., Lehrer, S., Elhanaty, E., Sabo, T., Brodt, P., Lachmi, B., Katz, D., Levin, R., Grosfeld, H., Velan, B. and Shafferman, A. 1990. Serologically defined linear epitopes in the E2 envelope glycoprotein of Semliki Forest virus. Arch. Virol. **113:** 99-106.

7

DNA VACCINES FOR BACTERIA AND VIRUSES

J. B. Ulmer, R. R. Deck, A. Yawman, A. Friedman, C. Dewitt,
D. Martinez, D. L. Montgomery, J. J. Donnelly, and M. A. Liu

Merck Research Laboratories
West Point, Pennsylvania 19486

1. INTRODUCTION

DNA vaccines are nonreplicating plasmids encoding genes from pathogens. The antigenic proteins are thus expressed in **the cells of** the vaccinated host and result in the generation of both antibody and cell-mediated immune responses. The ability to generate proteins with native conformation contrasts with certain recombinant protein or inactivated viral vaccines, and offers the means to generate antibodies against the relevant epitopes. Because the desired proteins are synthesized **within the host**, cell-mediated immune responses can be generated, without the inherent risks of **certain** viral vectors or of attenuation of **certain** attenuated viruses (**e.g., HIV**) and bacteria.

2. INFLUENZA

Protective immunity induced by a DNA vaccine was first demonstrated in a mouse model of influenza. DNA encoding influenza nucleoprotein (NP) induced high-titer antibodies and **cytotoxic T lymphocytes** (CTL), and cross-strain protection against a lethal challenge with virus (Ulmer *et al*, 1993). Anti-NP antibodies were detected by an ELISA and endpoint titers of $>10^6$ were measured, indicating that DNA vaccination is a very effective means of generating polyclonal antibodies without the need for purified protein. Both primary CTL (non-specifically stimulated with concanavalin A and IL-2) and antigen-restimulated CTL (restimulated with peptide-pulsed or virus-infected syngeneic spleen cells) were detected *in vitro*. The cross-strain protection was conferred by cell-mediated immune responses, since adoptive transfer of anti-NP antibodies into naive mice did not protect them from challenge (Ulmer *et al*, 1993), and depletion of T-cells *in vivo* prior to challenge abrogated NP DNA-induced protection (unpublished observations). Humoral (unpublished observations) and cell-mediated immune responses to NP are long-lived and have been detected two years after immunization of mice with NP DNA (Fig. 1).

Novel Strategies in Design and Production of Vaccines
Edited by S. Cohen and A. Shafferman, Plenum Press, New York, 1996

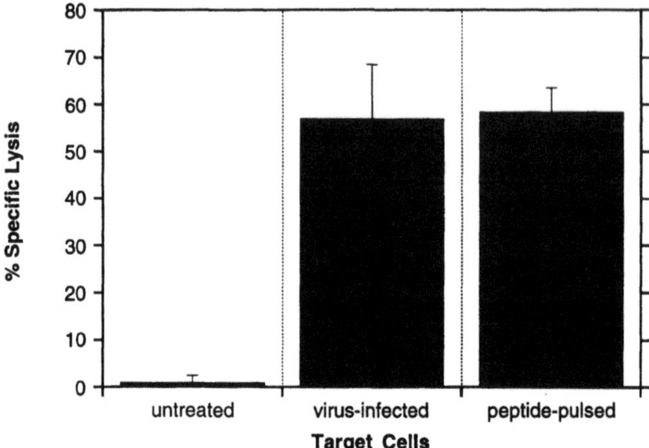

Figure 1. CTL responses in mice 2 years after injection of NP DNA. Female BALB/c mice (4-6 weeks) were injected with NP DNA (A/PR/8/34) at a dose of 6.25 μg/quadriceps three times at three-week intervals. CTL were obtained from mice 2 years after their third injection and restimulated *in vitro* with influenza virus (A/Victoria/73)-infected syngeneic spleen cells and IL-2. NP-specific CTL were assayed against P815 target cells infected with influenza virus (A/Victoria/73) or pulsed with NP peptide at an E:T of 25:1. Data **are** represented as % specific lysis ± sd for n=3.

DNA constructs encoding influenza hemagglutinin (HA) also are effective at generating protective immunity in mice. Injection of HA DNA induced high-titer antibodies, as measured by an ELISA and a hemagglutination inhibition (HI) assay. The latter assay measures antibodies that bind virus thereby inhibiting red blood cell agglutination, and is used as a surrogate indicator of neutralizing antibodies **and quantifying vaccine immunogenicity in clinical trials**. These antibodies confer complete protection against a lethal challenge of homologous virus (Montgomery *et al*, 1993), as indicated by a lack of morbidity and mortality and a substantial suppression of virus replication (unpublished observations). As little as 1 μg of DNA administered by i.m. injection is sufficient to protect mice from such a lethal challenge (Ulmer *et al*, 1994).

Influenza DNA vaccine efficacy also has been demonstrated in a ferret model. An advantage of this model over that of the mouse is the susceptibility of ferrets to infection by human clinical isolates of influenza virus. In contrast, mice are more resistant to disease caused by strains of virus that have not been adapted for mice. Therefore, one can test vaccine efficacy using recent **clinical** virus strains in the ferret model. Using this model, we have demonstrated that **an HA** DNA vaccine induces HI antibodies and protects ferrets from homologous virus challenge, as judged by limited virus shedding in the nasal passages (Donnelly *et al*, 1995a). To compare a DNA vaccine with a corresponding clinically available inactivated whole virus vaccine, a DNA vaccine was prepared containing constructs encoding HA, NP and matrix protein from A/Beijing/89. This combination reflects the contents of the reassortant inactivated virus vaccine. This DNA vaccine was significantly more effective at protecting ferrets challenged with a drifted virus strain (A/Georgia/93) than was the inactivated virus vaccine. Moreover, the level of protection induced by the combination DNA vaccine was comparable to that after injection of HA DNA from the homologous strain (A/Georgia/93). Therefore, a DNA vaccine has the ability to protect against challenge with an antigenically drifted strain of influenza virus, in part because of the added benefit of cell-mediated immunity against the conserved internal proteins of the virus. **This is significant in that the identity of future drifted strains cannot be predicted, which is a shortcoming in current viral vaccines.**

Immune responses induced by DNA vaccines also can be measured in nonhuman primates. A DNA vaccine containing HA (A/Beijing/89) in combination with other DNA constructs to mimic the components of the clinically available vaccines was compared to whole inactivated virus and subvirion vaccines. The DNA vaccine induced humoral immune responses that were as good as or better than **those induced by** the other vaccines. This was true in terms of both peak titer and duration of response (Donnelly *et al*, 1995a). A dose of 10 µg of HA DNA given twice was as effective as two doses of the full human dose of the inactivated virus vaccines (15 µg/strain).

3. HUMAN PAPILLOMA VIRUS

Human papilloma virus (HPV) is the etiologic agent responsible for the common wart, genital warts and cervical neoplasia. There are more than 30 strains, certain of which are associated with genital warts and cervical cancer (DeVilliers, 1989; Galloway *et al*, 1990). Neutralizing antibodies are directed against conformational epitopes of the major capsid protein L1 (Hagensee *et al*, 1994). Upon synthesis, this protein is directed to the nucleus of infected cells (Brown *et al*, 1994), and monomers associate to form virus capsids (Baker *et al*, 1991). Thus it was not clear that expression of L1 *in vivo* by a DNA vaccine would be capable of generating neutralizing antibodies against L1. Because human strains of papilloma virus cannot be grown *in vitro* or in animal models (with the exception of the subrenal capsular model for HPV type 11), our studies focused upon cottontail rabbit papilloma virus (CRPV). Utilizing plasmid DNA encoding CRPV L1, neutralizing and ELISA antibodies were generated, and immunized rabbits were protected from developing warts following challenge with CRPV (Donnelly *et al*, 1995b).

4. TUBERCULOSIS

Tuberculosis is a chronic infectious disease of the lung caused by the pathogen *Mycobacterium tuberculosis*, and is one of the most clinically significant infections world-wide, with an incidence of 3 million deaths and 10 million new cases each year (for review see Bloom and Murray, 1992). The only vaccine currently available is attenuated *M. bovis*. We have investigated the alternative approach of DNA vaccination using constructs encoding proteins of the antigen 85 complex. These proteins are secreted from mycobacteria and are targets for strong T-cell responses (Launois *et al*, 1994). Subunit vaccines comprised of the secreted antigens of *M. tuberculosis* have been shown to be protective in animal models of disease (Pal and Horowitz, 1992), and one of the protective antigens in this mixture is antigen 85 (Horowitz *et al*, 1995). Intramuscular injection of a DNA vaccine encoding antigen 85A generated high-titer antibodies and T-cells responses, including **specific** CTL and helper T-cells in mice (Fig. 2). The isotype profile of the antibody response was predominated by IgG2a, and the cytokines secreted from spleen cells restimulated *in vitro* with antigen were IL-2 and interferon-γ (unpublished observations). These results indicate that the phenotype of the helper T-cell response was T_h1 like. Immunity to disease caused by *M. tuberculosis* is thought to be conferred by T-cells and macrophages, including $CD4^+$ and $CD8^+$ cells, and T_h1 helper T-cells play a central role in their induction (for review see Orme *et al*, 1993). Therefore, DNA vaccines generate appropriate immune responses directed toward relevant antigen targets for immunity against mycobacterial disease and offer promise as an **improved** approach to the prophylaxis of tuberculosis.

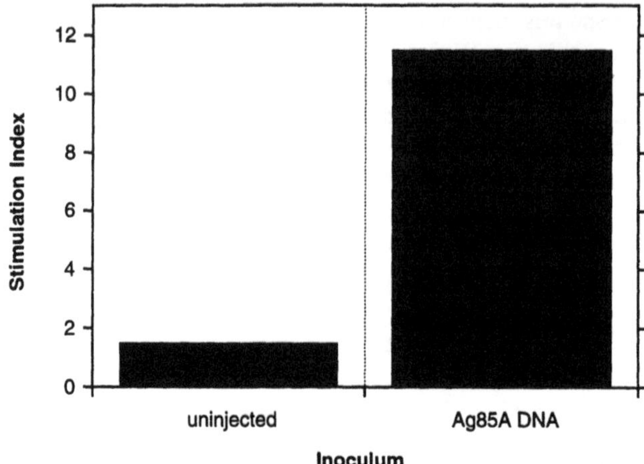

Figure 2. Lymphoproliferative responses in mice after injection of antigen 85A DNA. Female BALB/c mice (4-6 weeks) were uninjected or injected with DNA at a dose of 100 µg/leg three times at three-week intervals. Spleen cells from three mice from each group were prepared and pooled four months after injection and restimulated *in vitro* with *M. bovis* BCG culture filtrate proteins at a concentration of 1.5 µg/ml for five days. [^{3}H]thymidine was added at a concentration of 10 µCi/ml for the final 24 hr and radioactive incorporation was determined using a Tomtek harvestor. Data **are** presented as stimulation index, which is calculated as incorporation into restimulated spleen cells divided by that into cells incubated with medium.

5. CONCLUSIONS

Thus in preclinical studies, DNA vaccines generated effective protective immune responses based upon either neutralizing antibody (influenza and CRPV) or cellular immune responses (influenza, **tuberculosis**). In the case of **influenza**, cell-mediated immunity provided cross-strain protection by targeting epitopes of proteins which are highly conserved between different strains. In addition, strong helper T-cell responses were generated, as demonstrated here with plasmids encoding antigen 85A of *M. tuberculosis*. The safety profile of these vaccines needs to be thoroughly evaluated in order for DNA vaccines to reach clinical usage. Clearly, however, they are broadly efficacious in these animals modeled in their ability to generate various arms of the immune responses.

ACKNOWLEDGMENT

We gratefully acknowledge Drs. J. Content and K. Huygen, Institut Pasteur, Brussels, for the antigen 85A gene and assistance in cloning.

REFERENCES

1. Baker, T.S., Newcomb, W.W., Olson, N.H., Cowsert, L.M., Olson, C., and Brown, J.C. 1991. "Structures of bovine and human papillomaviruses. Analysis by cryoelectron microscopy and three- dimensional reconstruction". *Biophys. J.* 60, 1445-1456.
2. Bloom, B.R., and Murray, C.J.L. 1992. "Tuberculosis: Commentary on a reemergent killer". *Science* 257, 1055-1064.
3. Brown, D.R., Fan, L., Jones, J. and Bryan, J. 1994. "Colocalization of human papillomavirus type 11 E1^E4 and L1 proteins in human foreskin implants grown in athymic mice". *Virology* 201, 46-54

4. DeVilliers, E.M., 1989. "Heterogeneity of the human papillomavirus group". *J. Virol.* 63, 4898-4903.

5. Donnelly, J.J., Friedman, A., Martinez, D., Montgomery, D.L., Shiver, J.W., Motzel. S., Ulmer, J.B., Liu, M.A. 1995a. "Efficacy of a prototype clinical DNA vaccine: enhanced protection against antigenic drift in influenza virus". *Nature Med.* 1,583-587.

6. Donnelly, J.J., Martinez, D., Jansen, K.U., Ellis, R.W., Montgomery, D.L., and Liu, M.A. 1995b. "Protection against papillomavirus with a polinucleotide vaccine." *J. Infect. Dis.* (in press)

7. Galloway, D.A. and McDougall, J.K. 1989. "Human papillomaviruses and carcinomas. *Adv. Virus Res.* 37, 125-71.

8. Hagensee, M.E., Olson, N.H., Baker, T.S., and Galloway, D.A. 1994. "Three-dimensional structure of vaccinia virus-produced human papillomavirus type 1 capsids". *J. Virol.* 68, 4503-5.

9. Horwitz, M.A., Lee, B.W.E., Dillon, B.J., Harth, G. 1995. "Protective immunity against tuberculosis induced by vaccination with major extracellular proteins of *Mycobacterium tuberculosis*". *Proc. Natl. Acad. Sci. USA* 92, 1530-1534.

10. Launois, P., DeLeys, R., N'Diaye Niang, M., Drowart, A., Nadrien, M., Dierckx, P., Cartel, Sarthou, J.L., Van Nooren, J.P., and Huygen, K. 1994. "T cell epitope mapping of the major secreted mycobacterial antigen Ag85A in tuberculosis and leprosy". *Infect. Immunol.* 62, 3679-3687.

11. Montgomery, D.L., Shiver, J.W., Leander, K.R., Perry, H.C., Friedman, A., Martinez, D., Ulmer, J.B., Donnelly, J.J., and Liu, M.A. 1993. "Heterologous and homologous protection against influenza A by DNA vaccination: Optimization of vectors". *DNA Cell Biol.* 12, 777- 783.

12. Orme, I.M., Andersen, P., and Boom, W.H. 1993. "T cell responses to *Mycobacterium tuberculosis*". *J. Inf. Dis.* 167, 1481-1497.

13. Pal, P.G., and Horwitz, M.A. 1992. "Immunization with extracellular proteins of *Mycobacterium tuberculosis* induces cell-mediated immune responses and substantial protective immunity in a giunea pig model of pulmonary tuberculosis". *Infect. Immun.* 60, 4781-4792.

14. Ulmer, J.B., Deck, R.R., DeWitt, C.M., Friedman, A., Donnelly, J.J., and Liu, M.A. 1994. "Protective immunity by intramuscular injection of low doses of influenza virus DNA vaccines". *Vaccine* 12, 1541-1544.

15. Ulmer, J.B., Donnelly, J.J., Parker, S.E., Rhodes, G.H., Felgner, P.L., Dwarki, V.J., Gromkowski, S.H., Deck, R.R., DeWitt, C.M., Friedman, A., Hawe, L.A., Leander, K.R., Martinez, D., Perry, H.C., Shiver, J.W., Montgomery, D.L., and Liu, M.A. 1993. "Heterologous protection against influenza by injection of DNA encoding a viral protein". *Science* 259, 1745-1749.

8

NEW VACCINES AGAINST BACTERIAL TOXINS

Rino Rappuoli,[1] Mariagrazia Pizza,[1] Gill Douce,[2] and Gordon Dougan[2]

[1] IRIS, Chiron Biocine Immunobiological Research Institute Siena
Via Fiorentina 1, 53100 Siena, Italy
[2] Department of Biochemistry
Imperial College
London, United Kingdom

1. INTRODUCTION

Chemically detoxified bacterial toxins are the main or the sole components of several vaccines such as diphtheria, tetanus, pertussis, and cholera. Other toxins are good candidates for novel vaccines, such as the vacuolating cytotoxin of *Helicobacter pylori*[1]. Recently, genetic manipulation of the toxin's genes has been used to obtain molecules that are already non toxic and do not require chemical treatment for detoxification. This approach has been successful for pertussis[2], diphtheria[3], cholera and LT toxins[4]. Preclinical and clinical studies have shown that these molecules have several advantages over the conventional chemically detoxified vaccines. Generally, they are much more immunogenic and induce an immune response, that recognizes better the native toxin molecules. Non toxic derivatives of cholera toxin and LT, in addition to being good candidates for antidiarrheal vaccines, are also mucosal adjuvants[5]. Therefore, genetically detoxified bacterial toxins not only are good candidates to improve existing vaccines, but they represent new tools for the development of innovative vaccines targeted to the mucosal system.

2. PERTUSSIS TOXIN AND THE DEVELOPMENT OF ACELLULAR VACCINES FOR WHOOPING COUGH

Pertussis, a disease that affects infants and young children, is caused by *Bordetella pertussis*, a Gram-negative bacterium that infects virtually all children that are not immune[6-8]. The disease is characterized by long-lasting paroxysmal cough, accompanied by whoops, vomiting, cynanosis and apnoea. The disease is most severe in the first few months of life. Of infants that get the disease in the first year of life, 50% are hospitalized and 1% die. After the first year of life, only 4% of children with the disease are hospitalized. Worldwide, pertussis is still responsible for over half a million deaths each year[9]. Vaccination is the only way to control pertussis. Mass vaccination using killed bacteria (cellular vaccine) was introduced in the 1950s and reduced by 99% the incidence of disease: in the United States of America, the incidence decreased from 150 cases per 100,000 population in the pre-vaccine era to 0.6 cases per 100,000 population in 1980. In spite of the efficacy of vaccination, in the United States alone pertussis is still responsible for over 30,000 cases, 3300 hospitalizations and 25 deaths per year[10-11]. The use of the cellular vaccine is controversial, mostly because of fear of the side-effects that have been associated with it[7].

The fear of adverse reactions has decreased the acceptance of pertussis vaccination in many Western countries such as Italy, Germany, the United Kingdom and Sweden, stressing the need for new, improved vaccines, possibly composed of non-toxic, purified components.

The first acellular vaccine was developed in Japan by Yuji and Hiroko Sato in the late 1970s[12]. They observed that partially purified culture supernants of *B. pertussis* containing mostly FHA and PT could be detoxified by formaldehyde treatment and used as vaccine. The first acellular vaccine against whooping cough was licensed in Japan in 1981 for use in 2-year-old children.

Pertussis toxin, the main component of all acellular vaccines that have been described so far, is a complex bacterial protein toxin composed of five non-covalently linked subunits named S1 through S5[13]. S1 is an enzyme which has a toxic effect upon eukaryotic cells by ADP-ribosylating their GTP-binding proteins. Subunits S2, S3, S4 and S5, present in a 1:1:2:1 ratio, bind the receptors on the surface of eukaryotic cells and facilitate the translocation of the S1 subunit across the cellular membrane so that it can reach the target proteins. For vaccine preparation, the toxin is usually purified from culture supernatants of *B. pertussis* and inactivated by a chemical treatment. Although chemical inactivation of toxins has been successfully used for the manufacturing of vaccines such as diphtheria and tetanus, we were unwilling to use a technology developed over 60 years ago to develop a modern vaccine. Therefore, we decided to use the modern technologies provided by molecular biology to clone the gene and to study and inactivate the pertussis toxin. The genes coding for the five subunits of pertussis toxin were cloned and sequenced in our laboratory[14], and in the laboratory of J. Keith at the Rocky Mountains Laboratory in Montana[15]. The five genes were found to be located in a 3.5 Kbp region. In order to make non-toxic mutants, the region of the S1 subunit containing aminoacids 2-180 was mutagenized *in vitro* on the basis of sequence homologies with other bacterial toxins and computer modelling to identify the essential aminoacids. After extensive mutagenesis, we found that a mutant (PT-9K/129G) containing two aminoacid substitutions (Arg9 → Lys and Glu129 → Glu), did not show any of the toxic properties typical of PT such as lymphocytosis, histamine sensitivity, potentiation of anaphylaxis (Table 1), but maintained intact the B- and T-cell epitopes of the wild-type toxin, and was able to protect mice from the intracerebral challenge with virulent *B. pertussis* in a dose-dependent fashion [16].

The safety and immunogenicity of the PT-9K/129G mutant was initally tested in adult volunteers[17-18]. Two vaccines were used: one containing only 10 µg of the mutant toxin PT-9K/129G, and the other containing 5 µg of the mutant toxin PT-9K/129G, 2.5 µg of filamentous hemagglutinin and 2.5 µg of pertactin.

The National Institute for Allergy and Infectious Diseases (NIAID) performed a clinical trial in the USA, to compare ten acellular pertussis vaccines containing chemically detoxified pertussis toxin, two acellular vaccines containing genetically detoxified pertussis toxin and two whole cell vaccines[19]. Three doses of each vaccine were given to 120 infants. The results of the trial showed that all acellular vaccines are less reactogenic than the whole-cell vaccines[20]. The immunogenicity of the acellular vaccines varied considerably from vaccine to vaccine. Table 2 reports the anti-pertussis toxin antibodies induced by the

Table 1. Toxic and non toxic properties of the wild-type pertussis toxin and the genetically inactivated mutant PT-9K/129G

PT properties	Wild-type PT	PT-9K/129G
Toxic		
CHO cell clustering	0.005	>5000[a]
ADP-ribosylation	0.001	>20
Histamine-sensitive	0.1-0.5	>50
Leukocytosis stimulation	0.02	>50
Anaphylaxis potentiation	0.04	>7.5
Enhanced insulin secretion		>25
Lethal dose (LD$_{50}$)	15	>1500
Non toxic		
T cell mitogenicity	0.3	0.3
Hemagglutination	0.5	0.5
Affinity for anti-PT antibodies	2.0×10^{10}	9.8×10^9
Affinity for anti-S1 monoclonal (1B7)	2.4×10^8	6.1×10^8
Mitogenicity for PT-specific T cells	0.3	0.3

[a] Means that no effect was observed at the highest dose reported.

vaccines in the trial[21]. As shown, the genetically detoxified PT had a clearly superior immunogenicity per microgram of protein: from five to ten times higher.

In conclusion, the data obtained in the laboratory, in animal models and in several clinical trials have shown in a definitive way that genetic detoxification of PT has produced a molecule that is superior to those obtained by chemical treatment. In addition to the superior immunogenicity, the introduction of this molecule in acellular vaccines will have several other advantages. First, it will ensure the presence of a pertussis toxin antigen that cannot revert to toxicity. The absence, even in minimal amounts, of active pertussis toxin is crucial in novel vaccines, because this toxin has been shown to cause anaphylaxis[22] and permanent modification of the nerve-mediated permeability of the intestine[23]. Chemical detoxification

Table 2. Antibody to pertussis vaccine

Vaccine	PT, μg/dose	GMT	Seroconversion%	Elisa units/μg protein
1	10	180	100	18.0
2	5	99	99	19.8
3	23.4	127	99	5.4
4	25	104	98	4.1
5	50	99	95	1.9
6	25	68	97	2.7
7	25	66	96	2.6
8	25	54	90	2.1
9	10	39	88	3.9
10	10	38	92	3.8
11	10	36	94	3.6
12	10	29	89	2.9
13	3.5	14	67	4.0
14	—	67	83	—

1-2: Genetically detoxified PT.
3-13: Chemically detoxified PT.
14: Whole-cell vaccine.

cannot ensure this and active pertussis toxin has often been reported in several acellular vaccine preparations[24].

3. NON TOXIC DERIVATIVES OF *E. COLI* HEAT-LABILE ENTEROTOXIN AND CHOLERA TOXIN FOR NEW ANTIDIARRHEAL VACCINES AND MUCOSAL ADJUVANTS

Heat-labile enterotoxin (LT) and cholera toxin (CT) are homologous proteins that cause intestinal fluid accumulation[25-27]. CT is produced by *Vibrio cholerae* and is responsible for cholera, an epidemic diarrheal disease causing over 150,000 deaths each year[28-29]. LT is produced by enterotoxigenic *Escherichia coli* strains (ETEC) that are responsible for approximately two episodes of diarrhea in each child per year[28].

CT and LT are composed of two subunits: a monomeric, enzymatically active A subunit that ADP-ribosylates GTP-binding proteins, causing an increase in the cAMP level in target eukaryotic cells, and a pentameric, non-toxic, B subunit that binds the GM1 gangliosides on the surface of eukaryotic cells and delivers the A subunit across the cells membrane[27]. Using site-directed mutagenesis we replaced the serine residue at position 63 of the A subunit with lysine in order to construct a non-toxic LT mutant which still assembles as a holotoxin. The mutant protein, named LTK-63, has been purified and tested for ADP-ribosyltransferase and toxic activity in several assays. LTK-63 is still able to bind to GM1 ganglioside receptor, but shows a complete loss of enzymatic activity[4].

LT-K63 and a similar mutant of cholera toxin were tested for their immunogenicity in animal models. In contrast to the existing literature reporting that only the B oligomer is able to induce toxin neutralizing antibodies, we found that both LT-K63 and CT-K63 were able to induce toxin neutralizing antbodies against the A subunit. This novel finding suggests that both live and killed vaccines for cholera and enterotoxicogenic *E. coli* may be improved by using LT-K63 and/or CT-K63 instead of the B subunit[4, 30].

Finally, the LT-K63 non toxic derivative of LT was tested for its ability to act as a mucosal adjuvant[5]. Mice were immunized intranasally either with an antigen alone (ovalbumin and tetanus fragment), or with the antigen mixed with 1 µg of LT-K63. As shown in

Table 3. Serum and mucosal immune response to ovalbumin (OVA) and tetanus toxin fragment C (tet C)

Immunogen	Route (subcutaneous, sc) (intranasal, in)	Serum IgG response to Ova	Local IgA response to Ova
OVA	sc	+	−
Tet C	sc	+	−
LT	in	−	−
LT-K63	in	−	−
OVA	in	−	−
Tet C	in	−	−
LT + OVA	in	+	+
LT + Tet C	in	+	+
LT-K63 + OVA	in	+	+
LT-K63 + Tet C	in	+	+

Table 3, all mice, developed high levels of antibodies to the antigen in their sera. The local secretory IgA antibody levels to Ova and tetanus were measured in both lung and nose lavages. Mice immunized subcutaneously or intranasally with Ova or tetanus fragment C alone contained no detectable Ova- or tetanus-specific IgA in the washings sampled. On the contrary, all individual mice immunized with Ova or tetanus fragment C in combination with CT, LT or LT-K63, showed detectable levels of anti-Ova IgA. Thus mucosal immunization using the non toxic LT-K63 induces serum and mucosal antibody response against coadministered antigens. This finding opens the possibility of starting human clinical trials with novel mucosal vaccines.

REFERENCES

1. Marchetti, M., Aricò, B., Burroni, D., Figura, N., Rappuoli, R., and Ghiara, P., 1995, Development of a mouse model of *Helicobacter pylori* infection that mimics human disease, *Science*, 267:1655-1658.
2. Pizza, M., Covacci, A., Bartoloni, A., Perugini, M., Nencioni, L., De Magistris, M.T., Villa, L., Nucci, D., Manetti, R., Bugnoli, M., Giovannoni, F., Olivieri, R., Barbieri, J.T., Sato, H., and Rappuoli, R., 1989, Mutants of pertussis toxin suitable for vaccine development, Science, 246:497-500.
3. Rappuoli, R., 1990, New and improved vaccines against diphtheria and tetanus. In: Woodrow G.C. and Levine M.M. (eds.). *New Generation Vaccines,* Marcel Dekker Inc., New York and Basel, pp.251-268.
4. Pizza, M.G., Fontana, M.R., Giuliani, M.M., Domenighini, M., Magagnoli, C., Giannelli, V., Nucci, D., Hol, W., Manetti, R., and Rappuoli, R., 1994, A genetically detoxified derivative of heat labile E. coli enterotoxin induces neutralizing antibodies against the A subunit, *J. Exp. Med.,* 180:2147-2153.
5. Douce, G., Turcotte C., Roberts, M., Pizza, M.G., Domenighini, M., Rappuoli, R. and Dougan, G., 1995, Mutants of Escherichia coli heat-labile toxin lacking ADP-ribosyltransferase activity act as non-toxic, mucosal adjuvants. *PNAS,* 92:1644-1648.
6. Moxon, R. and Rappuoli, R., 1990, Modern vaccines: *Haemophilus influenzae* infections and whooping cough, *Lancet,* i:1324-1324-1329.
7. Cherry, J.D., Brunell, P.A., Golden, G.S. and Karzon, D.T., 1988, Report of the task force on pertussis and pertussis immunization-1988, *Pediatrics,* 81:933-984.
8. Giammanco, A., Chiarini, A., Straffolini, T., De Mattia, D., Chiaramonte, M., Moschen, M.E. *et* al. Seroepidemiology of pertussis in Italy, 1991, *Rev. Infect. Dis.,* 13:1216-1220.
9. Muller, A.S., Leeuwenburg, J. and Pratt, D.S, 1986, Pertussis: epidemiology and control, *Bull. WHO,* 64:321-331.
10. Farizo, K.M., Cochi, S.L., Zeii, E.R., Brink, E.W., Wassilak, S.G. and Patriarca, P.A., 1992, Epidemiological features of pertussis in United States, 1980-1989, *Clin. Infect. Dis.,* 14:708-719.
11. Sutter, R.W., and Cochl, L.M., 1992, Pertussis hospitalization and mortality in the United States, 1985-1988, *J. Am. Med. Assoc.,* 267:386-391.
12. Sato, Y., Kimura, M. and Fukumi, H., 1984, Development of a pertussis component vaccine in Japan, *Lancet,* i:122-126.
13. Tamura, M., Nogimori, K., Murai, S., Yajima, M., Ito, K., Katada, T. Ui, M., and Ishii, S., 1982, Subunit structure of the islet-activating protein, pertussis toxin, in conformity with the A-B model, *Biochemistry,* 21:5516 5522.
14. Nicosia, A., Perugini, M., Franzini, C., Casagli, M.C., Borri, M.G., Antoni, G., Almoni, M., Neri, P., Ratti, G., and Rappuoli, R., 1986, Cloning and sequencing of the pertussis toxin genes: operon structure and gene duplication, *PNAS,* 83:4631-4635.
15. Locht, C. and Keith, J., 1986, Pertussis toxin gene: nucleotide sequence and genetic organization, *Science,* 232:1258-1264.
16. Nencioni, L., Pizza, M.G., Bugnoli, M., De Magistris, M.T., Di Tommaso, A., Giovannoni, F., Manetti, R., Marsili, I., Matteucci, G., Nucci, D., Olivieri, R., Pileri, P., Presentini, R., Villa, L., Kreeftenberg, H., Silvestri, S., Tagliabue, A., and Rappuoli, R., 1990, Characterization of genetically inactivated pertussis toxin mutants: candidates for a new vaccine against whooping cough, *Infect. Immun.,* 58:1308-1315.
17. Podda, A., Nencioni, L., De Magistris, M.T., Di Tommaso, A., Bossù, P., Nuti, S., Pileri, P., Peppoloni, S., Bugnoli, M., Ruggiero, P., Marsili, I., D'Errico, A., Tagliabue, A., and Rappuoli, R., 1990, Metabolic, humoral and cellular responses in adult volunteers immunized with the genetically inactivated pertussis toxin mutant PT-9K,129G, *J. Exp. Mad.,* 172:861-868.

18. Podda, A., Nencioni, L., Marsili, I., Peppoloni, S., Volpini, G., Donati, D., Di Tommaso, A., De Magistris, M.T., and Rappuoli, R., 1991, Phase I clinical trial of an acellular pertussis vaccine composed of genetically detoxified pertussis toxin combined with FHA and 69K, *Vaccine*, 9:741-745.
19. Edwards, K.M., 1993, Acellular pertussis vaccines - a solution to the pertussis problem?, *J. Infect. Dis.*, 168:15-20.
20. Decker, M.D., Edwards, K.M., Steinhoff, M.C., Rennels, M.B., Pichichero, M.E., Englund, J.A., Anderson, E.L., Deloria, M.A., and Reed, G.F., 1995, Comparison of thirteen acellular pertussis vaccines: adverse reactions, *Pediatrics*, 96(3):557-566.
21. Edwards, K.M., Meade, B.D., Decker, M.D., Reed, G.F., Rennels, M.B., Steinhoff, M.C., Anderson, E.L., Englung, J.A., Pichichero, M.E., Deloria, M.A., and Deforest, A., 1995, Comparison of thirteen acellular pertussis vaccines: overview and serologic response, *Pediatrics*, 96(3):548-557.
22. Munoz, J.J., Peacock, M.G., and Hadlow, W.J., 1987, Anaphylaxis or so-called encephalopathy in mice sensitisized to an antigen with the aid of pertussigen (pertussis toxin), *Infect. Immun.*, 55: 1004-1008.
23. Kosecka, U., Marshall, J.S., Crowe, S.E., Bienenstock, J., and Perdue, M.H., 1994, Pertussis toxin stimulates hypersensitivity and enhances nerve-mediated antigen uptake in rat intestine, *Gastrointest. Liver Physiol.*, 30:G745-G753.
24. Anonymous, 1995, *Compatibility of acellular pertussis with other vaccines in UK primary immunisation and boosting schedules*, PHLS, CAMR, and NIBSC.
25. Spangler, B.D., 1992, Structure and function of cholera toxin and related *Escherichia coli* heat-labile enterotoxin, *Microbiol. Rev.* 56:622-647.
26. Betley, M.J., Miller, V.L., and Mekalanos, J.J., 1986, Genetics of bacterial enterotoxins, *Annu. Rev. Microbiol.* 40:577-605.
27. Rappuoli, R., and Pizza, M., 1991, Structure and evolutionary aspects of ADP-ribosylating toxins. In *Sourcebook of Bacterial Protein Toxins.* J. Alouf and J. Freer, editors, Academic Press Ltd., London, 1-20.
28. Del Giudice, G., 1991, Research priorities for diarrhoeal disease vaccines: memorandum from a WHO meeting, *Bull. WHO*, 69:667.
29. Anonymous, 1994, Cholera-update, end of 1993, *Weekly Epidemiological Record*, 69(3):13-17.
30. Fontana, M.R., Manetti, R., Giannelli, V., Magagnoli, C., Marchini, A., Olivieri, R., Domenighini, M., Rappuoli, R., and Pizza, M.G., 1995, Construction of non toxic derivatives of cholera toxin and characterization of the immunological response against the A subunit, *Infect. Immun.*, 63:2356-2360.

9

PARAMETERS FOR THE RATIONAL DESIGN OF GENETIC TOXOID VACCINES

W. Neal Burnette

Molecular Pharmaceutics Corporation
1553 Falling Star Avenue, Westlake Village, California 91362

1. INTRODUCTION

Pertussis and cholera endure as major contributors to worldwide morbidity and mortality. Even with efficacious vaccines against pertussis long available, it was not until recently that a significant reduction in the global incidence of infant disease has been recorded as a result of the successes of national and global vaccine initiatives. In contrast, no meaningfully effective vaccine exists for cholera, with the result that more than eight million cases of this disease and 150,000 cholera-related deaths occur each year.

A group of pathogenic bacteria share the characteristic of elaborating exotoxins that exhibit ADP-ribosyltransferase activity (Table 1). In addition to their rôles as virulence factors for the parent bacteria, endogenous prokaryotic and eukaryotic ribosyltransferases may also serve important functions in cellular regulation. The bacterial transferases are represented by the exotoxins of *Bordetella pertussis*, *Vibrio cholerae*, enterotoxigenic *Escherichia coli*, *Corynebacterium diphtheriae*, and *Pseudomonas aeruginosa*. Pertussis toxin (PT), cholera toxin (CT), and the heat-labile toxins (LTs) of enteropathogenic *E. coli* are structurally classified as AB_5 multimeric proteins, comprised of a single catalytic (A) subunit and a pentameric cell binding (B) oligomer; the B oligomer may either be heteropentameric (PT) or homopentameric (CT and LT). The enzymatically-active A protomers have substrate specificity for individual residues in the α subunits of G proteins involved in the regulation of adenylyl cyclase; ADP-ribosylation of such G protein subunits causes uncontrolled formation of cAMP that results in the cellular consequences of intoxication. Laboratory investigations employing recombinant DNA technologies and x-ray crystallography have recently allowed a detailed examination of structure-function relationships in these bacterial toxins and facilitated the design of new strategies in vaccine development.

2. PERTUSSIS GENETIC TOXOIDS

B. pertussis is a Gram-negative microorganism possessing a number of virulence factors that confer its pathogenic potential. Of these, PT is considered to be a necessary if

Table 1. Bacterial ADP-ribosyltransferases and related toxins

Organism	Toxin	Toxin structure	Binding oligomer	Activity	Substrate
Bordetella pertussis	pertussis toxin (PT)	AB_5	heteropentameric	ADP-ribosyltransferase	$G_i\alpha$
Vibrio cholerae	cholera toxin (CT)	AB_5	homopentameric	ADP-ribosyltransferase	$G_s\alpha$
Escherichia coli	heat-labile enterotoxins (LTs)	AB_5	homopentameric	ADP-ribosyltransferase	$G_s\alpha$
Corynebacterium diphtheriae	diphtheria toxin (DT)	A_1	monomeric	ADP-ribosyltransferase	EF-2
Pseudomonas aeruginosa	exotoxin A (ETA)	A_1	monomeric	ADP-ribosyltransferase	EF-2
Shigella dysenteriae	Shiga toxin	AB_5	homopentameric	*N*-glycosidase	rRNA
Escherichia coli	verotoxins	AB_5	homopentameric	*N*-glycosidase	rRNA
Castor bean	ricin toxin	AB	monomeric	*N*-glycosidase	rRNA

not sufficient component for complete immunoprotection. Heat-treated or chemically-inactivated toxoids have been shown to elicit protection against both toxin and bacterial challenge in mice; and it is now becoming clear that toxoids can also protect against human disease (Rappuoli *et al.*, 1992).

Pertussis toxin is a remarkably active pharmacologic agent. Although its use appears cardinal to immunoprotection, the dilemma of a toxin-based vaccine is that PT may be responsible for the major untoward effects of pertussis vaccination. The goal of recent studies was to produce commercially-significant quantities of this vaccine component by recombinant DNA means, dissect its pharmacological and immunogenic characteristics, and design a "genetic toxoid" capable of evoking protective immune responses, yet powerless to cause adverse reactions.

Pertussis toxin has the classical A-B architecture (Tamura *et al.*, 1982). Its B oligomer is composed of four distinct polypeptide subunits: S2, S3, S5, and two copies of S4. Subunits S2 and S3 share more than 70% amino acid sequence homology, but contain distinct receptor recognition domains that specify adherence to different glycoconjugate-containing receptors on sensitive eukaryotic cells (Saukkonen *et al.*, 1992; van't Wout *et al.*, 1992). The A protomer, or S1 subunit in PT, is the only subunit of the toxin that is transported into the membrane of sensitive cells and accounts for the negative effects of pertussis infection and vaccination.

To create a new, safe and effective toxin-based vaccine, the dissection of PT was deemed essential in order to uncouple its detrimental functions from the facility to stimulate protective immunity. The operon containing the cistronic elements encoding the individual PT subunits had been molecularly cloned and sequenced in various laboratories (Locht and Keith, 1986; Nicosia *et al.*, 1986). Each of these elements was subcloned in our laboratory and inserted individually into a plasmid optimized for direct overexpression of proteins in recombinant *E. coli* (Burnette *et al.*, 1988b).

The subunits were produced in quantities occasionally exceeding 50% of total cell protein. Recombinant PT S1 had specific enzyme activity essentially identical to that of the native protein. Although each of the PT subunit species could elicit antibodies crossreactive with whole toxin, none were capable of evoking toxin-neutralizing antibodies or of protecting animals against bacterial challenge (Burnette *et al.*, 1988b); this suggested that the protective antigenic determinants might require induction through holotoxin assembly in order to display appropriate epitope conformations to the immune system.

The initial question confronted was whether the toxicity-related enzyme activity of the S1 subunit could be uncoupled from those domains involved in formation of the lone immunodominant neutralizing and protective epitope recognized to reside in this protein. In a series of experiments, a region lying between tyrosine-8 and proline-15 was identified as essential for establishment of both an important catalytic subsite and the dominant neutralizing antigenic determinant (Cieplak *et al.*, 1988); this region is one of a number that are highly conserved among pertussis, cholera, and *E. coli* heat-labile enterotoxin A protomers (Locht and Keith, 1986; Nicosia *et al.*, 1986). A selection of codon substitutions was made within this segment and the resultant analog polypeptides were analyzed for the effects of the site-specific modifications (Burnette *et al.*, 1988a). Of the original constructs examined, only the analog with the substitution at arginine-9 had lost essentially all of its catalytic potential without modification to its reactivity with a neutralizing monoclonal antibody; successive site-specific substitution experiments also demonstrated that substitutions at glutamate-129 had a comparable effect on S1 (Pizza *et al.*, 1989). When reassembled *in vitro* with native B oligomer and analog S1 subunits containing such substitutions, the resulting holotoxin molecules were impotent for intoxicating cultured cells (Bartley *et al.*, 1989) and provoking toxin-related effects *in vivo* (Arciniega *et al.*, 1991). Nevertheless, the analog holotoxins were indistinguishable from native toxin in their ability to protect mice against the effects of toxin challenge and against aerosol infection with *Bordetella pertussis* (Arciniega *et al.*, 1991). Interestingly, however, there also seemed to be no significant difference between holotoxin and B oligomer alone for immunoprotection of mice. Studies demonstrated that native B oligomer could provide immunoprotection in experimental animals essentially equivalent to that of whole toxoid (Arciniega *et al.*, 1991), implying that either the dominant neutralizing epitope of S1 was sufficient but not necessary for protection, that the small contaminating amount of S1-containing holotoxin was contributing an enzyme-related adjuvant effect, or that there was a combination of both effects.

In attempts to assemble holotoxin *in vitro* entirely from recombinant subunits, it was noted that an excess of a B subunit-containing multimer was obtained. Quaternary B oligomer was thus assembled *in vitro* from its constituent recombinant subunits in the absence of S1 (Burnette *et al.*, 1992). The resultant B oligomer product, having no possibility of possessing S1 as a contaminant, was entirely sufficient for eliciting toxin neutralizing antibodies (Burnette *et al.*, 1992); mice immunized with B oligomer were completely protected against toxin-mediated lymphocytosis and aerosol challenge with *Bordetella* organisms.

3. CHOLERA GENETIC TOXOIDS

Cholera remains a serious epidemic disease of global proportions. Although various vaccine compositions have been available for many years, none of these products have shown acceptable efficacy against disease. Unlike PT, cholera toxin contains five identical B subunits comprising a binding oligomer with specificity for G_{M1} ganglioside-containing receptors of the mucosal epithelium. The enzymatically-active A subunit is cleaved following translation to yield a catalytic A1 polypeptide and an A2 peptide held together by a single disulfide bond.

As accomplished with PT S1, it was desired to produce analog CT A protomers that retained any potentially critical structural epitopes, preserved the ability to associate with B oligomer, yet lacked the catalytic competence to intoxicate cells. Portions of the operon encoding the mature A region (Mekalanos *et al.*, 1983) were molecularly cloned and expressed to high levels in recombinant *E. coli* (Burnette *et al.*, 1991). The A subunits of PT, CT, and LT share a region of strong amino acid sequence homology near their amino termini (Locht and Keith, 1986; Nicosia *et al.*, 1986); this region contains the essential arginine at residue 9 in PT S1 (Burnette *et al.*, 1988a) that is equivalent in position to arginine-7 in CT A protomer, suggesting that this amino acid might similarly contribute to enzyme-mediated toxicity in cholera. The exchange of CT A arginine-7 residue for lysine was effected by site-directed mutagenesis (Burnette *et al.*, 1991) with the result that the competence of CT A to catalytically modify Gα subunit was completely eliminated. A candidate genetic toxoid containing this mutation has recently been prepared by homologous recombination (Häse *et al.*, 1994).

The catalytic properties of CT are thought by some investigators to be crucial for its adjuvant activity and abrogation of oral tolerance to heterologous antigens. It was therefore of interest to also effect a modulation of enzyme activity. Two regions of the CT A sequence containing histidine-44 and histidine-70 could be aligned with a histidine residue in PT S1 that is also important for ADP-ribosylating activity (Kaslow *et al.*, 1989). All substitutions made at histidine-44, however, resulted in completely inactive analogs (Burnette *et al.*, 1994), intimating that this residue may be essential for recognition of the common NAD donor substrate, but does not determine acceptor substrate specificity. On the other hand, substitutions at histidine-70 resulted in loss of activity for Gα, but not for other cellular substrates (Burnette *et al.*, 1994). This suggested that histidine-70 may contribute to aspects of the A subunit that specify recognition of acceptor substrate. An understanding of this type of structure-function relationship may facilitate the design of CT analogs that, when delivered orally, are unable to evoke diarrheal fluid loss while still capable of augmenting mucosal immunity.

4. FUNCTIONAL CORRELATION WITH THREE-DIMENSIONAL STRUCTURE

Models of the ribosylating toxins derived from biochemical parameters could not predict the detail divulged by the recent solutions of their crystal structures (Burnette, 1994). The general portrait of the toxins that emerges from these biophysical studies (Merritt *et al.*, 1994; Sixma *et al.*, 1991, 1992, 1993; Stein *et al.*, 1994) is one of small, elegant "lunar landers" plying their trade on the fertile surface and subsurface of sensitive eukaryotic target cells. The B oligomers, resembling docking platforms for the functional A protomers, are somewhat erect in CT and LT (Merritt *et al.*, 1994; Sixma *et al.*, 1991, 1993) while that of PT is more flattened in appearance (Stein *et al.*, 1994). The CT B and LT B recognition domains for the G_{M1} pentasaccharide receptor reside on each of the B subunits at their "landing" surfaces (Merritt *et al.*, 1994; Sixma *et al.*, 1992), whereas the carbohydrate receptor recognition domains of PT occupy lateral positions only on the S2 and S3 subunits (Saukkonen *et al.*, 1992; Stein *et al.*, 1994). Along their five-fold axes of symmetry, the B oligomers of CT and LT (Sixma *et al.*, 1991, 1993) display five identical subunits arranged in a circular disc with a central channel occupied by the A2 peptide portion of the dipartite A protomer; PT B is roughly triangular when observed along this axis and has a more "squashed" appearance perpendicular to its five-fold axis (Stein *et al.*, 1994). PT S1 is almost pyramidal in shape, the cleft for its active site opening on one face above the S3 subunit (Stein *et al.*, 1994). In contrast, the A subunit of CT and LT rests majestically atop its B oligomer, with the active site cleft residing on the upper surface of A1, opposite to its point of contact with B oligomer (Sixma *et al.*, 1991, 1993).

The A subunits of PT, CT, and LT share a common fold near their amino termini that constitutes the catalytic site (Stein *et al.*, 1994); this functional domain is also conserved in a number of secondary structural elements. NAD in the active site of PT could interact directly with glutamate-129 (glutamate-112 in CT) and the side chain of arginine-9 (arginine-7 in CT) (Stein *et al.*, 1994); within this region, glutamate-129 is within hydrogen-bonding distance of histidine-35. These relative coördinates provide ample structural explanation for the reduction in catalytic activity precipitated by substitutions at any of these residues.

An explicitly functional structure for the LT B binding domains and their interaction with the pentasaccharide moiety of the G_{M1} ganglioside receptor on the gut mucosal epithelium have likewise been determined (Sixma *et al.*, 1992; Merritt *et al.*, 1994). Receptor binding by PT B is more problematic because of the its heteropentameric complexity. However, studies with recombinant B subunits (Saukkonen *et al.*, 1992; van't Wout *et al.*, 1992) demonstrated that S2 exhibits preferential binding for lactosylceramide-containing glycolipids in ciliated respiratory epithelial cells, the site of bacterial adherence in the infectious process, whereas S3 displays exclusive specificity for ganglioside-containing glycolipids in monocytic cells, such as bronchoalveolar macrophages. Site-specific substitutions in S2 and S3 showed that carbohydrate recognition dwells in a region demonstrated by three-dimensional analysis to overlap helix $\alpha 2$ on the outside lateral surface of these subunits (Stein *et al.*, 1994; Sandros *et al.*, 1994). Selected amino aid substitutions and recombinant exchange of these domains (Saukkonen *et al.*, 1992; van't Wout *et al.*, 1992), which share structural and functional properties with the eukaryotic selectins (Rozdzinski *et al.*, 1993a, 1993b; Sandros *et al.*, 1994), results in a conversion of both glycoconjugate specificity and cellular recognition.

5. CONCLUSIONS

Three-dimensional structure analysis of the AB_5 toxins provide a confirmation for what had been deduced from molecular biological and biochemical studies, yet afford a fresh perspective more explicitly linking toxin functional attributes to secondary, tertiary, and quaternary organization. Further functional and structural evaluation of selectively engineered AB_5 molecules will allow the rational design of analog toxins with both modified receptor binding properties and substrate recognition characteristics that can improve upon the current generation of genetic toxoid vaccines for disease prevention. They should also have value for the elucidation and modulation of G protein-mediated signal transduction pathways implicated in critical metabolic pathways and pathogenesis.

REFERENCES

Arciniega, J.L., Shahin, R.D., Burnette, W.N., Bartley, T.D., Whiteley, D.W., Mar, V.L., and Burns, D.L., 1991, Contribution of the B oligomer to the protective activity of genetically attenuated pertussis toxin, *Infect. Immun.* 59:3407-3410.

Bartley, T.D., Whiteley, D.W., Mar, V.L., Burns, D.L., and Burnette, W.N., 1989, Pertussis holotoxoid formed *in vitro* with a genetically deactivated S1 subunit, *Proc. Natl. Acad. Sci. USA* 86:8353-8357.

Burnette, W.N., 1994, AB_5 ADP-ribosylating toxins: comparative anatomy and physiology, *Structure* 2:151-158.

Burnette, W.N., Arciniega, J.L., Mar, V.L., and Burns, D.L., 1992, Properties of pertussis toxin B oligomer assembled *in vitro* from recombinant polypeptides produced by *Escherichia coli*, *Infect. Immun.* 60:2252-2256.

Burnette, W.N., Cieplak, W., Mar, V.L., Kaljot, K.T., Sato, H., and Keith, J.M., 1988a, Pertussis toxin S1 mutant with reduced enzyme activity and a conserved protective epitope, *Science* 242:72-74.

Burnette W.N., Mar, V.L., Cieplak, W., Morris, C.F., Kaljot, K.T., Marchitto, K.S., Sachdev, R.K., Locht, C., and Keith, J.M., 1988b, Direct expression of *Bordetella pertussis* toxin subunits to high levels in *Escherichia coli*, *Biotechnology* 6:699-706.

Burnette, W.N., Cieplak, W., Jr., Kaslow, H.R., Rappuoli, R., and Tuomanen, E.I., 1994, Recombinant microbial ADP-ribosylating toxins of *Bordetella pertussis*, *Vibrio cholerae*, and enterotoxigenic *Escherichia coli*: structure, function, and toxoid vaccine development, *In* Murooka, Y., and Imanaka, T., Eds., *Recombinant microbes for industrial and agricultural applications*, Marcel Dekker, Inc., New York, pp. 185-203.

Burnette, W.N., Mar, V.L., Platler, B.W., Schlotterbeck, J.D., McGinley, M.D., Stoney, K.S., Rohde, M.F., and Kaslow, H.R., 1991, Site-directed mutagenesis of the catalytic subunit of cholera toxin: substituting lysine for arginine 7 causes loss of activity, *Infect. Immun.* 59:4266-4270.

Cieplak, W., Burnette, W.N., Mar, V.L., Kaljot, K.T., Morris, C.F., Chen, K.K., Sato, H., and Keith, J.M., 1988, Identification of a region in the S1 subunit of pertussis toxin that is required for enzymatic activity and that contributes to the formation of a neutralizing antigenic determinant, *Proc. Natl. Acad. Sci. USA* 85:4667-4671.

Häse, C.C., Thai, L.S., Boesman-Finkelstein, M., Mar, V.L., Burnette, W.N., Kaslow, H.R., Stevens, L.A., Moss, J., and Finkelstein, R.A., 1994, Construction and characterization of recombinant *Vibrio cholerae* strains producing inactive cholera toxin analogs, *Infect. Immun.* 62:3051-3057.

Kaslow, H.R., Schlotterbeck, J.D., Mar, V.L., and Burnette, W.N., 1989, Alkylation of cysteine 41, but not cysteine 200, decreases the ADP-ribosyltransferase activity of the S1 subunit of pertussis toxin, *J. Biol. Chem.* 264:6386-6390.

Locht, C., and Keith, J.M., 1986, Pertussis toxin gene: nucleotide sequence and genetic organization, *Science* 232:1258-1264.

Mekalanos, J.J., Swartz, D.J., Pearson, G.D.N., Harford, N., Groyne, F., and DeWilde, M., 1983, Cholera toxin genes: nucleotide sequence, deletion analysis and vaccine development, *Nature* 306:551-557.

Merritt, E.A., Sarfaty, S., Vandenakker, F., L'hoir, C., Martial, J.A., and Hol, W.G.J., 1994, Crystal structure of cholera toxin B-pentamer bound to receptor G_{M1} pentasaccharide, *Protein Sci.* 3:166-175.

Nicosia, A., Perugini, M., Franzini, C., Casagli, M.C., Borri, M.G., Antoni, G., Almoni, M., Neri, P., Ratti, G., and R. Rappuoli, R., 1986, Cloning and sequencing of the pertussis toxin genes: operon structure and gene duplication, *Proc. Natl. Acad. Sci. USA* 83:4631-4635.

Pizza, M., Covacci, A., Bartoloni, A., Perugini, M., Nencioni, L., De Magistris, M.T., Villa, L., Nucci, D., Manetti, R., Bugnoli, M., Giovannoni, F., Olivieri, R., Barbieri, J.T., Sato, H., and Rappuoli, R., 1989, Mutants of pertussis toxin suitable for vaccine development, *Science* 246:497-500.

Rappuoli, R., Pizza, M., De Magistris, M.T., Podda, A., Bugnoli, M., Manetti, R., and Nencioni, L., 1992, Development and clinical testing of an acellular pertussis vaccine containing genetically detoxified pertussis toxin, *Immunobiology* 184:230-239.

Rozdzinski, E., Burnette, W.N., Jones, T., Mar, V., and Tuomanen, E., 1993a, Prokaryotic peptides that block leukocyte adherence to selectins, *J. Exp. Med.* 178:917-924.

Rozdzinski, E., Jones, T., Burnette, W.N., Burroughs, M., and Tuomanen, E., 1993b, Antiinflammatory effects in experimental meningitis of prokaryotic peptides that mimic selectins, *J. Infect. Dis.* 168:1422-1428.

Sandros, J., Rozdzinski, E., Zheng, J., Cowburn, D., and Tuomanen, E., 1994, Lectin domains in the toxin of *Bordetella pertussis*: selectin mimicry linked to microbial pathogenesis, *Glycoconjugate J.* 11:501-506.

Saukkonen, K., Burnette, W.N., Mar, V.L., Masure, H.R., and Tuomanen, E.I., 1992, Pertussis toxin has eukaryotic-like carbohydrate recognition domains, *Proc. Natl. Acad. Sci. USA* 89:118-122.

Sixma, T.K., Kalk, K.H., Vanzanten, B.A.M., Dauter, Z., Kingma, J., Witholt, B., and Hol, W.G.J., 1993, Refined structure of *Escherichia coli* heat-labile enterotoxin, a close relative of cholera toxin, *J. Mol. Biol.* 230:890-918.

Sixma, T.K., Pronk, S.E., Kalk, K.H., Vanzanten, B.A.M., Berghuis, A.M., and Hol, W.G.J., 1992, Lactose binding to heat-labile enterotoxin revealed by X-ray crystallography, *Nature* 355:561-564.

Sixma, T.K., Pronk, S.E., Kalk, K.H., Wartna, E.S., Vanzanten, B.A.M., Witholt, B., and Hol, W.G.J., 1991, Crystal structure of a cholera toxin-related heat-labile enterotoxin from *E. coli*, *Nature* 351:371-377.

Stein, P.E., Boodhoo, A., Armstrong, G.D., Cockle, S.A., Klein, M.H., and Read, R.J., 1994, The crystal structure of pertussis toxin, *Structure* 2:45-57.

Tamura, M., Nogimori, K., Murai, S., Yajima, N., Ito, K., Katada, T., Ui, M., and Ishii, S., 1982, Subunit structure of the islet-activating protein, pertussis toxin, in conformity with the A-B model, *Biochemistry* 21:5516-5522.

van't Wout, J., Burnette, W.N., Mar, V.L., Rozdzinski, E., Wright, S.D., and Tuomanen, E.I., 1992, Role of carbohydrate recognition domains of pertussis toxin in adherence of *Bordetella pertussis* to human macrophages, *Infect. Immun.* 60:3303-3308.

10

PROTECTIVE IMMUNITY INDUCED BY *BACILLUS ANTHRACIS* TOXIN MUTANT STRAINS

C. Pezard., J-C. Sirard, and M. Mock

Laboratoire de Génétique Moléculaire des Toxines
Institut Pasteur
28, rue du Docteur Roux, 75724 - Paris Cédex 15, France

INTRODUCTION

Bacillus anthracis is the etiological agent of anthrax, a disease often fatal in humans and many animals species. Fully virulent strains of this pathogen harbor two plasmids, pXO1 and pXO2, coding for the production of two toxins and D-glutamic acid polymer capsule, respectively. The two toxins, edema and lethal toxin, are secreted by *B. anthracis* and are composed of three distinct proteins, protective antigen (PA; 85 kDa), lethal factor (LF; 83 kDa) and edema factor (EF; 89 kDa). PA combined with LF forms the lethal toxin (Beall *et al.*, 1962 ; Smith & Stoner, 1967), whereas edema toxin consists of PA and EF. Both toxins are organized according to the A-B type model (Gill, 1978). PA represents a common B component, with receptor-binding activity, and mediates entry of either LF or EF into target cells (Leppla, 1984). EF has been shown to be a calmodulin-dependent adenylate cyclase (Leppla, 1982). By sequence comparison, it has been suggested that LF is a metalloprotease (Klimpel *et al.*, 1994).

The role of PA as a protective antigen against anthrax was established soon after discovery of the toxin. Livestock is commonly vaccinated with a suspension of viable, virulence-attenuated spores of the Sterne strain, which lacks pXO2. This uncapsulated strain still carries pXO1 and therefore produces the three toxin factors. The efficacy and duration of the protection conferred by the Sterne strain in experimentally vaccinated animals are much greater than those of that obtained with cell-free PA vaccines, despite the fact that antibody titers against PA induced by live vaccines are often lower than those induced by cell-free vaccines. We have constructed Sterne strain-derived *B. anthracis* mutants that are deficient in the production of one or two toxin components (Pezard *et al.*, 1991 ; Pezard *et al.*, 1993). These strains were used to study the contribution of *in vivo*-produced PA, EF, and LF to the immune response. Antibody response to each toxin component and its respective role in immunoprotection were analyzed.

Novel Strategies in Design and Production of Vaccines
Edited by S. Cohen and A. Shafferman, Plenum Press, New York, 1996

RESULTS AND DISCUSSION

Antibody response to toxin components after infection with *B. anthracis* mutants

In mice immunized with mutants producing EF (RP31), LF (RP4), or EF and LF (RP8), the response to these proteins was weak, and low specific antibody titers were found (Fig. 1). In contrast, when LF or EF were produced from strains which also produced PA (RP9 and RP10) a significant increase in the response against LF or EF was observed. As shown in Fig. 1, sera obtained after RP9 immunization exhibited high titers to LF, whereas, the titers were significantly lower ($p < 0.009$) after RP4 immunization. A similar effect was found for EF when comparing titers obtained with strains RP31 and RP10 ($p < 0.04$). The fact that titers to EF were always lower than those observed for PA and LF, might be a consequence of the weaker expression of the *cya* gene with respect to that of *pag* or *lef*, as it was demonstrated by the use of transcriptional gene fusions (Sirard *et al.*, 1994). This intriguing observation that antibody titers to EF and LF were significantly higher in animals immunized with bacteria also producing PA is probably not a consequence of differences in toxin expression by the mutant strains. The six mutant strains used

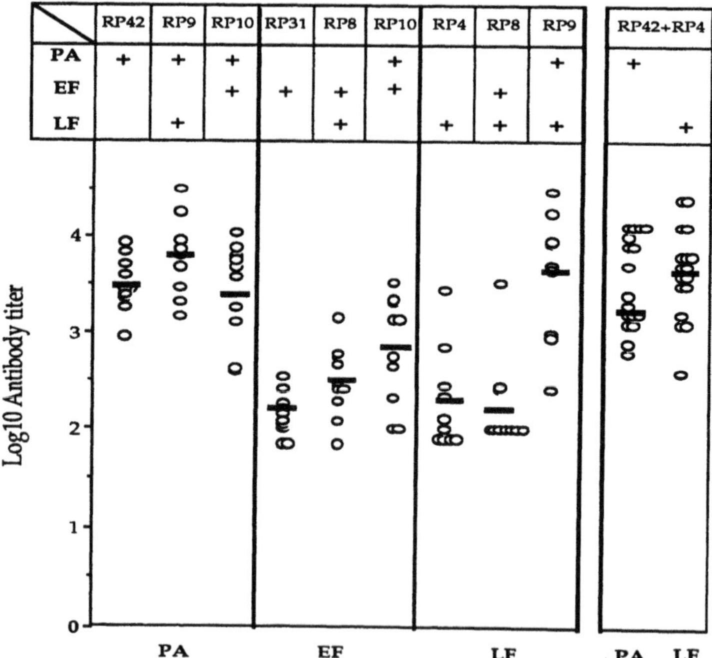

	RP42	RP9	RP10	RP31	RP8	RP10	RP4	RP8	RP9		RP42+RP4
PA	+	+	+			+			+		+
EF			+	+	+	+		+			
LF		+			+		+	+	+		+

Figure 1. ELISA-detected antibodies to PA, EF, and LF in mice immunized with *B. anthracis* mutant strains. Mice (10 per group) were immunized with 5.10^7 spores of the appropriate *B. anthracis* strain and bled six weeks after immunization. Circles represent individual animal titers and the black bar represents the arithmetic mean of log titer of the group. Strains used for immunization and the respective toxin components produced are indicated on the top of the figure. At the bottom are indicated each toxin component against which the antibody titers were determined. The right panel represents the titers to PA and LF in animals immunized with a mixture of strains RP42 + RP4.

in this study have been characterized in a previous work, and we determined that PA, LF, EF were synthesized *in vitro* in amounts similar to those obtained from the parental Sterne strain (Pezard *et al.*, 1993). However, to rule out possible differences in *in vivo* toxin production mice were immunized with a mixture of RP42 and RP4 spores and the resulting titers compared to those from mice receiving RP9 (Fig. 1). A lethal effect was observed as 4 mice in a group of 20 died after immunization. From these experiments, it appears that spores of RP42 and RP4 are able to reconstitute *in vivo* the biological effects of an active lethal toxin through the independant production of PA and LF. Analysis of sera showed that antibody titers to LF in animals immunized with RP42 and RP4 were significantly higher than in those receiving only RP4 ($p <$ *0,003*) and were similar to those found in RP9 immunized animals. This result suggests that the increased immunogenicity of LF originates from a protein complementation mechanism. Thus, the ability of PA to bind to cell surface receptors, and facilitate the internalization and intracellular processing of EF or LF, may be a prerequisite for the higher antibody response to these two proteins. In contrast, when EF and LF are produced from strains deficient for PA production, these two toxin components may not have the opportunity to interact with the appropriate effector cells.

In order to define a common marker for all strains we also evaluated the humoral response against other bacterial antigens unrelated to the toxins. For this purpose, antibody titers against extracellular antigens, present in the culture medium of the plasmidless strain 7700, were determined by ELISA (data not shown), (Pezard *et al.*, 1995). It clearly appeared that the six mutant strains induced a similar antibody response to extracellular antigens. This supports the notion that the mutants are able to develop similarly in the host. In contrast, spores of the plasmidless strain 7700 did not induce an antibody response to extracellular antigens, indicating that they may not have germinated or that the resulting bacteria did not multiply, or did so only poorly. These results point out for the first time a possible role of pXO1 in bacterial survival in the host. In addition to the toxin structural and regulatory genes (Leppla, 1991 ; Mock & Ullmann, 1993 ; Uchida *et al.* 1993), this large virulence plasmid may also carry other determinants involved in spore germination and/or bacterial multiplication *in vivo*.

Protection of mice with B. anthracis mutants. In order to compare the antibody response with the protective efficacy of the strains, protection experiments were conducted.

Table 1. Protective efficacy of *B. anthracis* mutant strains. Swiss mice (10 or 20 per group) were immunized subcutaneously with a single dose (0.5 ml) of spores at different concentrations (2×10^6-2×10^8/ml) of the appropriate *B. anthracis* strain. A group of 50 control mice received 0.5 ml physiological saline. Six weeks after immunization, mice were challenged subcutaneously with 10^9 spores of the Sterne strain of *B. anthracis* (1000 times the LD_{50} for Swiss mice). Two of control mice (4%) survived the challenge.

Immunizing strain	Toxin factor(s) produced	No of survivors/no challenged(%)
7700	—	0
RP31	EF	23
RP42	PA	43
RP4	LF	47
RP8	EF, LF	30
RP10	PA, EF	58
RP9	PA, LF	74

The protection provided by the various *B. anthracis* mutants against a lethal challenge with the Sterne strain was tested in mice six weeks after a single immunization. Spore doses, (10^6, 10^7 and 10^8) were studied. Table 1 represents the cumulative data obtained with the three spore doses.

The six mutant strains were capable of protecting to a greater or lesser extent. Immunization at higher doses ($\geq 10^7$) with any of the three strains producing PA, as either a single component or in combination with LF or EF provided protection and confirmed the role of PA as a major protective antigen involved in humoral response (Pezard *et al.*, 1995). This study also suggests that both EF and LF contribute to immunoprotection.

The control strain, 7700, never protected. This observation is in agreement with the serological data suggesting that this strain, lacking pXO1, may not be able to develop normally *in vivo*. Moreover this hypothesis is supported by the fact that in contrast to 7700 the three mutant strains deficient in PA production are still able to provide protection to some extent. It is unlikely that the weak antibody response to toxin components elicited by these strains could account for their protective effect. It seems rather that this protection results from some cellular or humoral responses to *B. anthracis* unrelated to toxin production.

ACKNOWLEDGMENTS

This work was supported by the I.N.S.E.R.M. (CRE 910612).

REFERENCES

Beall, F.A., Taylor, M.J., and Thorne, C.B., 1962, Rapid lethal effects in rats of a third component found upon fractionating the toxin of *Bacillus anthracis. J. Bacteriol.* 83:1274-1280.

Gill, D.M., 1978. Seven toxic peptides that cross cell membranes. Bacterial Toxins and Cell Membranes. Academic Press. New York, Eds. J. Jeljaszewicz and T. Wadstrom. 291-332.

Klimpel, K.R., Arora, N., and Leppla, S.H., 1994, Anthrax toxin lethal factor contains a zinc metalloprotease consensus sequence which is required for lethal toxin activity. *Mol. Microbiol.* 13:1093-1100.

Leppla, S.H., 1982, Anthrax toxin edema factor : A bacterial adenylate cyclase that increases cyclic AMP concentrations in eukaryotic cells. *Proc. Natl. Acad. Sci. U.S.A.* 79:3162-3166.

Leppla, S.H., 1984, *Bacillus anthracis* calmodulin-dependent adenylate cyclase : Chemical and enzymatic properties and interactions with eucaryotic cells. *Adv. Cycl. Nucl. Prot. Phospho. Res.* 17:189-198.

Leppla, S.H., 1991, The anthrax toxin complex, In J.E. Alouf and J.H. Freer (ed.), Sourcebook of bacterial protein toxins, *Academic Press, London.* 14:277-302.

Mock, M., and Ullmann, A., 1993, Calmodulin-activated bacterial adenylate cyclases as virulence factors. *Trends Microbiol.* 1:187-192.

Pezard, C., Berche, P., and Mock, M., 1991, Contribution of individual toxin components to virulence of *Bacillus anthracis. Infect. Immun.* 59:3472-3477.

Pezard, C., Duflot, E., and Mock. M., 1993, Construction of *Bacillus anthracis* mutant strains producing a single toxin component. *J. Gen. Microbiol.* 139:2459-2463.

Pezard, C., Weber, M., Sirard, J-C., Berche, P., and Mock., M., 1995, Protective immunity induced by *Bacillus anthracis* toxin-deficient strains. *Infect. Immun.* 63:1369-1372.

Sirard, J.-C., Mock, M., and Fouet, A., 1994, The *three Bacillus anthracis* toxin genes are coordinately regulated by bicarbonate and temperature. *J. Bacteriol.* 176:5188-5192.

Smith, H., and Stoner, H.B., 1967, Anthrax toxin complex. *Fed. Proc.* 26:1554-1557.

Uchida, I., Hornung, J.M., Thorne, C.B., Klimpel, K.R., and Leppla, H., 1993, Cloning and characterization of a gene whose product is a trans-activator of anthrax toxin synthesis. *J. Bacteriol. 175:5329-5338.*

11

BACTERIAL OUTER MEMBRANE PROTEIN VACCINES

The Meningococcal Example

Jan T. Poolman

National Institute of Public Health and Environmental Protection (RIVM)
Laboratory of Vaccine Development and Immune Mechanisms
Antonie van Leeuwenhoeklaan 9, P.O. Box 1, 3720 BA Bilthoven, The
Netherlands

With respect to bacterial vaccines, a number of approaches were found successful by way of empirical research, trial and error.

Attenuated or killed whole bacterial vaccines are used on a large scale with some difficulty. The killed whole-cell pertussis vaccine is efficacious in protecting against whooping cough, albeit with the presence of some, mostly local, side-effects. Efforts to develop subunit pertussis vaccines have led to the availability of a few possible combinations of antigens, the pertussis toxoid being present in all. Surface proteins like filamentous hemagglutinin, pertactin and fimbriae also have been incorporated in subunit pertussis vaccines [28]. With respect to protection against pertussis, antibody mediated toxin neutralization and bactericidal effects by way of complement and phagocytic cells are likely to play a major role. It will take longitudinal surveillance in order to determine the effects on disease, carriage and transmission by the old whole-cell vaccine as compared to the new acellular vaccines. The spectrum of immune responses, *i.e.* effector antibody (subclasses, isotypes, affinities) and T-cell mediated immunity as well as B- and T-cell memory, against various antigens will certainly differ between the cellular and acellular vaccines. It is unknown if T-cell mediated immunity, besides help for B-cells, plays an important role with regard to pertussis. If survival within macrophages amongst other cell types is important, T-cell mediated immunity (most likely MHC class II restricted $CD4^+$-T-cells) which activates macrophages can be relevant. Considering pertussis, research indicated that outer membrane proteins are able to mimick the potency of the whole cell vaccine, when presented in an outer membrane vesicle (OMV) formulation [24].

With respect to the attenuated BCG (Baccillus Calmette Guérin) vaccine that is being used on a large scale to prevent tuberculosis and leprosy, it has become clear that the potency varies from poor to reasonable and that safety (local side-effects) deserves attention. Since the dominant protective immune responses appear to rely upon $CD4^+$, MHC class II-restricted T-cell responses activating intracellular (macrophage) killing mechanisms, this opens ways for development of new vaccines. Extracellular proteins from *Mycobacterium tuberculosis* are able to protect mice against tuberculosis challenge [17].

Attenuated or killed whole cell vaccines given orally appear efficacious against diseases such as typhoid and cholera, although improvement still is being sought [12].

Toxoid vaccines have a good record with respect to potency and safety, tetanus and diphtheria being the classical examples. Genetic detoxification using site-directed mutagenesis or deleting the active sites/subunits can replace the chemical detoxification processes. Pertussis toxoid is close to realization, the B (binding) subunit of cholera toxin is used with success [12]. The principle of toxoid vaccines can be improved further by rDNA technology such as heterologous expression and other applications (*Helicobacter pylori*, pneumococci, others) are within reach.

Polysaccharide-protein conjugate vaccines have recently come to large scale application. This is a major breakthrough in vaccinology, *i.e.* the science that deals with the induction of immune responses to prevent or treat infectious and/or chronic diseases. The chemical conjugation of polysaccharides to proteins ensures the involvement of protein (peptide) specific T helper lymphocytes with regard to the induction and activation of saccharide specific B cells. The practical consequence of this principle is the possibility to induce long-lasting immunity in infants against a number of bacterial infectious diseases. Field studies in Finland have demonstrated that a conjugate vaccine derived from the capsular polysaccharide of *Haemophilus influenzae* type b (Hib) does protect infants. Conjugate vaccines against meningococcal, pneumococcal and other diseases (*Pseudomonas aeruginosa*, group B streptococcus, others) are now under development.

However, for a number of bacterial diseases neither whole cells, toxoids nor conjugates will suffice as a vaccine. For such diseases, outer membrane proteins are interesting vaccine candidates in case of gramnegative bacterial diseases. Development of vaccines on the basis of outer membrane proteins has reached the stage of large-scale field testing with respect to group B meningococcal OMP vaccines [12]. It was demonstrated that OMP vaccines have intermediary efficacies. However, infants were not protected and duration of immunity was unsatisfactory [3,5]. A number of reasons could explain these results such as epitope specificity and isotype/subclass of the antibodies induced. The quality and quantity of T helper-lymphocytes stimulating activities can also be of critical importance [38]. A proper presentation/conformation is critical for OMP, the native conformation was determined to be a cylindric transmembrane structure exposing a few surface loops [10]. These surface loops represent targets for protective immune responses [33]. Ideally, short peptides representing such epitopes would be sufficient for the induction of protective immune responses. Neither synthetic peptides nor purified OMP were found very efficient inducers of protective antibodies as compared to membrane bound OMP [25]. The potency of peptide vaccines can be greatly improved by cyclization or by preparing multiple antigen peptide constructs [4,6,7,16]. In our hands, direct comparisons are in favour of membrane bound complete OMP [16,25].

An elegant way to prepare membrane bound native OMP is the purification of excreted and/or extracted outer membrane vesicles (OMV) [11]. This uses the property of meningococci to excrete large quantities of outer membrane blebs, which are treated with detergents to partially remove the lipopolysaccharide (endotoxin), to reduce toxicity without destroying the vesicle structure [26,27]. Out of a practical vaccine perspective, the **OMV principle** represents an easy production procedure leading to high yields. By applying recombinant DNA technology, vaccine strains can be constructed to contain an OMP composition suitable for vaccine production [4,34-36]. This will enable the deletion of nonprotective OMP and simultaneous expression of multiple serotype dependent OMP. At the same time, potentially hazardous components because of structural identity with the host can be deleted. With respect to the group B meningococcus, the biosynthesis of the capsular polysaccharide (homopolymer of α2-8 sialic acid) and the lacto-N-neotetraose structures, both being identical to host structures, were deleted in this way [36]. Potential side-effects due to auto-immune responses can be avoided in this way. Consequently, multivalent OMP-containing OMV vaccines can be developed which cover most serotypes [8]. Clinical studies with such vaccines have started.

Because of the above mentioned activities, meningococcal OMP-containing vaccines have become the prototype for bacterial OMP vaccines. The OMV vaccine principle using rDNA technology for construction of tailor-made vaccine strains has come close to application. Synthetic peptide, particularly cyclic peptide constructs, are being investigated thoroughly. Another option to develop vaccines relates to incorporation of purified OMP into membrane-like structures such as liposomes [18]. Heterologous expression in Bacillus will avoid potential side-effects due to residual endotoxin. It still needs to be determined which OMP are the best vaccine candidates. The meningococcal PorA is a prime candidate [26]; other OMP of interest are the Fe-limitation inducible OMP [20-22,27].

Once it has been worked out how to prepare efficacious meningococcal OMP vaccines, this will have a great impact on bacterial OMP vaccine development in general. Examples are nontypable *Heamophilus influenzae* [2,14,30,31], *Chlamydia trachomatis* [1,9,23,29], *Neisseria gonorrhoeae* [37], *Moraxella catarrhalis* [15] and possibly others [12,19,29]. The development of the OMV vaccine principle for gramnegative bacteria in general will depend upon the possibility to induce blebbing, the release of outer membrane blebs. *E.coli* mutants missing the major lipoprotein as well as OmpA are coccoid and bleb [32], which opens ways to generalize the OMV principle.

REFERENCES

1. Baehr, W, Zhang, Y. Z., Joseph, T., Su, H., Nano, F. E., Everett, K. D. E. Caldwell, H. D., 1988, Mapping antigenic domains expressed by *Chlamydia trachomatis* major outer membrane genes, *Proc. Natl. Acad. Sci. USA*, 85:4000-4004.

2. Bell, J., Grass, S., Jeanteur, D., Munson, R. S. jr., Diversity of the P2 protein among nontypeable *Haemophilus influenzae* isolates, *Inf. Immun.* 62:2639-2643.

3. Bjune, G., Høiby, E. A., Grønnesby, J. K., Arnesen, Ø., Fredriksen, J. H., Halstenen, A., Holten, E., Lindbak, A. K., Nøkleby, H., Rosenqvist, E, Solberg, L. K., Closs, O., Eng, J., Frøholm, L. O., Lystad, A., Bakketeig, L. S., Hareide, B., 1991, Effect of outer membrane vesicle vaccine against group B meningococcal disease in Norway, *Lancet* 338:1093-1096.

4. Brugghe, H. F., Timmermans, J. A. M., Van Unen, L. M. A., Ten Hove, G. J., Van de Werken, G.., Poolman, J. T. and Hoogerhout, P., 1994, Simultaneous multiple synthesis and selective conjugation of head-to-tail cyclized peptides, derived from a surface-loop of a meningococcal class 1 outer membrane protein, *Int. J. Pept. Prot. Res.* 43:166-172.

5. Cassio de Moraes, J., Perkins, B.A., Camargo, M.C.C., Rossetto Hidaldo, N.T., Aparecida Barbosa, H., Tavares Sacchi, C., Landgraf, I. M., Gattas, V. L., Vascondcelos, H. de G., Plihaytis, B. D., Wenger, J. D., Broome, C. V., 1992, Protective efficacy of a serogroup B meningococcal vaccine in Sao Paulo, Brazil, *Lancet* 340:1074-1078.

6. Christodoulides, M., McGuinness, B. T., Heckels, J. E., 1993, Immunization with synthetic peptides containing epitopes of the class 1 outer membrane protein of *Neisseria meningitidis*: production of bactericidal antibodies on immunization with a cyclic peptide, *J. Gen. Microbiol.* 139:1729-1738.

7. Christodoulides, M., Heckels, J.E., 1994, Immunization with a multiple antigen peptide containing defined B- and T-cell epitopes: production of bactericidal antibodies against group B *Neisseria* meningitidis, *Microbiology* 240:2951-2960.

8. Claassen, I., Meylis, J., Van der Ley, P., Peeters, C., Brons, H., Robert, J., Borsboom, D., Van der Ark, A., Van Straaten, I., Roholl, P., Kuipers, B., Poolman, J., Production, characterization and control of a hexavalent Class 1 Outer Membrane protein containing vesicle vaccine made from tailor-made *Neisseria meningitidis* strains, *Vaccine* submitted.

9. Conlan, J. W., Clarke, I. N., Ward, M. E., 1988, Epitope mapping with solid-phase peptides: identification of type-, subspecies-, species- and genus-reactive antibody binding domains on the major outer membrane protein of *Chlamydia trachomatis*, *Mol. Microbiol.* 2:673-679.

10. Cowan, S. W., Schirmer, T., Rummel, G., Steiert, M., Ghosh, R., Pauptit, R. A., Jansonius, J. N., Rosenbusch, J. P., 1992, Crystal structures explain functional properties of two *E.coli* porins, *Nature*, 358:727-733.

11. Fredriksen, J. H., Rosenqvist, E., Wedege, E., Bryn, K., Bjune, G., Frøholm, L. O., Lindbak, A. K., Møgster, B., Namork, E., Rye, U., Stabbetorp, G, Winsnes, R., Aase, B., Closs, O., 1991, Production, characterization and control of MenB-vaccine helsa: an outer membrane vesicle vaccine against group B meningococcal disease, *NIPH annals* 14:67-80.

12. Frontiers in medicine: Vaccines, 1994, *Science* 265:1371-1404.

13. Gilleland, H. E. jr., Parker, M. G., Matthews, J. M., Berg, R.D., 1984, Use of a purified outer membrane protein F (porin) preparation of *Pseudomonas aeruginosa* as a protective vaccine in mice, *Inf. Immun.* 44:49-54.

14. Haase, E. M., Yi, K., Morse, G. D., Murphy, T. F., 1994, Mapping of bactericidal epitopes of the P2 porin protein of nontypeable *Haemophilus influenzae*, *Inf. Immun.* 62:3712-3722.

15. Helminen, M. E., Maciver, I., Latimer, J. L., Cope, L. D., McCracken, G. M. jr., Hansen, E. J., 1993, A major outer membrane protein of *Moraxella catarrhalis* is a target for antibodies that enhance pulmonary clearance of the pathogen in an animal model, *Inf. Immun.* 61:2003-2010.

16. Hoogerhout P., Donders, E. M. L. M., Van Gaans-van den Brink, J. A. M., Kuipers, B, Brugghe, H. F., Van Unen, L. M. A., Timmermans, H., Ten Hove, G. J., De Jong, A. P. J. M., Peeters, C. C. A. M., Wiertz, E. J. H. J., Poolman. J. T., Conjugates of synthetic cyclic peptides elicit bactericidal antibodies against a conformational epitope on a class 1 outer membrane protein of *Neisseria meningitidis*, *Inf. Immun.* 63: 3473-3478.

17. Horwitz M. A., Lee, B. W. E., Dillon, B. J., Harth, G., 1995, Protective immunity against tuberculosis induced by vaccination with major extracellular proteins of *Mycobacterium tuberculosis*, *Proc. Natl. Acad. Sci. USA* 92:1530-1534.

18. Idänpään-Heikkilä, I., Muttilainen, S., Wahlström, Saarinen, L., Leinonen, M., Sarvas, M., Mäkelä, P. H., The antibody response to a prototype liposome vaccine containing *Neisseria meningitidis* outer membrane protein P1 produced in *Bacillus subtilis*, *Vaccine* in press.

19. Isibasi, A., Ortiz-Navarrete, V., Paniagua, J., Pelayo, R., Gonzalez, C. R., Garcia, J. A., Kumate, J., 1992, Active protection of mice against *Salmonella typhi* by immunization with strain-specific porins, *Vaccine* 10:811-813.

20. Lissolo, L., Maitre-Wilmotte, G., Dumas, P., Mignon, M., Danve, B., Quentin-Millet, M. J., 1995, Evaluation of transferrin-binding protein complex as a potential antigen for future meningococcal vaccines, *Inf. Immun.*, 63:884-900.

21. Pettersson, A., Kuipers, B., Pelzer, M., Verhagen, E. P. M., Tiesjema, R. H., Tommassen, J., Poolman, J. T., 1990, Monoclonal antibodies against the 70-kilodalton iron-regulated protein of *Neisseria meningitidis* are bactericidal and strain-specific, *Infect. Immun.* 58:3036-3041.

22. Petterson, A., Van der Ley, P. A., Poolman, J. T., Tomassen, J., 1993, Molecular characterization of the 98kDa non-regulated outer membrane protein of *Neisseria meningitidis*, *Inf.Immun.* 61:4724-4733.

23. Poole, E., Lamont, I., 1992, Serovar differentiation of *Chlamydia trachomatis* by direct sequence analysis of the variable segment 4 region of the major outer membrane protein gene, *Inf. Immun.* 60:1089-1094.

24. Poolman, J. T., Hamstra, H. J., Barlow, A. K., Kuipers, A. J., Loggen, H., Nagel, J., 1990, Outer membrane vesicles of Bordetella *pertussis* are protective antigens in the mouse intracerebral challenge model. *In: Manclark, C.R.(ed.). Proc.VI International Pertussis Symposium, US Public Health Service, Bethesda, Maryland, DHHSPubl. no. (FDA)90-1164*, pp 148-156.

25. Poolman, J. T., Van der Ley, P. A., Wiertz, E. J. H. J., Hoogerhout, P., 1991, Second generation meningococcal OMP-LPS vaccines, *NIPH Annuals* 14:233-241.

26. Poolman, J. T., 1995, Development of a meningococcal vaccine, *Infect. Agents Dis.* 4:13-28.

27. Poolman, J. T., Van der Ley, P. A., Tomassen, J., 1995, Surface structures and secreted products of meningococci, *In: Meningococcal Disease, Publ. John Wiley & Sons, Ed. K. Cartwright;* pp 21-34.

28. Rappuoli, R., Pizza, M., Podda, A., 1991, Towards third-generation whooping cough vaccines, *Tibtech.* 9:232-238.

29. Roy, S., Das, A. B., Ghosh, A. N., Biswas, T., 1994, Purification, pore-forming ability, and antigenic relatedness of the major outer membrane protein of *Shigella dysenteride* type 1, *Inf. Immun.* 62:433-4338.

30. Sikkema, D. J., Murphy, T. F., 1992, Molecular analysis of the P2 porin protein of nontypeable *Haemophilus influenzae. Inf. Immun.* 60:5204-5211.

31. Skrikumar, R., Dahan, D., Gras, M. F., Ratcliffe, M. J. H., van Alphen, L., Coulton, J. W., 1992, Antigenic sites on porin of *Haemophilus influenzae* type b: mapping with synthetic peptides and evaluation of structure presictions, *J. Bacteriol.* 174:4007-4016.

32. Sonntag, I., Schwartz, H., Hirota, Y., Henning, U., 1978, Cell envelope and shape of *Escherichia coli*: multiple mutants missing the outer membrane lipoprotein and other major outer membrane proteins, *J. Bacteriol.* 136:280-285.

33. Van der Ley, P. A., Heckels, J. E., Virji, M., Hoogerhout, P., Poolman J. T., 1991, Topology of outermembrane porins in pathogenic Neisseria spp, *Infect. Immun.* 59:2963-2971.

34. Van der Ley, P. A., Poolman, J. T., 1992, Construction of multivalent class 1 OMP expressing meningococcal vaccine strain, *Infect. Immun,* 60:3156-3161.

35. Van der Ley, P., Van der Biezen, J., Peeters, C. C. A. M., Poolman, J. T., 1993, Use of transformation to construct antigenic hybrids of the class 1 outer membrane protein in *Neisseria meningitidis*, *Inf. Immun.* 61:4724-4733.

36. Van der Ley, P. A., Van der Biezen, J., Poolman, J. T, 1995, Construction of *Neisseria meningitidis* strains carrying multiple chromosomal copies of the porA gene for use in the production of a multivalent outer membrane vesicle vaccine, *Vaccine* 13:401-407.

37. Wetzler, L. M., Blake, M. S., Barry, K., Gotschlich, E. C., 1992, Gonococcal porin vaccine evaluation: comparison of Por proteosomes, liposomes, and blebs isolated from *rmp* deletion mutants, *J. Infect. Dis.*, 166:551-555.

38. Wiertz, E.J.H.J., Van Gaans-van den Brink, J.A.M., Gausephol, H., Prochnicka-Chalufour, A., Hoogerhout, P., Poolman, J.T., 1992, Identification of T cell epitopes occurring in a meningococcal class 1 outer membrane protein using overlapping peptides assembled with simultaneous multiple peptide synthesis, *J. Exp. Med.*, 176:79-88.

39. Zhong, G., Berry, J., Brunham, R. C., 1994, Antibody recognition of a neutralization epitope on the major outer membrane protein of *Chlamydia trachomatis*, *Inf. Immun.* 62:1576-1583.

12

CHANGING PARADIGMS FOR AN HIV VACCINE

Alan M. Schultz

Vaccine and Prevention Research Program, Division of AIDS
National Institute of Allergy and Infectious Disease
National Institutes of Health
Bethesda, Maryland 20852

More than ten years have passed since the discovery of HIV[1,2], the virus which initiates the poorly understood cascade of events resulting in immunodeficiency and the clinical progression of AIDS. Enthusiasm for developing and testing prophylactic HIV vaccines has waxed and waned repeatedly in the intervening decade. Expectations of what the vaccine should do, and consequently how it should be designed, have evolved during that period. From the perspective of 1995, it is worthwhile to review that intellectual progression, take stock of current status of HIV vaccine development, and peer into the future of further development and possible actual human efficacy trials of candidate HIV vaccines.

1. BACKGROUND

In the mid-1980s there was no lack of pessimism about eventual success in the search for an effective HIV vaccine. HIV variation, potential immunopathogenesis, lack of an animal model for HIV disease, and uncertainty about any potential correlate of protective immunity contributed to the malaise[3-6]. And the anticipated difficulty of blocking sexual transmission, with the implication that infection would be carried across the vaginal or rectal mucosa via HIV-infected cells, was proposed as an additional barrier[7].

Unfortunately for everyone, the vast majority of HIV-infected individuals proceed to immunodeficiency disease and death, despite easily measurable humoral and cellular anti-HIV responses[8-10]. A consequence of this sobering observation is that a clearly identifiable population that has recovered from HIV infection is lacking. For other diseases, examination of convalescent patients and comparison to those who suffered severe disease consequences from the same pathogen frequently provided essential clues to the relevant immune responses needed for protection. The lack of an agreed-upon correlate of immunity has provided no guidance for AIDS vaccine design. All these facts together led to the first paradigm for an HIV vaccine.

Novel Strategies in Design and Production of Vaccines
Edited by S. Cohen and A. Shafferman, Plenum Press, New York, 1996

2. STERILIZING IMMUNITY

The initial sentiment was that a vaccine would have to totally prevent HIV infection if there were to be any hope of preventing AIDS. There are immediate corollaries of this paradigm having implications for vaccine design. First, *a priori*, neutralizing antibody is the only relevant immune response. Second, HIV envelope proteins gp120 and gp41, which contain the neutralization epitopes [11-13], are the only relevant antigens for the vaccine. Third, because of the extravagant variability found in the envelope protein, and especially in the V3 principal neutralizing domain[14], breadth of protection based on neutralization as the active principle is going to be a challenge. Either very high neutralization titers will have to be attained (which then might provide sufficient cross-reactivity and thus cross-neutralization), or cross-reactive epitopes will have to be defined and antibodies to them selectively and strongly induced, or a multivalent approach employing envelope proteins of multiple strains from different serotypes (which are as yet undefined) will have to be attempted. In any case, neutralization titers will have to be maintained at high levels in order for the vaccine to be effective.

2.1 First Generation Vaccines in Humans

Several types of vaccines, designed in accord with the paradigm, have been created and given initial testing in humans (Figure 1). Different genetically engineered expression systems (insect cell, yeast, or mammalian cell) have been used to produce envelope subunit proteins, either the mature surface gp120 or the gp160 precursor protein also containing the transmembrane glycoprotein. These proteins have been formulated in alum or in novel adjuvants. A second vaccine concept, inserting the HIV *env* gene into live vectors (first vaccinia and more recently canarypox), has the advantage of endogenous production of the HIV antigens in the volunteer after immunization. This approach hopes to mimic the effective immunogenicity of attenuated, live vaccines. Thirdly, peptide epitope vaccines are designed to eliminate irrelevant epitopes and force the immune system to focus on the neutralization epitopes.

Human safety and immunogenicity testing of first generation vaccines began in 1988 and has slowly continued as new products became available. All products induced persistent proliferative responses, and binding antibody responses were dose-dependent and transient. Anamnestic responses were observed, indicating that immunologic memory was established. In a minority of volunteers, CD4-cell-mediated cytotoxicity was observed with some vaccines. CD8-cell-mediated cytotoxic activity was not found with recombinant subunits, which is not surprising since the vaccines were not specifically intended to do so, and such activity was present in 25% or less of vectored poxvirus vaccine recipients.

Recombinant subunits produced in yeast and insect cell systems were found to be very poor at inducing neutralizing antibody in human volunteers. Likewise, the recombinant poxvirus vectors by themselves are poor inducers of neutralizing antibody. In contrast, gp120 vaccines produced in mammalian cells could induce such antibodies in virtually 100% of volunteers, and these antibodies also cross-neutralized HIV strains other than that used to make the vaccine. However, the cross-neutralizing titers were low and the antibodies

Subunit gp160 or gp120
Vaccinia containing *env*
Canarypox containing *env*
V3-peptide conjugates

Figure 1. 1st generation HIV vaccines.

declined significantly over a period of months. The so-called prime/boost combination, recombinant live vector first then followed by a subunit protein boost, gave titers of neutralizing antibody equivalent to the gp120 vaccines, but this occurred in only a little more than 60% of volunteers. Analysis of the peptide epitope vaccines in humans has only recently begun.

2.1.2. Primary HIV Isolate Neutralization. Most distressingly, the first generation vaccine-induced antibodies that neutralized laboratory strains proved to be totally ineffective against clinical isolates of HIV[15,16]. Neutralization tests against recent isolates of HIV were performed to predict whether the first generation vaccines could induce antibodies effective against HIV currently circulating in populations suitable for efficacy testing. It became apparent that freshly isolated HIV strains which grow only in PBMC are much more difficult to neutralize *in vitro* than the HIV laboratory strains adapted to grow in cell lines previously used. The reasons for this are still being determined, and it is far from certain that *in vitro* neutralization is a necessary prerequisite for a successful vaccine. Nonetheless, for first generation vaccines, designed to rely solely on neutralization as the active principle, this failure was a severe blow and was a major factor among many in the decision not to advance them beyond Phase II testing into efficacy trials[17].

2.1.2. Improving First Generation Vaccines. We know that primary HIV isolates are neutralizable, for their growth is inhibited by sera from those few infected subjects who remain symptom-free and with low virus loads for ten years or more [18] and by some monoclonal antibodies[19,20]. Is something missing from the first generation vaccines? The glycoprotein surface spikes of HIV are multimers of gp120/gp41, whereas the subunit vaccines are monomeric. Binding to the CD4 receptor molecule by these recombinant proteins is relatively weak; gp120 produced in mammalian cells has the best CD4-binding activity among them and also induces the best neutralizing antibody (as measured against laboratory-adapted strains of HIV) of all vaccines tested so far. The term "native", implying that they contain conformational determinants similar to virus glycoprotein *in situ*, has been applied to these products, in contrast to proteins produced from other expression systems[21]. However, there is no evidence that the monomeric gp120s are truly "native" structures.

Experiments that concentrated by 100-fold IgG purified from immunized volunteers have suggested that the failure to neutralize primary HIV is not simply one of titer; these concentrated antibodies still do not effectively neutralize primary HIV *in vitro* nor do they protect reconstituted SCID mice from primary HIV challenge[22]. However at least one of the vaccine products appears to contain the epitopes against which antibodies capable of neutralizing primary HIV isolates are directed. Adsorption of sera that neutralize primary HIV with gp120 removed the neutralizing activity. This is a classic illustration of antigenicity vs. immunogenicity. The vaccine preparation contains the relevant antigen(s), but is not sufficiently immunogenic to induce the antibodies to them.

Several approaches are being tried to improve the immunogenicity of envelope-only (i.e. - first generation) vaccines, especially subunit vaccines. A variety of novel adjuvants have been formulated with gp120 and tested in humans. Early analysis of these trials indicates that acceleration of antibody response and up to 4-fold boosts in titer may be achieved, over formulation of those same antigens in alum. However, it appears unlikely that these modestly higher titers will result in neutralization of primary HIV. It has been observed that envelope proteins containing the entire external gp120 region plus only part of gp41 will form oligomeric structures [23]. It is hoped that these proteins will more closely mimic the truly "native" conformation of viral spikes and therefore be more immunogenic. Also, there is some evidence that envelope glycoproteins from primary HIV, especially macrophage-tropic isolates, may be intrinsically more immunogenic with respect to neutralizing antibody. And finally, there is the possibility that antigens produced from nucleic acid vaccines may have more efficient access to antigen-presenting cells, and therefore be an improvement over recombinant live vector vaccines. It is too early to evaluate the utility of any of these last approaches, which are only now beginning primate studies and may be years away from initial human testing.

2.2 Preclinical Studies

The "sterilizing Immunity" paradigm initially seemed to be upheld in chimpanzees and in the SIV model. Passive transfer of neutralizing monoclonal or polyclonal antibodies showed that high circulating titers could indeed prevent infection with HIV_{IIIB}[26-27]. After some early failed active immunization experiments in chimpanzees, a few successful protections against intravenous, homologous HIV challenge were observed[28,29]. And hundreds of macaques were protected against pathogenic SIV challenge in many experiments using whole-inactivated vaccines[30]. In these experiments there were no signs of any transient infection at all, not even anamnestic boosts of antibody titers upon challenge. These vaccines appeared to totally prevent infection. However, neutralizing antibody titers, though tending to correlate with protection in chimpanzees, did not correlate at all with protection in the SIV/macaque experiments.

The apparent success of whole-inactivated vaccines in the SIV model unravelled when it developed that the most relevant antigens in the preparations were not the SIV proteins at all, but rather antigens from the cells used to produce the vaccine. It had been convenient to use human cells to make both large-scale virus production runs for the SIV vaccine, as well as for the titered SIV challenge stocks. Immunized macaques made responses to human antigens found in membrane fragments in the vaccine preparations and incorporated into the virions themselves. The fact that protection was due to such xeno-antigens common to the vaccine and the challenge virus was demonstrated by challenge with SIV grown in macaque cells. Animals exhibiting sterilizing immunity against challenge with SIV from human cells were completely susceptible to infection when subsequently challenged with the very same virus grown in macaque PBMC[31,32]. It was now obvious that neutralizing antibody did not correlate with protection induced by whole-inactivated vaccines in the SIV model because SIV envelope was not the relevant antigen!

These disappointing results did not obviate the fact that protection against pathogenic SIV was clearly obtainable by vaccination, although the success in this model could not be transferred easily to a human vaccine because HIV to which humans are exposed contains human cellular antigens, not xeno-antigens.

2.2.1 Primate Disease Models for AIDS. Other candidate vaccines rarely met the sterilizing immunity criteria. Envelope subunit vaccines were complete failures in the SIV model[33,34]. Subunit vaccines showed promise in the HIV/chimpanzee model[28,29], culminating in the first demonstration of cross-protection, protecting chimpanzees against the SF2 strain of HIV using a vaccine made from the MN strain[35]. The challenge virus, maintained in human PBMC since isolation, was not neutralized by chimp sera on the day of challenge, although these sera would neutralize SF2 adapted to growth on T-cell lines. However, this protection in the absence of neutralization of the challenge virus was ultimately not considered convincing, because virus loads of SF2 in chimpanzees are low, and chimpanzees do not become ill from any strain of HIV. At the present time, without disease, protection in primates is not taken as strong evidence of the protective potential of a vaccine.

Success of other vaccine concepts in primates was demonstrable only against the *mne* strain of SIV. Vaccinia prime/boost combinations [36], and a peptide epitope vaccine[37] protected macaques against homologous challenge with this virus. In fact, evidence of recovery from infection after challenge was seen in one of the vaccinated macaques receiving the peptide vaccine. Although the *mne* virus causes immunodeficiency and is lethal, animals survive for years before dying. Since similar vaccine concepts tested against the *mac* or *sm* strains of SIV, in which most animals die within 18 months of infection, were not successful, these results with the *mne* strain have been accorded minimal relevance.

2.2.2 Attenuated Live Vaccines for SIV. Whole-inactivated HIV has never been seriously attempted as a human vaccine, in large part because of the grave consequences should any lot of vaccine fail to be completely inactivated. There are also technological problems in retaining sufficient, immunogenic gp120 in such preparations, as was demonstrated in a single chimpanzee experiment employing such a vaccine[38]. The rationale for the whole-inactivated vaccine experiments in the SIV model was to empirically test a methodology, proven for vaccines against other pathogens, irrespective of concerns about safety. These had initiated as conceptual studies, aimed at exploring the limits of immune protection against an immunodeficiency virus.

When whole-inactivated vaccines failed against SIV, the same logic then was applied to the attenuated, live vaccine approach. Attenuated viral vaccines are the most immunogenic and successful vaccines in use today. Safety issues with respect to their actual use in humans for HIV would be enormous. However, in an animal model, it is possible to test the limits and parameters of immune protection against SIV (and by implication, HIV), again irrespective of safety concerns. If such a vaccine would work against SIV, the fact that it worked, and discovering how it worked, could bolster the development of an HIV vaccine. On the other hand, if such a vaccine also failed, as did the whole-inactivated vaccine approach, then the path to a successful HIV vaccine was likely to be long, slow, and tortuous, and perhaps even unattainable.

A live SIV vaccine, attenuated by deleting the *nef* gene, indeed demonstrated the most impressive protection against SIV that has been seen[39]. Macaques challenged more than two years after immunization were protected, even against 1000 animal infectious doses of uncloned SIVmac251 grown in rhesus PBMC, which is among the most pathogenic simian immunodeficiency viruses known. This result was encouraging, in that active immunization provided protection in a stringent, disease model of simian AIDS. Elucidating a correlate of protection from such a complex vaccine is a daunting task. Neutralizing antibodies induced by this vaccine were not obviously more potent than those induced by prime/boost protocols in the SIV model. A property of this vaccine, in contrast to "traditional" attenuated live vaccines for other pathogens which appear to be cleared by the host immune response, was that it was not eliminated but persisted as a replicating entity, albeit at barely detectable levels.

A curious observation in the initial report of protection was that SIV was isolated from a single sample, the first blood sample taken post-challenge, of one of the four protected macaques. No attempt was made to examine the virus, and discrimination between the challenge virus or reactivation of the vaccine virus was not possible. But in a subsequent experiment, in which other attenuated SIV vaccines were tested and in which challenge occurred within months rather than years of the initial immunization with the attenuated vaccine, the significance of this observation became clearer.

Although most of the macaques in this large experiment were clearly protected and a few became infected after challenge with pathogenic SIVmac251, several showed definite signs of transient infection. PCR analysis of the *nef* gene can discriminate between the full-length wild-type and the deleted version found in the vaccine. In these several macaques, virus loads in PBMC rose sharply after challenge but then dropped to very low levels. PCR proved that wild-type challenge virus was present but then disappeared from circulating PBMC; persistence of the attenuated vaccine virus was noted[40].

3. RECOVERY FROM INFECTION

The second paradigm for an HIV vaccine represents the confluence of several threads of analysis derived from the intervening years of research since 1984. Although new for HIV, this paradigm is the common one for vaccines, *viz.* that after exposure to the pathogen, an infection begins but is contained and then often ultimately actually cleared. The previous observations of the persistence of HIV despite HIV-specific immune responses had been interpreted to mean that HIV always prevails. This lead to the first paradigm, requiring sterilizing immunity.

What has changed? One development is the very recent discovery that the virus levels detectable in the plasma reflect a steady-state balance between daily production and clearance of enormous amounts of HIV[41]. In this context, there is now an appreciation of how close the immune system comes to success against HIV. It copes for a very long time, about ten years on average, losing to HIV only after a titanic battle. The description of long-term non-progressors, a small but significant number of patients infected with HIV for more than 8 years, who are not merely still alive but have barely detectable virus, suggests that immune containment of HIV may be possible[42-44].

A second thread culminating in the second paradigm comes from the primate experiments just described. Many vaccines that fail to protect against SIV infection nevertheless reduce virus loads after challenge and in some cases seem to increase survival times[45]. And the transient infection seen occasionally in attenuated, live SIV vaccine experiments is the best evidence that the traditional vaccine paradigm, recovery from infection, can be operant for SIV (and by analogy, HIV).

This paradigm has corollaries as well. First, mechanistically speaking, cytotoxic responses will need to be induced, as they are essential for killing HIV-infected cells. Second, non-*env* proteins should be included for two reasons: [a] the presence of core proteins may improve native conformation of *env* proteins and therefore induce better quality neutralizing antibody; [b] cytotoxic T-cells tend to be directed to non-*env* proteins. Third, since core proteins tend to be more conserved, HIV variation may be less of a problem for the vaccine to overcome.

3.1. Second Generation Human Vaccines

In accord with this paradigm, a series of second generation vaccine candidates is entering human safety and immunogenicity trials (Figure 2). Vaccinia and canarypox vectors, which in the first generation contained only HIV *env*, now include the *gag* and protease genes, with varying amounts of the *pol* gene in addition. A genetically inactivated HIV (pseudovirion) product, which should be a completely non-infectious and safe form of whole-inactivated virus, is in a small primate trial and awaits initial human testing. Finally, synthetic peptide vaccines, when conjugated to certain lipid moieties, have been shown to induce CTL in mice if he proper epitopes are chosen. Some products of this type are entering human testing, and may eventually comprise part of combination vaccines designed to induce both neutralizing antibody and cytotoxic cells.

Pseudovirion
Canarypox containing *gag-pro; env*
Vaccinia containing *gag-pol; env*
Lipidated peptide conjugates
Ty-gag Virus-like Particles

Figure 2. 2nd generation HIV vaccines.

It is much too early to tell if the second generation of vaccines represents a quantum leap in HIV vaccine design. Obtaining by active immunization polyclonal sera that will neutralize primary HIV remains a lofty goal, and such an accomplishment would vault any vaccine that caused it into contention for rapid inauguration of a phase 3 efficacy trial. However, failure to attain this particular goal will not be so damning as it has been for first generation vaccines, for the second generation vaccines provide a full array of epitopes, conformational as well as linear, with the potential to induce a variety of responses. A combination of immune responses, the exact complexity of which may vary from vaccinee to vaccinee depending on their genetic make-up, is more likely to be effective than reliance on a single immune response.

3.2. Abortive Infection vs Suppressed Infection

What exactly is meant by recovery from infection by HIV? Reference to an idealized graph of virus load as a function of time after infection (Figure 3) will help in the description. This graph focuses on the trough of virus load after the initial peak of viremia, which is intentionally off-scale in the Figure. Curve [1] represents rapidly progressing patients, whose virus load falls somewhat after the initial peak but never becomes truly low. Virus load then steadily increases, and the clinical picture worsens; in the pathogenic SIV model, about 25% of macaques pursue this course and die within 6 months of infection. Curve [2] traces the more usual course of virus load in the majority of HIV infections. The initial viremia is brought under control and remains at a low but persistent level. After a period of years, virus load begins to rise again and clinical symptoms begin.

The concept of vaccine-induced suppressed infection is also consistent with curve [2]. However, vaccine "success" is defined as modifying the parameters of curve [2] so that all vaccinees who become infected experience an increased length of the low virus load plateau, and survival extends significantly beyond the 10-11 year average now observed for HIV infection in unvaccinated subjects. Vaccine "success" also includes preventing any curve [1] cases among vaccinees. According to this scenario, the virus load in vaccinees that become infected will be substantially lower than if they had not been immunized. The patient is still likely to die with immunodeficiency, but to live substantially longer than if not vaccinated. This scenario may have been demonstrated in some SIV vaccine experiments already[45]. One would not specifically design a vaccine to attain only this degree of "success". However, it is important to remember that vaccines are used to protect populations, and that interrupting transmission is the goal. If a reduced virus load caused by the vaccine reduces

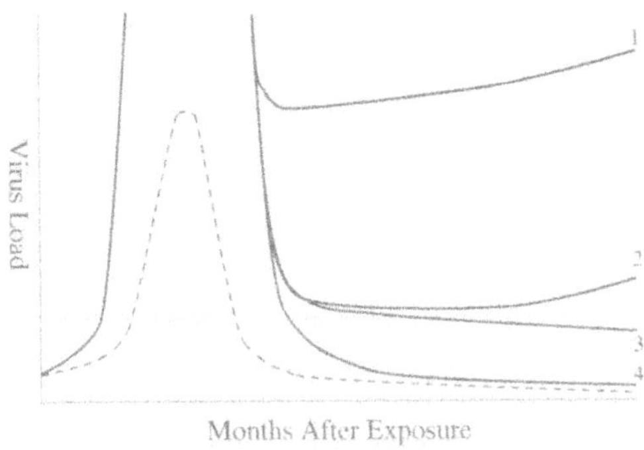

Figure 3. Months after infection.

the likelihood of transmission, the vaccine may have real benefit, even if the infected vaccinee nonetheless eventually succumbs to the disease.

Abortive infection, which is an unproven outcome at present for HIV, is the true goal of the second paradigm. If infection can occur but be contained, then a vaccinee who becomes infected will be protected from AIDS and live a normal life-span. The chain of transmission will also be broken. Two possibilities for abortive infection are shown as curves [3] and [4] in Figure 3. The dotted line in Figure 3 represents a hypothetical threshold virus load level below which continued HIV infection becomes unsustainable and comes to an end, or "aborts". Curve [4] shows an abrupt ablation of virus load induced by a hypothetical successful vaccine, and curve [3] is intended to imply a less robust immune response which nevertheless eventually succeeds in reducing the virus load below the hypothetical threshold level. The dashed curve in the initial viremia period reflects a common view that the vaccine, in order to be successful and result in either curve [3] or curve [4], will have to induce an immune response which blunts the initial viremic peak.

Whether outcomes [3] or [4] (Figure 3) are possible will require further detailed analysis of longitudinal virus load in more primate vaccine experiments and in human natural history studies. Attenuated, live vaccines in the SIV model may have exhibited abortive infection, although longer observation periods of "recovered" macaques is needed to gain confidence in the outcome. With respect to human disease, a recent publication shows that survival after HIV infection, with a median of 8.3 years of follow-up, is highly correlated with plasmavirus load soon after infection is established[46]. A human example may be the infant born with HIV infection who apparently is now HIV-free[47]. Conceptually, abortive infection turns all vaccinees who become infected vaccinees into long-term non-progressors who maintain very low virus loads and potentially normal life spans; the suppressed infection outcome produces long-term survivors, who live longer than expected in the absence of pre-immunization but die with immunodeficiency.

If this paradigm is fulfilled, efficacy trials of vaccines will need to be monitored not only for infection, but for virus load. A reasonable expectation of this paradigm, coupled with the biology of retroviruses, is that a vaccinee may become PCR-positive but virus isolation negative, with very low plasmavirus levels and incapable of transmission. Much more data is needed from macaque studies before secondary endpoints of human trials can be designed and relied upon.

4. PREVENTING SEXUAL TRANSMISSION

A third paradigm for HIV has developed, based on the premise that mucosal transmission may present a special problem for an HIV vaccine. According to this paradigm, vaccines must be designed to induce mucosal immunity because transmission occurs across rectal or vaginal mucosa. The primary mode of HIV transmission is sexual, with heterosexual transmission predominating in the developing world.

Some vaccine approaches designed according to this paradigm are listed in Figure 4. A major premise in these designs is the concept of the common mucosal system[48], so that antigen delivery to one portion of the system (oral or nasal portals) will be effective at physically remote

Adenovirus recombinants
Poliovirus recombinants
Rhinovirus recombinants
Oral formulations

Figure 4. 3rd generation HIV vaccines.

regions (rectum and vagina). Obvious delivery vehicles for immunizing the mucosal surfaces are viruses which replicate there: adenovirus, poliovirus, rhinovirus. Each of these has been modified to express HIV genes[49-51], or to display HIV epitopes on the surface of the virion[52,53]. Ideas about inducing mucosal immunity with non-replicating proteins abound, including various adjuvants and formulated for oral administration. Most of these approaches are in very early development.

What is meant by mucosal immunity? Relying on secreted IgA or transudated IgG in the local region as the essential immune response for blocking transmission runs the risk of repeating the sterilizing immunity fallacy. However, IgA secretion could be a marker for some kind of regional immunity.

4.1. Infection Across the Mucosa in Primates

Previous experiments in the SIV model had shown that intramuscularly administered whole-inactivated vaccine, which previously had been an effective immunogen, was ineffective against vaginal challenge[54]. This result could suggest that sexual transmission is indeed an especial challenge for an HIV vaccine. However, the converse has also now been shown. Whole-inactivated SIV formulated in slow-release form and administered orally and tracheally was shown to protect against vaginal challenge but not against intravenous challenge with homologous SIV[55].

This last experiment is not compelling, as it is compromised by the presence of human cellular antigens and by the high doses of SIV required to achieve infection in this model. However, it does hint that protection depends on formulation and route of administration as much as it does on the actual antigens used. Subtle difference in immune responses in macaques, depending on the route of administration, have been observed[56]. This may mean that a single vaccine may not be protective against both intravenous and sexual transmission, but it does not mean that preventing sexual transmission will be an especially difficult task.

Is infection via the mucosa different in some way from infection directly into the blood? That the answer is yes is suggested by intriguing observations with vaginal transmission of SIV in macaques and HIV in chimpanzees. Infection of these primates can be achieved if sufficiently high doses of virus are used[57]. When lower doses are used by the vaginal route, in naive animals, transient infection is observed. In both chimpanzees[58] and macaques[57], virus was detectable in the circulation by PCR, and even occasionally by virus isolation, but the infection never became established, and seroconversion was not observed. With time, the PCR signal disappeared from the circulation.

If transient infection with low-dose vaginal exposure in un-immunized primates is frequently observed, then vaccine-induced protection against sexual transmission may not be a special problem. Attempts to infect primates vaginally using SIV-infected cells have been unsuccessful[59]. Although it is clear that modelling sexual transmission in primates is not well-developed and can not yet be a predictor of the human condition, it is a hopeful sign that mucosal transmission may not be a highly efficient process.

5. THE ELUSIVE CORRELATE OF IMMUNITY

In the interest of improving vaccines, the designs are being changed to include more antigens. More attention is being paid to a variety of responses to an array of epitopes. It is now appreciated from natural history studies that anti-HIV immune responses are not futile, and that their rapid induction in response to early infection may provide the additional advantage needed for success. Thus the strategy is to engage the whole armamentarium of immune responses and to recover from infection. If the primate results just discussed are relevant to the human condition, preventing sexual transmission may need just a little extra help.

In contrast to this full-scale approach, focus on subtleties of Th1/Th2 responses has been proposed[60]. Whether the distinction between Th1 and Th2 responses is clear enough to drive vaccine design is too early to say, and lies far beyond the scope of this article. However, it is an active area of research. The use of adjuvants to control specific cytokine levels is a fascinating subject for the future. Populations who are apparently exposed to HIV but remain uninfected are becoming better defined[61]. The failure to identify a significant population that has recovered from HIV infection may have been a consequence of using seroconversion to HIV as the starting point for the search. The exposed but uninfected populations may be the human equivalent of the primates who experience transient infection after vaginal exposure but do not establish infection and do not seroconvert. Whether this exposure induces protective immunity, according to a new Th1/Th2 paradigm, remains to be seen.

Will the initiation of phase 3 trials await a defined correlate? Certainly if any vaccine would induce antibodies that could neutralize a range of primary HIV, there would be strong enthusiasm for proceeding. But the newer paradigms may not easily translate into entry criteria for a large-scale trial. Cytotoxic T-cells are difficult to measure, and CTL "activity" may not be a sufficient response on which to make judgments. More specificity with respect to specific epitopes or to a multiplicity of epitope responses is likely to be required before CTL alone will be considered sufficient. Assessing protective mucosal immunity is even more problematic. Empiric challenge results from primate models, especially with the lack of an HIV disease model, will probably not be totally convincing. Such a decision will be very complex, involving a multiplicity of factors.

6. CONCLUSION

Vaccines have long been an essential weapon in the worldwide fight against morbidity and mortality caused by infectious disease. When they are successful, they provide a low-cost and effective barrier, protecting entire populations against epidemic spread of infectious agents. A vaccine against AIDS is thus desperately needed to intervene in this global pandemic. As designs for HIV vaccines become more complex, there must be a greater reliance on an empiric approach to testing. The true value of any vaccine will not be known until it is evaluated in expanded human testing under field conditions.

REFERENCES

1. Barre-Sinnoussi F, Chermann JC, Rey F, ET AL (1983) Isolation of a T-lymphotropic retrovirus from a patient at risk for acquired immune deficiency syndrome (AIDS). Science 220:868-871.
2. Popovic M, Sarngadharan MG, Read E, ET AL (1984) Detection, isolation, and continuous production of cytopathic retroviruses (HTLV-III) from patients with AIDS and pre-AIDS. Science 224:497-500
3. Francis DP, Petricciani JC (1985) The prospects for and pathways towards a vaccine for AIDS. N Engl J Med 313:1586-1590
4. Koff WC, Hoth DF (1988) Development and testing of AIDS vaccines. Science 241:426-432
5. Ada GL (1988) Prospects for HIV vaccines. J Acquir Immune Defic Syndr 1:295-303
6. Hoth DL (1993) Issues in the development of a prophylactic HIV vaccine. Ann NY Acad Sci 685:777-783
7. Sabin AB (1992) Improbability of effective vaccination against human immunodeficiency virus because of its intracellular transmission and rectal port of entry. Proc Natl Acad Sci USA 89:8852-8855y
8. Lui KJ, Darrow WW, Rutherford GW (1988) A model-based estimate of the mean incubation period for AIDS in homosexual men. Science 240:1333-1335
9. Lyerly HK, Reed DL, Matthews TJ, ET AL (1987) Anti-gp120 antibodies from HIV seropositive individuals mediate broadly reactive anti-HIV ADCC. AIDS Res Hum Retr 3:409-422
10. Walker BD, Chakrabarti S, Moss B, ET AL (1987) HIV-specific cytotoxic T lymphocytes in seropositive individuals. Nature 328: 345-348

11. Robey WG, Arthur LO, Matthews TJ, ET AL (1986) Prospect for prevention of human immunodeficiency virus infection: purified 120 kDa envelope glycoprotein induces neutralizing antibody. Proc Natl Acad Sci USA 83:7023-7027

12. Ho DD, Sarngadharan MG, Hirsch MS, ET AL (1987) Human immunodeficiency virus neutralizing antibodies recognize several conserved domains on the envelope glycoproteins. J Virol 61:2024-2028

13. Dalgleish AG, Chanh TC, Kennedy RC, ET AL (1988) Neutralization of diverse HIV-1 strains by monoclonal antibodies raised against a gp41 synthetic peptide. Virology 165:209-215

14. Myers G, Korber B, Wain-Hobson S, ET AL (eds) (1993) Human Retroviruses and AIDS 1993 I-II: A compilation and analysis of nucleic acid and amino acid sequences. Los Alamos NM: U.S.Department of Energy (Theoretical Biology and Biophysics Group T-10), Los Alamos National Laboratory Publication Number LA-UR93-3063

15. Mascola J, Weislow O, Snyder S, ET AL (1994) Neutralizing antibody activity in sera from human immunodeficiency virus type-1 vaccine recipients from the AIDS Vaccine Clinical Trials Network [abstract]. AIDS Res Hum Retr 10 (suppl 1):S55

16. Matthews T, McDanal C, Greenwell T, ET AL (1994) Serological reactivity from HIV-1 vaccine recipients in the AIDS Vaccine Clinical Trials Network [abstract]. AIDS Res Hum Retr 10 (suppl 1):S55

17. Cohen J (1994) U.S. panel votes to delay real-world vaccine trials [News & Comment]. Science 264:1839

18. Cao Y, Qin L, Zhang L, ET AL (1995) Virologic and Immunologic characterization of long-term survivors of human immunodeficiency virus type 1 infection. N Engl J Med 332:201-208

19. Burton DR, Pyati J, Koduri R, ET AL (1994) Efficient neutralization of primary isolates of HIV-1 by a recombinant monoclonal antibody. Science 266:1024-1027

20. Purtscher M, Trkola A, Gruber G, ET AL (1994) A broadly neutralizing human monoclonal antibody against gp41 of human immunodeficiency virus type 1. AIDS Res Hum Retr 10:1651-1658

21. Haigwood NL, Nara PL, Brooks E, ET AL (1992) Native but not denatured recombinant human immunodeficiency virus type 1 gp120 generates broad spectrum neutralizing antibody in baboons. J Virol 66:172-182

22. Steimer KS, Sinangil F, Kahn J, ET AL (1994) Primary isolate neutralizing activity of human antibodies directed to recombinant, native HIV-SF2 gp120 [abstract]. AIDS Res Hum Retr 10 (suppl 1):S55 and personal communication

23. Broder CC, Earl PL, Long D, ET AL (1994) Antigenic implications of human immunodeficiency virus type 1 envelope quaternary structure: oligomer-specific and -sensitive monoclonal antibodies. Proc Natl Acad Sci USA 91:11699-703

24. Emini EA, Schlief WA, Nunberg JH, ET AL: Prevention of HIV-1 infection in chimpanzees by gp120 V3 domain-specific monoclonal antibody. Nature 1992, 355:728-730.

25. Prince AM, Horowitz B, Shulman RW, ET AL (1990) Apparent prevention of HIV infection by HIV immunoglobulin given prior to low-dose HIV challenge. In Vaccines '90 edited by Brown F, Chanock R, Ginsberg H, Lerner R. Cold Spring Harbor, Cold Spring Harbor Laboratory Press, pp. 347-351.

26. Prince AM, Reesink H, Pascual D, ET AL: Prevention of infection by passive immunization with HIV immunoglobulin. AIDS Res Hum Retroviruses 1991, 7:971-973

27. Putkonen P, Thorstensson R, Ghavamzadeh L, ET AL (1991) Prevention of HIV-2 and SIVsm infection with passive immunization in cynomolgus monkeys. Nature 352:436-438

28. Berman PW, Gregory TJ, Riddle L, ET AL: Protection of chimpanzees from infection by HIV-1 after vaccination with recombinant glycoprotein gp120 but not gp160. Nature 1990, 345:622-625

29. Girard M, Kieny MP, Pinter A, ET AL: Immunization of chimpanzees confers protection against challenge with human immunodeficiency virus. Proc Natl Acad Sci USA 1991, 88:542-546.

30. Warren JT, Dolatshi M (1993) First updated and revised survey of worldwide HIV and SIV vaccine challenge studies in non-human primates: progress in first and second order studies. J Med Primatol 22:203-205

31. le Grand R, Vasin B, Vogt G, ET AL (1992) AIDS vaccine developments [letter]. Nature 355:684

32. Cranage MP, Ashworth LA, Greenaway PJ, ET AL (1992) AIDS vaccine developments [letter]. Nature 355:685-686

33. Planelles V, Giavedoni L, Marthas M, ET AL (1992) Vaccine studies with SIVmac1A11 recombinant gp130: Lack of protection from SIVmac251 challenge. In "Vaccines '92", edited by Brown F, Chanock R, Ginsberg H, Lerner R. Cold Spring Harbor, Cold Spring Harbor Laboratory Press, pp. 123-129

34. Mills KHG, Page M, Chan WL, ET AL (1992) Protection against SIV challenge in macaques. J Med Primatol 21:50-58

35. Berman PW, Eastman D, Nakamura G, ET AL (1995) Apparent protection of MN-rgp120-immunized chimpanzees from infection with a primary isolate of HIV-1. In "Vaccines '95", edited by Brown F, Chanock R, Ginsberg H, Lerner R. Cold Spring Harbor, Cold Spring Harbor Laboratory Press, in press

36. Hu S-L, Stallard V, Abrams K, ET AL (1993) Protection of vaccinia-primed macaques against SIVmne infection by combination immunization with recombinant vaccinia virus and SIVmne gp160. J Med Primatol 22:92-99

37. Shafferman A, Jahrling PB, Benveniste RE, ET AL (1991) Protection of macaques with a simian immunodeficiency virus envelope peptide vaccine based on conserved human immunodeficiency virus type 1 sequences. Proc Natl Acad Sci USA 88:7126-7130

38. Neidrig M, Gregerson J-P, Fultz PN, ET AL (1993) Immune responses of chimpanzees after immunization with the inactivated whole immunodeficiency virus (HIV-1), three different adjuvants and challenge. Vaccine 11:67-74

39. Daniel MD, Kirchhoff F, Czajak SC, ET AL (1992) Protective effects of a live attenuated SIV vaccine with a deletion in the nef gene. Science 258:1938-1941

40. Garcia-Moll M, Wyand M, Desrosiers RC; personal communication

41. Wei X, Ghosh SK, Taylor ME, ET AL (1995) Viral dynamics in human immunodeficiency virus type 1 infection. Nature 373:117-122

42. Ho DD, Neumann AU, Perelson AS, ET AL (1995) Rapid turnover of plasma virions and CD4 lymphocytes in HIV-1 infection. Nature 373:123-126

43. Buchbinder SP, Katz MH, Hessol NA, ET AL (1994) Long term HIV-1 infection without immunologic progression. AIDS 8:1123-1128

44. Pantaleo G, Menzo S, Vaccareeza M, ET AL (1995) Studies in subjects with long-term non-progressive human immunodeficiency virus infection. N Engl J Med 332:209-216

45. Hirsch V, Goldstein S, Hynes NA, ET AL (1993) Immunization with inactivated human cell-culture-derived SIV vaccine prolongs survival of monkeys subsequently infected with simian cell-associated SIV. In "Vaccines '93", edited by Ginsberg H, Brown F, Chanock R, Lerner R. Cold Spring Harbor, Cold Spring Harbor Laboratory Press, pp. 63-69

46. Mellors JW, Kingsley LA, Rinaldo CR, ET AL (1995) Quantitation of HIV-1 RNA in plasma predicts outcome after seroconversion. Ann Intern Med 122:573-579

47. Bryson YJ, Pang S, Wei LS, ET AL (1995) Clearance of HIV infection in a perinatally infected infant. N Engl J Med 332:833-838

48. Mestecky J (1987) The common mucosal immune system and current strategies for induction of immune responses in external secretions. J Clin Immunol 7:265-278

49. Natuk RJ, Lubeck MD, Chanda PK, ET AL (1992) Immunogenicity of recombinant human adenovirus-human immunodeficiency virus vaccines in chimpanzees. AIDS Res Hum Retr 9:395-404

50. Alexander L, Lu HH, Gromeier M, ET AL (1994) Dicistronic polioviruses as expression vectors for foreign genes. AIDS Res Hum Retr 10 (suppl 2):S57-S60

51. Andino R, Silvera D, Suggest SD, ET AL (1994) Engineering poliovirus as a vaccine vector for the expression of diverse antigens. Science 265:1448-1451

52. Dedieu JF, Ronco J, van der Werf S, ET AL (1992) Poliovirus chimeras expressing sequences from the principal neutralization domain of human immunodeficiency virus type 1. J Virol 66:3161-3167

53. Resnick DA, Smith AD, Geisler SC, ET AL (1995) Chimeras from a human rhinovirus 14-human immunodeficiency virus type 1 (HIV-1) V3 loop seroprevalence library induce neutralizing responses against HIV-1. J Virol 69:2406-2411

54. Sutjipto S, Pedersen NC, Miller CJ, ET AL (1990) Inactivated simian immunodeficiency virus vaccine failed to protect rhesus macaques from intravenous or genital mucosal infection but delayed disease in intravenously exposed animals. J Virol 64:2290-2297

55. Marx PA, Compans RW, Gettie A, ET AL (1993) Protection against vaginal SIV transmission with microencapsulated vaccine. Science 260:1323-1327

56. Lehner T, Tao L, Panagiotidi C, ET AL (1994) Mucosal model of genital immunization in male rhesus macaques with a recombinant simian immunodeficiency virus p27 antigen. J Virol 68:1624-1632

57. Miller CJ, Marthas M, Torten J, ET AL (1994) Intravaginal inoculation of rhesus macaques with cell-free simian immunodeficiency virus results in persistent or transient viremia. J Virol 68:6391-6400

58. Girard M (1992) HIV-1 genital infection: a chimpanzee model. In "7e Colloque des Cent Gardes", edited by Girard M, Valette L. Fondation Marcel Merieux, Lyon, pp. 75-79

59. Miller CJ; personal communication

60. Salk J, Bretscher PA, Salk PL, ET AL (1993) A strategy for prophylactic vaccination against HIV. Science 260:1270-1272

61. Rowland-Jones S, Sutton J, Ariyoshi A, ET AL (1995) HIV-specific cytotoxic T-cells in HIV-exposed but uninfected Gambian women. Nature Medicine 1:59-64

13

COMPLEXED HIV ENVELOPE AS A TARGET FOR AN AIDS VACCINE

J. M. Gershoni,* G. F. Denisova, D. Raviv, B. Stern, and J. Zwickel

Department of Cell Research and Immunology
George S. Wise Faculty of Life Sciences
Tel Aviv University
Ramat Aviv, Tel Aviv 69978, Israel

1. INTRODUCTION

The AIDS epidemic has been threatening us for over a decade and despite the enormous research effort, we are still unable to cope with HIV. Neither cure, treatment nor prophylactic-vaccine have emerged that might provide real efficacy against this "stealth virus".

The object of our research has been to study the HIV envelope structure and function with the intent to apply new knowledge to the development of AIDS vaccines, therapeutics and diagnostics. The working hypothesis of our laboratory is based on two assumptions:

1. *Vaccination is possible*; if indeed this is the case then it is necessary to identify cross reactive neutralizing epitopes of the virus and to exploit these structures for the production of effective subunit vaccines.
2. *HIV is ancient*; thus it has evolved over thousands and possibly millions of years during which it has developed answers to most of our natural immune defenses.

The experimental approach adopted by us therefore, has been to subject HIV to situations evolution may not have been able to anticipate. This idea would for example argue that there may exist epitopes that are critical to the virus and can not tolerate molecular modification. Such epitopes may be normally buried in the depth of the envelope protein, gp120 and become exposed only transiently during the course of pathogenesis. Thus possibly complexation of gp120 with its corresponding receptor, CD4, may elicit conformational rearrangements in these proteins revealing structures that previously may not have been noticed or exploited. A second complex of gp120 that might be of interest and use is the immunocomplex of this protein.

A major epitope that has undergone extensive examination is the variable loop V3 of gp120 (residues 295-300) [1]. We have prepared an immunocomplex of gp120/M77. The

---

*Tel: 972-3-640-8981 Fax: 972-3-642-2046.

Novel Strategies in Design and Production of Vaccines
Edited by S. Cohen and A. Shafferman, Plenum Press, New York, 1996

latter, M77, is a commercially available murine monoclonal antibody directed against the tip of the V3 loop [2]. The logic behind these experiments is that this complex may more effectively present epitopes that have normally been less immunogenic in gp120 alone.

The following report summarizes some of our results derived from experiments in which novel panels of monoclonal antibodies (mAbs) have been prepared from mice immunized with complexes of HIV-1$_{IIIB}$ gp120.

2. MATERIALS AND METHODS

2.1. Preparation of mAbs

Balb/C mice were immunized with recombinant gp120 (purchased from Intracel Corporation, Boston, MA) or gp120 complexed with either recombinant soluble CD4 or with the anti-V3 loop mAb; M77 (Advanced BioScience Laboratories Inc., Rockville MD). The splenocytes of the mice that acquired relatively high anti-gp120 titers were fused with NS/O myeloma cells (kindly provided by Milstein, Cambridge). The hybridomas were screened by ELISA either against the original antigen or its components separately.

2.2. Analyses of mAbs

Once hybridomas were cloned their corresponding mAbs were either purified from spent media or from ascites fluids by standard procedures [3]. The mAbs were then analyzed in competitive ELISA assays, Scatchard analyses or used in Western blots of *S. aureus* V8 proteolyzed gp120. For these studies it was often necessary to either biotinylate or radioiodinate the mAbs as per described previously [3].

2.3. Epitope Mapping

In order to map the position of the epitopes of the mAbs isolated, a combinatorial phage display epitope library was prepared [see 4-6]. A totally randomized 20 amino acid sequence was inserted into the N-terminal of the pIII of the filamentous bacteriophage (the vector fuSE5 was kindly provided by George Smith [4]). The library was screened using the mAbs individually and isolating plaques after one round of panning. For this a solid phase slot blot assay was developed in order to identify those plaques that responded to the relevant mAb. The inserts of the phages selected were then sequenced and areas of homology common to the phages and gp120 were identified.

3. RESULTS

As can be seen in Figure 1 proteolysis of gp120 with *S. aureus* V8 protease generates a pattern of proteolytic fragments that can be recognized by the polyclonal sera of mice immunized with gp120 or its complexes. Each immunization scheme generates a distinct, unique and reproducible response illustrated by the fact that different fragments are recognized in each mouse.

The mice were then used for fusions and production of mAbs. Table 1 summarizes five fusion experiments (two for gp120, two for gp120/CD4 and one for gp120/M77). In total, 62 mAbs were isolated and characterized. The ELISA assays were performed using either gp120 in its native form or denatured gp120. In both cases the total amount of antigen in each well was kept the same as the denaturation step was done only after plating. Such an

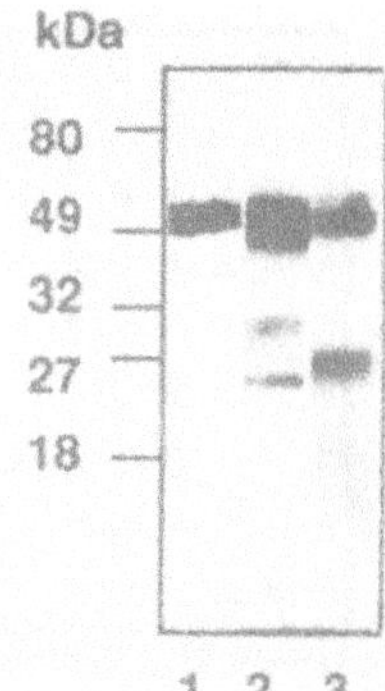

Figure 1. Western blot analysis of anti-gp120 polyclonal sera. Mice were immunized with gp120 (lane 1); gp120 complexed with CD4 (lane 2) or gp120 complexed with M77 (lane 3). In all cases the same amount of gp120$_{IIIB}$ (30µg/mouse/injection) was used and each animal was boosted 3 times over 2 months. Serum samples were obtained and used to probe Western blots of *S. aureus* V8 protease treated gp120, immobilized on nitrocellulose filters. ECL (Amersham Co., IL) was used to visualize the immunocomplexed bands. Note the qualitatively different response for each mouse.

analysis indicated the availability of the epitopes and their sensitivity to denaturation, a measure of the conformational nature of the epitopes in question. From these studies it became apparent that for gp120 and gp120/CD4 the vast majority of mAbs were "conformational" rather than "linear". Complexation with M77 on the other hand led to the appearance of numerous mAbs that recognized "linear" epitopes.

Further analysis of the mAbs by Western blot could provide insight as to the location of the epitope within the gp120 molecule. This was accomplished by systematically probing the blots of proteolyzed gp120 with mAbs of known epitopes and thus identifying specific fragments as either NH$_2$-terminal, COOH-terminal or central parts of the molecule. Obviously this type of analysis of the mAbs was only possible for those that were least sensitive to denaturation. Nonetheless, it appeared that the majority of the response to the gp120/M77 complex was to the NH$_2$-terminal aspects of the gp120.

More detailed epitope mapping was accomplished using the mAbs to screen a phage display library. For this selected mAbs were reacted with the library and panned using goat anti-mouse Fc as the immobilizing reagent placed in the petri dishes. Individual plaques were subsequently isolated and tested for their ability to bind the different mAbs. Those that had

Table 1. mAbs prepared against gp120 and its complexes

ELISA tests were performed using native gp120 plated in the wells. The wells were then either incubated 15min with 1%SDS+5%2-mecaptoethanol at 55°C (denatured gp120) or not (native gp120). Subsequently, the gp120 samples were reacted with the mAbs followed by goat anti-mouse immunoglobulin conjugated with alkaline phosphatase and enzymatically detected. The mAbs were divided into three groups according to their relative responses to the native vs denatured antigen. Strongly conformationally dependent mAbs are those with a >2.5 ratio whereas linear epitopes have <1.0 ratio. Previous results using the *S. aureus* V8 proteolyzed gp120 allow us to determine that the majority of the linear epitopes recognized by the mAbs in this study are within the NH$_2$ terminal third of the protein

		native:denatured ELISA (OD$_{405}$)			V$_8$-gp120 protein blot		
	# of mAbs	>2.5	2.5-1.0	<1.0	NH$_2$- term.	Central part	COOH-term.
gp120	7	4	3	—	—	—	1
gp120/CD4	12	10	2	—	—	—	—
gp120/M77	36	13	13	10	10	1	3

The values represent the numbers of mAbs produced for each category.

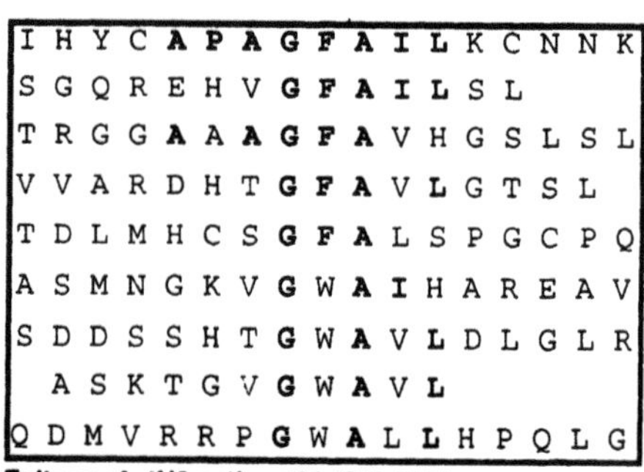

Epitope of 1A8 anti-gp120 (105-115)   **Epitope of 4D3 anti-gp120 (91-100)**

Epitope of 1G2 anti-gp120 (494-499)   **Epitope of 4H3 anti-gp120 (219-226)**

Figure 2. Epitope mapping of 4 mAbs using a phage display library. Four mAbs derived from a gp120/M77 immunized mouse were analyzed using a combinatorial phage display library containing a randomized 20 amino acid insert. For each mAb a collection of phages was selected and the insert of each phage was sequenced and compared with the most homologous sequence in gp120 (top line in each panel).

substantial affinity for a specific mAb were then further analyzed by sequencing their corresponding inserts.

Figure 2 illustrates the analyses of four different mAbs. In each panel the upper most sequence is that of gp120$_{IIIB}$ and the other sequences are those of a collection of phages arranged for their best alignment with the gp120. As can be seen, a unique gp120 sequence has been identified for each of the mAbs (see also Table 2). Moreover, some of the mAbs (e.g., 1G2 and 4H3) show high linear contiguous homology to their corresponding gp120 epitope. By ranking the phages for homology one can realize that there are some residues that are apparently critical for the recognition by the mAb whereas others are amenable to variation. Interesting are the mAbs 1A8 and 4D3 for which there is no distinct block of contiguous homology but rather a motif. Thus for example, in the case of 1A8 it appears that a positive residue followed by any two amino acids preceding an aliphatic methyl contributed by any of the residues; V, L, I or A followed by any two residues followed by a LW would suffice. This type of requirement implies a secondary configuration in this area of gp120. An alpha helix would place the residues HILW of the motif HxxIxxLW on one contiguous surface of the helix.

The selected phages were then used to screen other mAbs obtained from the fusions so to test whether they map to the same sites or not. At least six other mAbs could be shown to bind these selected phages containing the epitope-mimics previously identified (see Table 2). Interesting is the fact that 1A8 and 7A4 are IgG1 and IgM respectively. This would

Table 2. Linear epitopes of gp120$_{IIIB}$. The gp120 epitopes of the mAbs described in Figure 2 are shown in the table. Three of the epitopes have been previously reported to be T-cell epitopes. The epitope of 4D3 also satisfies the theoretical requirements for a typical T-cell epitope [12]

mAb	Position	Sequence	Homologous mAbs	Reference
1A8	105-115	*HEDIISLWDQS*	7A4, 5H5	7, 8
4D3	91-100	*ENFNMWKNDM*	4H4, 5F9	—
1G2	494-499	*LGVAPT*	12F6, 3H1	7, 8
4H3	219-226	*APAGFAIL*		9

therefore imply that these mAbs are derived from two distinct B-cell clones rather than simply being two daughter cells produced from one common parent clone.

4. DISCUSSION

Our analyses of the mAbs produced for the gp120 complexes has provided insights to structure and function of HIV envelope epitopes. Clearly, by complexing gp120 with specific counterparts one is able to modify the immune response to this protein and reveal various aspects that are otherwise less immunogenic. Of interest are the linear epitopes that appear to be particularly well presented in the immune-complexed gp120/M77. It appears that not only immune-complexation increases the exposure of these linear sequences it turns out that these precise structures have previously been recognized as T-cell epitopes (see Table 2, [7, 8, 9]).

One explanation for this phenomenon could be that binding of M77 to the V3 loop causes structural rearrangements with gp120 thus exposing these otherwise buried and less accessible sequences. Alternatively, one could argue that by masking the dominant V3 loop new previously silent epitopes are rendered more immunogenic. However, we believe that the more efficient presentation of these structures is due to the opsonization of the antigen. Thus gp120 when bound to M77 can be readily recognized by macrophage Fc receptors and internalized. The gp120 is then processed and its peptides presented via MHC class II restriction. Should this be the case, one must evaluate the ramifications of immunization with immunocomplexed gp120 with the intent of *primary* presentation via antigen presenting cells. Does such an approach enhance the T-cell immunity and prime a vaccinee more effectively towards exposure to a genuine insult? Does the humoral response towards the T-cell epitopes provide advantages? These are some of the questions we are concerned with.

Finally the analyses presented here are but examples of the strategy we have developed in our laboratory which have led us to the following general conclusions:

1. Through the use of the combinatorial phage display library and the approach of analyzing a spectrum of phages rather than striving to isolate the best fit phage we have realized that one can define four classes of epitopes. In essence one should not refer to linear vs conformational but rather consider primary, secondary, tertiary and quaternary epitopes. Each class relates to protein domains that are recognized by the immune system (thus being epitopes) that are the direct result of primary, secondary, tertiary and quaternary protein structures. Thus for example the epitope of 1G2 (see figure 2) is a primary epitope and that of 1A8 is a secondary epitope. It is clear that the region of residues 90-115 in the C1 domain of gp120 must therefore be in an extended alpha helical configuration. This is not predicted through computer algorithm analyses but rather a conclusion based on experimen-

tal data derived from mAb analyses of combinatorial phage display libraries. In our laboratory we have isolated mAbs that satisfy tertiary and quaternary epitopes as well [9].

2. In the introduction we stated that a prerequisite for an effective vaccine would be its cross reactivity with the variety of HIV variants. This study has shed new light on the different mechanisms of cross reactivity. Obviously, it would be useful to identify highly conserved neutralizing epitopes and indeed the T-cell epitopes described in Figure 2 are rather well conserved. Yet through the epitope library analyses we discover that each mAb can be promiscuous and interact with genuinely different peptide sequences. Thus one might want to devise immunization schemes that increase the degree of poly-reactive antibodies that may neutralize different viruses due to their ability to interact with variable epitope sequences. Lastly, a new type of cross reactivity has been identified, namely inducible cross reactivity by which we have been able to illustrate that immunomodulation of the immune response can enhance the efficacy of pre-existing neutralizing antibodies (see reference 10).

REFERENCES

1. Rusche, J. R., Javaherian K., McDanal C., Petro, J., Lynn, D. L., Grimaila R., Langlois, A., Gallo, R. C., Arthur, L. O. & Fischinger, P. J. (1988) Antibodies that inhibit fusion of human immunodeficiency virus-infected cells bind a 24 amino-acid sequence of the viral envelope, gp120. *Proc. Natl. Acad. Sci. USA* **85**:3198-3202.

2. Pal, R., Veronese, FD., Nair, B.C., Rahman, R.,Hoke, G., Mumbauer, S.W., Sarngadharan, M.G. (1992) Characterization of a neutralizing monoclonal antibody to the external glycoprotein of HIV-1. *Intervirology* **86**:86-93.

3. Harlow, E., and Lane, D. (1988) Antibodies. A laboratory manual, Cold Spring Harbor Laboratory

4. Smith, G.P., and J.K. Scott. 1993. Libraries of peptides and proteins displayed on filamentous phage. *Methods in Enzymology* **217**:228-257.

5. Haas, S.J., and G.P. Smith. 1993. Rapid sequencing of viral DNA from filamentous bacteriophages. *Biotechniques* **15**:422-431.

6. Cwirla, S.E., Peter, E.A., Barrett, R.W., and Dower, W.J. (1990) Peptides on Phages: A Vast Library of Peptides for Identifying Ligands. *Proc. natl. Acad. Sci. USA* **87**:6378-6382.

7. Clerici, M., Lucey, D.R., Zajac, R.A., Boswell, R.N., Gebel, H.M., Takahashi, H., Berzofsky, J.A. and Shearer, G.M. (1991) Detection of cytotoxic T-lymphocytes specific for synthetic peptides of gp160 in seropositive individuals. *J. Immunol.* **146**:2214-2219.

8. Falk, K., Rotzchke, O., Stevanovic, S., Joung, G., and Rammensee, H.-G. (1991) Identification of normally processed viral nonapeptides allows their quantification in infected cells and suggest an allele-specific T-cell epitope forecast. *J. Exp. Med.* **174**:425-435.

9. Manca, F., Habeshaw, J. and Dalgleish, A. (1991) The naive repertoire of human T helper cells specific for gp120, the envelope glycoprotein of HIV. *J. Immunol.* **146**:1964-1969.

10. Gershoni, J.M., Denisova, G., Raviv, D., Smorodinsky, N.I., & Buyaner, D. (1993) HIV binding to its receptor creates specific epitopes for the CD4/gp120 complex. *FASEB J.* **7**:1185-1187.

11. Denisova, G., Zwickel, J., and Gershoni, J.M. (1995) Binding of HIV-1 gp120 to an anti-V3 loop antibody reveals novel antigen-induced epitopes. *FASEB J.* **9**:126-132.

12. Berzofsky, J.A. (1993) Human Immunodeficiency Virus: Structural Features of T-Cell Epitopes and Their Use in Vaccine Development. *in* "Viruses and the Cellular Immune Response" (ed. by Thomas, D.B.) National Institute for Medical Research London, United Kingdom, pp101-126.

14

HIV–PEPLOTION VACCINE

A Novel Approach to Vaccination against AIDS by Transepithelial Transport of Viral Peptides and Antigens to Langerhans Cells for Induction of Cytolytic T Cells by HLA Class I and CD1 Molecules for Long Term Protection

Yechiel Becker[*]

Department of Molecular Virology
Institute of Microbiology, Faculty of Medicine
The Hebrew University of Jerusalem
Jerusalem, Israel

1. INTRODUCTION

1.1. The Immune Response in HIV-Infected Individuals

Two properties of the human immunodeficiency virus (HIV) make the control of HIV spread in the human population difficult: a) infection of T cells and dendritic cells and macrophages, the professional antigen-presenting cells and b) transmission from donor to recipient by HIV-1-infected cells. The rapid spread of HIV infection in the human population in epidemic form was enhanced by the transmission of infected cells from infected individuals to non-infected partners as part of human sexual behavior, and due to exposure of intravenous drug users to infected syringes. Despite attempts to educate the human population in safe sexual behavior, the spread of HIV infection continues and the end of the HIV epidemic is not in sight.

HIV-1 infection starts as a regular virus infection, namely, the cellular and humoral arms of the immune response react to viral antigens processed by the infected cells. Viral peptides derived from various viral proteins are presented by HLA class I peptide binding grooves to CD8[+] T cells to prime cytotoxic T cells (CTLs) (Schultz *et al.*, 1991) and by HLA class II molecules to CD4[+] T cells to prime the antibody response. After several weeks the CTL response declines, antiviral antibodies persist in the serum of the infected individual and it seems that the virus infection is contained. Nevertheless, it was reported that

---

[*]Member, UNESCO European Network "Man Against Virus."

Novel Strategies in Design and Production of Vaccines
Edited by S. Cohen and A. Shafferman, Plenum Press, New York, 1996

replication of HIV-1 virus in the immune system's CD4$^+$ cells (T cells, dendritic cells and macrophages) continues in the lymph nodes and virus is continuously shed into the bloodstream. Years after the initial HIV-1 infection, virus replication is markedly stimulated, due to an unknown signal, and very high virus titers are reached concomitantly with the disappearance of antiviral antibodies from the serum. At this stage non-CD4$^+$ cells (e.g., in the gut epithelium) are also infected, probably due to the binding of virus-antibody complexes with Fc receptors on cells. This stage of the virus infection precedes the decline and collapse of the immune system.

The deterioration of the immune system allows the development of virus infections due to activation of latent viruses which were kept under control by the immune response. Infection by viruses, bacteria and fungi, as well as cancer (Burkitt's lymphoma, Kaposi's sarcoma), take hold of the HIV-infected individual with AIDS. The development of AIDS in an individual seems to be affected by HLA haplotypes. Cameron *et al.* (1990) indicated that "several alleles at multiple HLA loci have been found to be associated with HIV-1 infection: HLA A1, B8, B35, Cw7; DR1, DR3, and DQ 1, which are associated with disease manifestation and/or disease progression". The molecular basis for the HLA-related increased risk of developing AIDS is not understood. My suggestions for blocking the deterioration of an HIV-1- infected individual into an AIDS patient were presented (Symposium - Concepts in Virology From Ivanovsky to the Present (Becker, 1993)).

The world population can be divided into two categories: a) the majority of human beings who are uninfected and need protection against HIV-1 infection, and b) the HIV-1-infected population who needs to be cured and saved from AIDS. The cure can be achieved possibly by treatment with effective nontoxic antiviral drugs or by modulating the still-existing immune system to eradicate the slow virus infection. It is possible to envision that utilization of the residual immune response in HIV-1-infected individuals prior to AIDS by stimulation of the CTL response to delay or prevent the signals for rapid HIV-1 replication and acquired immune deficiency (Becker, 1993). Therefore, there is a need to develop an anti-HIV vaccine to prime CD8$^+$ cytotoxic T cells.

1.2. Attempts to Develop Protective Vaccines to Prevent AIDS

The current efforts to develop anti-AIDS vaccines are concentrated on a vaccine that will stimulate the humoral immune response in the vaccinee after injection of viral antigens (Haynes, 1993). Albert Sabin (1992), in his last analysis of the approach to immunization against HIV-1-caused AIDS, indicated that "The main challenge is to find a way to kill cells with chromosomally integrated HIV cDNA without harming normal cells." Indeed, HIV-1 cDNA integrated into the infected cell chromosomal DNA without expression of the viral genes may be a threat to the infected individual when the latent HIV-1 genome is activated by viral gene transcription and the synthesis of viral proteins. All cells in the body express HLA class I molecules and present nonameric peptides within the HLA class I peptide binding grooves to T cell receptors of CD8$^+$ cytotoxic T cells. There is a good possibility that when a latent HIV-1 cDNA will be activated to synthesize viral proteins and viral peptides, the proteolytic cleavage products will be presented to the CD8$^+$ CTLs by HLA class I molecules. Therefore, if the HIV-infected individual will have memory CD8$^+$ cytotoxic T cells which were primed to recognize HIV-1 peptides by a CD8$^+$ CTL vaccine, there may be a chance that in this individual the cells harboring the activated latent HIV-1 will be destroyed by the antiviral CTLs prior to the synthesis of the infectious virus. This analysis is in agreement with the suggestions of Dr. Jonas Salk (1993) that "A prophylactic vaccine against Human immunodeficiency virus (HIV) infection represents the best hope for controlling the continuing and devastating worldwide AIDS epidemic" and that "a vaccination strategy which will induce a stable Th1 predominant memory state will favor the induction of a strong

CTL response upon subsequent exposure to live HIV even if such responses are not induced by primary immunization". Recently, Desrosiers (1994) reported that an attenuated apathogenic HIV was able to immunize monkeys against challenge with HIV, but newborn monkeys were susceptible to the attenuated vaccine virus and succumbed to the virus infection (Bolognesi, 1994)

2. "HIV PEPLOTION VACCINE": TRANSPORT OF ANTIGENS TO EPITHELIAL LANGERHANS CELLS TO INDUCE ANTIVIRAL CYTOLYTIC T CELLS

2.1. The Concept

The idea presented here is to change the current vaccination strategy, the priming of the humoral immune response by directing viral proteins to professional antigen-presenting cells (dendritic cells and macrophages), to the priming of antiviral $CD8^+$ CTLs. The new vaccination procedure for primary immunization of uninfected individuals and of individuals immediately after infection with HIV-1 (after the decline of the primary anti-HIV CTL response) with HIV proteins or peptides in adjuvants will direct the peptide antigens to the cytoplasm of the professional antigen-presenting dendritic cells in the skin and other epithelia. In these cells processing and antigen presentation of the viral peptides to $CD8^+$ CTLs via HLA class I molecules will take place in the draining lymph nodes. In addition, nonpeptide antigens can be processed and presented to $CD4^-$, $CD8^-$ cytolytic T cells by CD1 molecules. Such a novel vaccine will be introduced in the form of a lotion to the skin, or to the gut, anal and genital epithelia to allow for transepidermal transport of HIV proteins, peptides and lipid antigen to epidermal Langerhans cells (LC) that will allow cytoplasmic processing of the viral antigens, and subsequent travel to the draining lymph nodes to stimulate the antiviral CTL response. An effective CTL response can be achieved since the entire LC layer in skin and epithelia may be exposed to the viral antigens.

2.2. LC/Dendritic Cells Efficiently Present Peptide Antigens and Nonpeptide Antigens to Cytolytic T Cells

The LCs present in the skin are generated from a bone marrow progenitor stem cell defined as dendritic/LC colony-forming unit. It was found that macrophages and dendritic/LC share a common bone marrow stem cell (Reid *et al.*, 1990). The extraordinary capacity of allogeneic epidermal LC, at a dose of ten LC-primed allospecific T cells was reported by McKinney and Streilein (1989). Epidermal LCs utilize two different pathways to present antigens to $CD8^-$ T cells: 1) HLA class I molecules present peptides, and 2) the CD1a,b,c molecules present nonpeptide antigens. Thus, epidermal LC which take up foreign antigens migrate to the draining regional lymph nodes and present the processed foreign antigen via HLA class I to $CD8^+$ or CD1 molecules to $CD8^-$ T cells which are primed to become specific cytolytic T cells.

2.3. Presentation of Peptide Antigen by HLA Class I Molecules

The current knowledge of the motifs of nonapeptides presented by different types and haplotypes of HLA class I molecules revealed that the amino acid sequence of the HLA class I peptide binding groove, especially around "pocket B" in the groove, determines the ability of a peptide to interact with the groove (reviewed in Becker, 1994a). There is thus a need to understand the nature of the peptides presented by human LC on the basis of the reported motifs of presented peptides and on the basis of the known HLA class I atomic coordinates derived from the X-ray crystal analysis of these proteins (Bjorkman *et al.*, 1987).

Mutations in the HLA class I genes result in human ethnic variation. Thus, making the use of synthetic peptides with motifs to fit all the HLA class I variants difficult. Therefore, transepidermal transport of HIV proteins or synthetic peptides to LC and DC for processing and presentation by HLA class I molecules will enhance the development of the CD8+ cytotoxic T cells with α/β T cell receptors.

2.4. Presentation of Nonpeptide Antigens by CD1 Molecules

Skin LC were characterized as having CD1 (cluster of diffentiation 1, defined by monoclonal antibody T 6) molecules on their cell membrane (Porcelli *et al.*, 1989). CD1 is a family of cell surface glycoproteins (the homologous proteins CD1a, b and c have been defined serologically) transcribed from CD1 gene locus on human chromosome 1 which contains five potential CD1 genes. Analysis of the predicted amino acid sequence of the CD1 protein revealed a low, but significant level of homology to HLA class I and II. Similar to HLA class I α polypeptide, CD1 polypeptide associates non-covalently with β2-microglobulin, suggesting the ability to present antigens to cytolytic T cells. Specific recognition of CD1a is by a CD4$^-$CD8$^-$ α/β T - cell receptor (TCR) expressing cytolytic T lymphocyte (CTL) line. Specific recognition of CD1c is by a CD4$^-$CD8$^-$ γ/δ TCR CTL line. The interaction of CD1-specific cells with CD1+ target cells appeared to involve the CD3-TCR complex and did not show evidence of MHC restriction (Porcelli *et al.*, 1989). CD1b was reported to restrict the response of human CD4$^-$ CD8$^-$ α/β T lymphocytes to a microbial (*Mycobacterium tuberculosis*) antigen (Porcelli *et al.*, 1992). Beckman *et al.* (1994) reported that a purified CD1b-restricted antigen of *M.tuberculosis* presented to α/βTCR T cells is mycolic acid, indicating that α/β TCR+ T cells recognize a broader range of antigens and at least one member of the CD1 family has evolved the ability to present lipid antigens. These authors indicated that "a unique processing pathway for CD1 glycoproteins, the divergence of CD1 structure from that MHC molecule and the nature of the antigens recognized by this system indicates that antigen presentation should be viewed as separate from MHC - encoded presentation. Presumably, CD1-restricted responses to lipids or hydrophobic antigens other than mycolic acid also may be found. By including CD1 as a non-protein antigen-presenting molecule, the immune system appears to have extended the potential repertoire of foreign antigens recognized by α/β T cells beyond the realm of those peptides that can bind to MHC class I, Ib and II molecules".

Thus, introduction of HIV peptides and lipid-peptide complexes may be useful in the induction of CD4$^-$CD8$^-$ cytolytic T cells not only against HIV-1 infected cells in HIV-infected patients, but also against opportunistic infections by viruses, bacteria and fungi especially in patients with AIDS.

2.5 The Aim: Development of a "HIV Peplotion Vaccine" for Application as a Lotion Containing HIV Peptides/Proteins/Lipidic and Nonpeptide Antigens to LC in Epithelial Surfaces of Skin, Gut and Genitalia Which Will Prime the CTL Responses in Lymph Nodes

The development of a vaccine to induce anti-HIV-1 CTL response calls for a new approach for targeting antigens to LCs in epithelia of the skin, sexual organs and the gut, the site of HIV infection. It must be considered that individuals in the human population which are predisposed to a rapid disease (like those individuals who have HLA Class I B8 or B35 haplotypes) may need continuous applications of the peplotion vaccine to stimulate the antiviral CD4$^-$8$^+$ CTL response. The use of HIV peptide antigens, which will be processed via the HLA class I antigen pathway and HIV lipid antigens, which will be processed via the CD1 antigen pathway, to induce CD4$^-$8$^-$ α/β TCR or γ/δ TCR cytolytic T cells, will provide a defense mechanism against HIV infection in uninfected individuals as well as HIV-infected people prior to and after the start of AIDS symptoms. The possiblity of including in the "HIV peplotion vaccine" lipid-containing antigens from opportunistic bacteria, fungi or enveloped viruses may extend the immune coverage of HIV-infected patients. This consideration excludes the need for injection of the vaccine by trained personnel and the use of disposable syringes. When very large populations in the developed and developing parts of the world are concerned, the present vaccination approach may be needed. Alloreactivity of the individual may be enhanced by including alloantigens in the "HIV vaccine peplotion".

The skin, gut anal, genital and vaginal epithelia in humans are the port of entry of HIV-1 to the human body during sexual encounters and LC here are accessible for treatment. The idea of the "HIV peplotion vaccine" is supported by the following experimental data: 1) HIV-1 gp160 in ISCOM induces MHC class I CTL response (Takahashi *et al.* 1990) suggesting that an anti-HIV-1 CTL response results when HIV-1 proteins are applied to the skin LC with an adjuvant; 2) mixing of cationic lipids with viral proteins forms complexes which are delivered to the cytoplasm and the degradation peptides stimulate CTLs by an HLA class I mechanism (Walker *et al.*,1992); 3) a viral protein encapsulated in pH-sensitive liposomes induced primary antiviral CTL response after administration to dendritic cells (Nair *et al.*, 1993) and 4) the bioreactive peptide enkephalin in nonionic surfactant at pH 5.0 permeated through hairless mouse skin (Choi *et al.*, 1990).

The use of ISCOM containing the adjuvant glycoside Quil A (Morein *et al.*, 1984) may enhance the selection of the MHC class I molecules for peptide presentation to CD8$^+$ T cells (Rabinovich *et al.*, 1994). It was recently reported that mixing viral proteins with cationic lipids induces complex formation which, when taken up by antigen-presenting cells, directs the proteins to the cytoplasm of the cells. At this site the proteins are processed by the cellular proteasomes and the resulting peptides are transported to the endoplasmic reticulum and associate with HLA class I molecules (Walker *et al.*, 1992).

The combination of adjuvant, a nonionic surfactant at pH 5.0 that will prevent proteolytic degradation of the HIV-1 peptides or proteins present in the "HIV-1 peplotion vaccine", complexed with a cationic lipid, may lead to efficient vaccination of uninfected humans, and possibly recently infected individals, by priming anti-HIV-1 CTL responses and memory cells. The use of "HIV-1 peplotion vaccine" may, except in specific medical skin conditions, be repeated to provide long-term and possibly life-long protection.

3. EXPERIMENTAL STEPS IN THE RESEARCH AND DEVELOPMENT OF HIV PEPLOTION VACCINE

3.1 Computer Simulation to Predict the Availability of HIV Peptides with Known HLA Class I Motifs for Presentation by HLA Class I Molecules

The computer program "Findpatterns" was applied to the search for linear amino acid sequences in HIV-1 structural, enzymatic and regulatory proteins which were obtained from the GCG data bank. The combination of HLA class I binding motifs and the cleavage pattern allowed a prediction of the putative availability of virus peptides which may bind the peptide binding grooves of different HLA class I haplotypes. Seven peptides were found in the HIV-1 gag polypeptide with the HLA A2 motif. Three of these peptides (aa151-159, aa345-353 and aa362-370) were reported by Buseyne *et al.* (reviewed in Becker, 1995) as HIV-1 p24 gag epitopes with HLA A2 CTL specificity and, interestingly, are hydrophobic. One of the four putative peptides predicted by the computer program to fit HLA A68 aa322-331 was also reported by Buseyne *et al.* However, the gag peptide used by Falk *et al.* (reviewed in Becker, 1995) was not found by computer analysis. It is also of interest that the number of putative peptides with HLA A motifs in the HIV-1 gag polypeptide are more abundant than putative peptides with HLA-B haplotypes. Yet, the computer analysis did not identify the gag aa265-274 peptide reported by Parker *et al.* (reviewed in Becker, 1995) with HLA B27 motif. Computer analysis of HIV-1 polymerase polypeptide also revealed an abundance of putative peptides with motifs to fit HLA A2 and 68 and few putative peptides to HLA B27 and B35. It was reported by Falk *et al.* (reviewed in Becker, 1995) that peptide aa461-485 arising from the reverse transcriptase has an HLA A2 binding motif. This peptide was predicted as a putative peptide aa476-484.

The computer analysis of HIV-1 gp160 envelope amino acid sequence revealed the putative peptides which may be generated from the env proteins by cytosolic proteasome proteolysis and by ER-associated signal peptidase proteolysis in the ER lumen. The abundance of putative peptides with binding motifs to HLA class I A molecules, relative to peptides with HLA B motifs, was also noted with HIV-1 env.

Computer analysis of HIV-1 proteinase and the regulatory proteins vpu, nef, rev and tat revealed that putative peptides with HLA class I motifs can be found in these proteins. Importantly, three peptides predicted by the computer program were found in nef polypeptide. The polypeptide aa69-77 was already reported by Hadida *et al.* (reviewed in Becker, 1995) as an HLA A1-related peptide, while the same peptide was considered to be with the HLA A68 motif in the present computer analysis. Nef peptide (aa178-187) was reported by Riviere *et al.* (reviewed in Becker, 1995), while nef peptide aa134-142 was reported by Culmann *et al.* (reviewed in Becker, 1995) as an HLA B18-restricted peptide. Yet, the computer program did not identify additional published nef epitopes which have been reported in the literature and summarized by Riviere *et al.* (reviewed in Becker, 1995).

It was reported that the HLA class I B8 and B35 haplotypes may serve as risk factors for an enhanced HIV-1-related diseases in HIV-1 individuals with these specific HLA class I haplotypes. As seen here only peptides (aa486-aa494) and (aa608-aa617) from the HIV-1 gp160 envelope glycoprotein, which have HLA class I B8 and HLA B35 motifs, respectively, were detected in all the viral structural and nonstructural proteins.

4. CONCLUSIONS

4.1 Transepidermal Transport of Peptides in Antigens

Experiments to test the effect of commercially available antigen carriers on the activity and function of mouse skin LCs are in progress.

4.2 Utilization of Nonpeptide Antigens for Presentation by CD1 Molecules

The idea that introduction of HIV antigens into the epithelium to the resident LCs for priming anti-HIV-1 $CD4^-8^+$ $\alpha/\beta TCR$ CTLs by transepithelial transport using HIV peptides may be extended to include antigens presentation by CD1a,b,c molecules to induce $CD4^-8^-$ cytolytic α/β or γ/δ TCRs cytolytic T cells to destroy HIV-infected $CD4^+$ cells, as well as against opportunistic infections by bacteria, viruses and fungi during the AIDS phase of the disease. An additional advantage of this novel approach is that the cellular immune response is utilized and the synthesis of anti-HIV-1 antibodies may be surpassed. This will avoid the identification of people using "HIV-1 peplotion vaccine" as HIV-1-positive in the regular immunotests to diagnose HIV-1 infection. However, it should be considered that the induction of HIV-1 neutralizing antibodies to one critical HIV-1 gp120 epitope in the V3 loop of gp120 may be needed and HIV peptide antigen designed for presentation by epithelial LC cells can be included in the "HIV peplotion vaccine" for presentation by the HLA class II molecules to $CD4^+$ helper cells to induce just the neutralizing antibodies.

Another advantage of the "HIV peplotion vaccine" is the ease of application to the skin or genitals and to the gut to allow LCs to stimulate CTLs in all lymphnodes which drain the antigen-treated epithelia. Application of the "HIV peplotion vaccine" to gut epithelium and to genital and anal epithelia may lead to the development of memory $CD4^-8^+$ CTLs in the organs which serve as the port of entry for HIV. The addition of lipidic antigens to the "HIV peplotion vaccine" for presentation by LC CD1 molecules extends the potential repertoire of foreign antigens recognized by α/β and γ/δ TCRs of cytolytic T cells (Beckman et al., 1994) and broadens the protection against HIV and opportunistic microorganisms.

It may be especially important to develop the "HIV peplotion vaccine" for treatment of HIV-infected individuals prior to and during the AIDS stage to recruit the residual $CD8^+$ and $CD4^-8^-$ cytolytic T cells to overcome or reduce the number of infected $CD4^+$ cells and to relieve AIDS patients from enhanced HIV replication and destruction of white blood cells and from opportunistic infections.

ACKNOWLEDGMENTS

The work in the author's laboratory is continuously supported by the Foundation for Molecular Virology and Cell Biology (Mrs. Ronnie Bendheim, President, Phoenix, Arizona). The studies on the Langerhans and dendritic cells are based on the work of Drs. Eli Sprecher, Cheryl Berkowitz-Balshayi and Dan David. These studies were supported by grants from the USA-Israel Binational Science Foundation and from A.I.D.

The work is also supported by a grant from UNESCO ROSTE, Venice, Italy in the framework of UNESCO Network "Man Against Virus".

The author is indebted to Prof. Raymond Daudel, President, European Academy of Arts, Sciences and Humanities, Paris, for stimulating discussions, to Dr. Claude Rosenfeld, Science Division UNESCO and to Dr. V.A. Kouzminov, Chief of ROSTE, UNESCO, for their interest and support.

REFERENCES

Becker, Y., 1993, From the discovery of poliovirus vaccinia virus mRNAs and polyribosomes to computer analysis of HIV-1 and 2 glycoproteins, in Concepts in Virology (B.W.J. Mahy and D.K. Lvov, editors) pp 77-79, Hardwood Academic Publishers.

Becker, Y., 1994a, HIV-1 proteins in infected cells determine the presentation of viral peptides by HLA class I and class II molecules and the nature of the cellular and humoral antiviral immune responses - a review, Virus Genes, 8:249-270.

Becker, Y., 1994b, An analysis of the role of skin Langerhans cells (LC) in the cytoplasmic processing of HIV-1 peptide after "peplotion" transpidermal transfer and HLA class I presentation to $CD8^+$ CTLs - an approach to immunization of humans, Virus Genes, 9:133-147.

Becker, Y., 1995, Computer simulations to predict the availability of peptides with known HLA class I motifs possibly generated by proteolysis of HIV-1 proteins in infected cells, Virus Genes 10:in press.

Beckman, E.M., Porcelli, S.A., Morita, C.T., Behar, S.M., Furlong, S., and Brenner, M.B., 1994, Recognition of a lipid antigen by CD1 restricted α/β^+ T cells, *Nature*, 37: 691-694.

Bjorkman, P.J., Saper, M.A., Samaraoni, B., Bennet, W.S., Strominger, J.L., and Wiley, D.C., 1987, The foreign antigen binding site and T cell recognition regions of class I histocompatibility antigens, *Nature* 329:512-518, 1987.

Bolognesi, D., 1994, Not Yet, it is too early to use a live attenuated virus vaccine against HIV-1, *J. NIH Res.* 6:55, 59-62.

Cameron, P.U., Mallal, S.A., French, M.A.H., and Dawkins, R.L. 1990, Central MHC genes between HLA-B and complement C4 confer risk for HIV-1 disease progression, *Human Immunology* 29:282-295.

Choi, H.K., Flynn, G.L., and Amidon, G.G., 1994, Transdermal delivery of bioactive peptides: the effect of n-decylmethyl solfoxide, pH and inhibitors of enkephalin metabolism and transport, *Pharm. Res.* 7:1099-1106, 1990.

Desrosiers, R.C., 1994, Yes, it is time to consider use of a live-attenuated virus vaccine against HIV, *J. NIH Res.* 6:54,56-59.

Haynes, B.F., 1993, Scientific and social issues of human immunodeficiency virus vaccine development, *Science* 260:1279-1286.

McKinney, E.L., and Streilein, J.W., 1989, On the extraordinary capacity of allogeneic epidermal Langerhans cells to prime cytotoxic T cells in vivo, *J. Immunol.* 143:1560-1564.

Nair, S., Babu, J.S., Dunham, R.G., Kanda, P., Burke, R.L., and Rouse, B.T., 1993, Induction of primary, antiviral cytotoxic, and proliferative responses with antigens administered via dendritic cells, *J. Virol.* 67:4062-4069.

Porcelli, S., Brenner, M.B., Greenstein, J.L., Balk, S.P., Terhorst, C. and Bleicher, P.A., 1989, Recognition of cluster of differentiation 1 antigens by human CD4⁻CD8⁻ cytolytic T lymphocytes, *Nature* 341:447-450.

Porcelli, S., Morita, C.T., and Brenner, M.B., 1992, CD1b restricts the response of human CD4⁻8⁻ T lymphocytes to a microbial antigen, *Nature* 360:593-597.

Rabinovich, N.R., McInnes, P., Klein, D.L., and Hall, B.F.,1994, Vaccine technologies: view to the future, *Science* 265:1401-1404.

Reid, C.D.L., Fryer, P.R., Clifford, C., Kirk, A., Tikerpae, J., and Knight, S.C., 1990, Identification of hematopoietic progenitors of macrophages and dendritic Langerhans cells (DL-CFU) in human bone marrow and peripheral blood, *Blood* 76:1139-1149.

Sabin, A.B., 1992, Improbability of effective vaccination agaoinst human immunodeficiency virus because of its intracellular transmission and rectal portal of entry, *Proc. Natl. Acad. Sci. USA* 89:8852-8855.

Salk, J., Bretscher, P.A., Salk, P.L., Clerici, M., and Shearer, G.M., 1993, A strategy for prophylactic vaccination against AIDS, *Science* 260:1270-1272.

Schultz, M., Zinkernagel, R.M., and Hengartner, H., 1991, Peptide-induced antiviral protection by cytotoxic T cells, *Proc. Natl. Acad. Sci. USA* 88:991-993.

Takahashi, H., Takeshita, T., Morein, B., Putney, S., Germain, R.N., and Berzofsky, J.A., 1990, Induction of CD8⁺ cytotoxic T cells by imunization with purified HIV-1 envelope protein in ISCOMs, *Nature* 34:873-875.

Walker, C., Selby, M., Erickson, A., Do, D.C., Valensi, J-P., and Van Nest, G., 1992, Cationic lipids direct a viral glycoprotein into class I major histocompatibility complex antigen-presentation pathway, *Proc. Natl. Acad. Sci. USA* 89:7915-7918.

15

THE ROLE OF ADJUVANTS AND DELIVERY SYSTEMS IN MODULATION OF IMMUNE RESPONSE TO VACCINES

Rajesh K. Gupta, Paul Griffin, Jr., An-Cheng Chang, Rachel Rivera, Roger Anderson, Bradford Rost, Douglas Cecchini, Mary Nicholson, and George R. Siber

Massachusetts Public Health Biologic Laboratories
State Laboratory Institute
Boston, Massachusetts 02130

1. INTRODUCTION

Adjuvants have been used to augment the immune response to antigens in experimental immunology and vaccination purposes for 70 years (Ramon, 1925, 1926; Glenny et al., 1926). Traditionally, adjuvants have been used with routine human vaccines to elicit an early, high and long lasting immune response. But in recent years adjuvants received much attention because of: 1) poor immunogenicity of newly developed purified, subunit and synthetic vaccines which need adjuvants to evoke the immune response, and 2) selective modulation of immune response by adjuvants with regard to major histocompatibility complex (MHC) class (I or II) and T-helper cell type (Th1 or Th2) which is very important for protection against diseases caused by intracellular pathogens such as viruses, parasites and bacteria (Gupta and Siber, 1995a). Additionally, with the use of adjuvants, less antigen may be required to stimulate the immune response which would not only be a saving on cost of vaccines, it would be useful in the development of combination vaccines, thus reducing the complications due to antigen competition and carrier specific epitope suppression. In this paper, an overview on the role of adjuvants in modulation of immune response to vaccine antigens is presented.

2. MODULATION OF ANTIBODY RESPONSE

Adjuvants have been used to modulate the antibody response to vaccine antigens in humans as well as in animals. The major advantage of using adjuvants (aluminum compounds and calcium phosphate) with routine human vaccines was the development of earlier, higher and longer-lasting immunity especially after primary immunization

Novel Strategies in Design and Production of Vaccines
Edited by S. Cohen and A. Shafferman, Plenum Press, New York, 1996

Table 1. Antibody response of mice (outbred, CD-1, female 4 weeks old, 10 mice per group) to tetanus toxoid and diphtheria toxoid as soluble or adsorbed onto aluminum phosphate and calcium phosphate adjuvants. Each mouse was injected with 0.5 Lf of tetanus toxoid or 1 Lf of diphtheria toxoid subcutaneously at 0 and 30 days. The mice were bled 4 weeks after first dose and 2 weeks after 2nd injection

| | Antibody levels (per ml of serum) after | | | |
| | First dose | | Second dose | |
Adjuvant	TN (IU)*	GM IgG†	TN (IU)*	GM IgG†
Tetanus toxoid				
Aluminum phosphate	0.75	2.36 EIU	20.0	14.8 EIU
Calcium phosphate	0.15	1.13 EIU	12.0	10.9 EIU
None	0.03	0.27 EIU	11.0	10.0 EIU
Diphtheria toxoid				
Aluminum phosphate	0.24	87.00 µg	4.80	1082.4 µg
Aluminum hydroxide	0.12	114.00 µg	4.80	1144.3 µg
Calcium phosphate	0.01	1.01 µg	2.00	163.0 µg
None	<0.01	0.05 µg	<0.01	0.8 µg

* Toxin neutralization (TN) titers in International units (IU) were determined on pooled sera, for tetanus antitoxin in mice at L+/1000 level of tetanus toxin (Gupta and Siber, 1994a, b) and for diphtheria antitoxin in Vero cells at Led/1000 level of diphtheria toxin (Gupta et al., 1994a).

† IgG antibodies were determined by ELISA on individual serum samples and results expressed as geometric mean on antibody levels determined against reference sera. Tetanus toxin IgG antibodies are expressed in ELISA International units (EIU) (Gupta and Siber, 1994a,b) and diphtheria toxin IgG antibodies are in µg/ml (Gupta and Siber, 1995b).

compared to soluble vaccines (Aprile and Wardlaw, 1966; Gupta et al, 1993a; 1995a; Gupta and Siber, 1994a; 1995a). In many studies aluminum-adsorbed vaccines did not show any advantage over soluble preparations for the booster or secondary response (Aprile and Wardlaw, 1966; Gupta et al., 1995a; Gupta and Siber, 1995a). Table 1 shows that tetanus toxoid adsorbed to aluminum phosphate and calcium phosphate elicited higher tetanus antitoxin and tetanus toxin IgG antibodies than soluble tetanus toxoid after first dose whereas there were no differences among various preparations after second injection. This is particularly true with good immunogens like tetanus toxoid. But with poor immunogens like diphtheria toxoid, the adsorbed preparations showed higher antibody levels in mice after second dose also (Table 1). The antibody levels elicited with adjuvanted preparations persist longer than those elicited by soluble preparations (Gupta et al., 1995a).

2.1. Controlled Release of Vaccine Antigens

The only adjuvants used widely with routine human vaccines are aluminum adjuvants (Gupta et al., 1995a; Gupta and Siber, 1995a). At least 2 to 3 doses of vaccines adsorbed to aluminum adjuvants are required for primary immunization to achieve protection. The logistics of delivering 2-3 doses, particularly in developing countries, are difficult and compliance is frequently inadequate. Therefore, in recent years efforts have been made to develop controlled release vaccines using biodegradable polymer microspheres (Eldridge et al., 1991; Singh et al., 1992; O'Hagan et al., 1993; Gupta et al., 1993b; Alonso et al., 1994; Morris et al., 1994). Biodegradable polymer microspheres have mainly been used: 1) as vehicle to target antigens to microfold (M) cells on mucosal

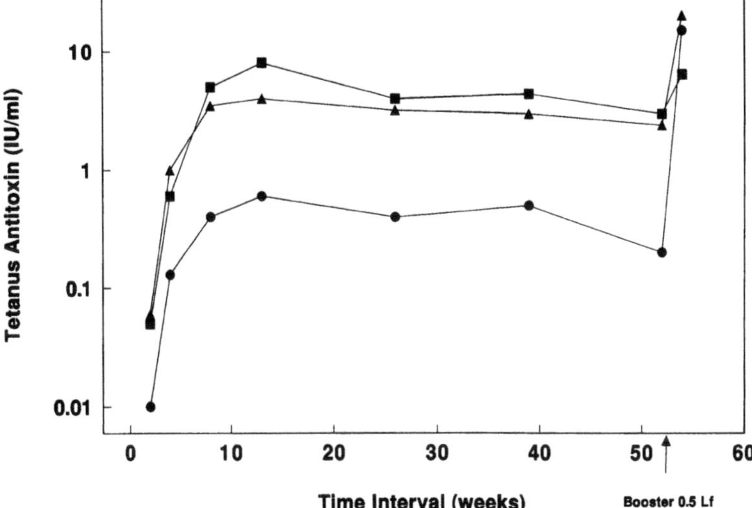

Figure 1. Tetanus antitoxin levels in sera of mice (outbred, CD-1, 4 week, 6-8 mice per group) injected with soluble tetanus toxoid (●—●), aluminum phosphate adsorbed preparation (■—■) and tetanus toxoid encapsulated in microspheres (▲—▲) composed of poly (D,L lactic glycolic) acid, mw 100,000 (average size 50 μm) (Gupta et al., 1993b). Each mouse was injected with 5 Lf of tetanus toxoid at day 0 and boosted with 0.5 Lf at 1 year after first injection. The mice were bled at different intervals. The individual serum samples were assayed for tetanus toxin IgG antibodies by ELISA (Gupta and Siber, 1994a,b) and pooled sera were assayed for tetanus antitoxin by toxin neutralization test at L+/1000 dose of tetanus toxin (Gupta and Siber, 1994a,b). As tetanus toxin IgG antibodies and tetanus antitoxin titers showed a good correlation (Gupta and Siber, 1994b), IgG antibody data are not shown here.

surfaces or to antigen presenting cells by parenteral route (Eldridge et al., 1989; Morris et al., 1994); and 2) for controlled release of vaccine antigens with an aim to reducing the number of doses required for primary immunization (Eldridge et al., 1991; Singh et al., 1992; O'Hagan et al., 1993; Gupta et al., 1993b; Alonso et al., 1994; Morris et al., 1994).

For mucosal immunization, microspheres protect antigen from extreme conditions of gut (extreme pH and enzymes) and maternal antibodies and deliver antigen efficiently to M cells as particulate antigen without inducing tolerance. For parenteral immunizations, several human vaccine antigens encapsulated in microspheres elicited antibody levels in animals similar to those obtained with potent adjuvants such as aluminum compounds and complete Freund's adjuvant (Eldridge et al., 1991; Singh et al., 1992; O'Hagan et al., 1993; Gupta et al., 1993b; Alonso et al., 1994; Morris et al., 1994). We found that tetanus toxoid encapsulated in poly (D,L-lactic glycolic) acid (PLGA) microspheres elicited high levels of tetanus toxin IgG antibodies and tetanus antitoxin in mice and guinea pigs after a single injection (Fig. 1). The antibody levels were similar to those elicited by aluminum phosphate adsorbed tetanus toxoid and were significantly higher than those elicited by soluble tetanus toxoid (Gupta et al., 1993b; Alonso et al., 1994). Recently, we encapsulated conjugate vaccine composed of capsular polysaccharide of *Haemophilus influenzae* type b (Hib) and tetanus toxoid in PLGA microspheres. A single injection of these microspheres into mice elicited antibody levels to both Hib capsular polysaccharide and tetanus toxoid. The antibody levels were similar to those elicited in mice after 2 doses of the conjugate.

Table 2. IgG subclass antibodies in sera of mice (outbred, CD-1 for tetanus toxoid and inbred, C57 black mice for diphtheria toxoid, 4 week old, 6-10 mice in each group) injected with tetanus toxoid (0.3-0.5 Lf per mouse) or diphtheria toxoid (0.5 Lf per mouse) with different adjuvants. Each mouse was injected subcutaneously at 0 and 30 days. The mice were bled 4 weeks after first dose and 2 weeks after 2nd injection. The IgG subclass antibodies to specific antigens were determined on the pooled sera of mice by ELISA (Gupta and Siber, 1994a; 1995b)

| | | IgG subclass antibodies (µg/ml) after | | | | | |
| | | First dose | | | Second dose | | |
Adjuvant	Strain of mice	IgG1	IgG2a	IgG2b	IgG1	IgG2a	IgG2b
Tetanus Toxoid							
Aluminum phosphate	CD-1	73.3	0.07	0.70	375.5	0.73	6.39
Calcium phosphate	CD-1	62.3	0.04	0.37	387.6	1.99	13.43
Stearyl tyrosine	CD-1	11.2	0.14	0.54	360.2	3.78	37.79
None	CD-1	9.7	0.02	0.14	500.4	1.01	13.88
Aluminum phosphate*	CD-1	110.5	0.34	2.05	317.7	0.65	6.61
Liposome*	CD-1	71.7	0.18	2.33	399.1	1.48	12.17
Liposome-squalene/MPL*	CD-1	171.4	1.33	5.72	603.9	7.51	39.25
Liposome-squalene*	CD-1	143.6	1.06	4.41	488.7	4.10	16.40
None*	CD-1	0.6	0.03	0.18	243.2	0.75	7.50
Diphtheria Toxoid							
Aluminum phosphate	C57	18.4	0.03	0.20	200.8	0.06	0.72
Aluminum hydroxide	C57	11.7	0.03	0.22	240.9	0.03	1.90
γinulin	C57	11.0	0.04	0.40	256.5	6.91	8.73
Algammulin	C57	31.9	0.07	0.89	775.4	6.41	16.79
None	C57	0.03	0.03	0.03	10.2	0.03	0.19

* From (Gupta et al., 1995c)

2.2. Modulation of Antibody Isotypes and Subclasses

The adjuvants have been used to modulate the response to different antibody isotypes. For example, oral adjuvant, cholera toxin modulated immune response to elicit IgA, IgG and IgE antibodies whereas delivery of antigen by a live vector such as *Salmonella typhimurium* elicited mainly IgG antibodies (Staats et al., 1994). Antigens injected with *Bordetella pertussis* and aluminum adjuvants elicit IgG1 and IgE antibodies (Dahlback et al., 1983; Gupta and Siber, 1994a) and those injected with stearyl tyrosine, γ inulin and certain liposome formulations elicited relatively higher levels of IgG2a antibodies in mice (Table 2). The antibody isotype and IgG subclass switch has been explained by selective modulation of T helper cell types (discussed below).

3. MODULATION OF T-HELPER CELL TYPES

It is now well recognized that adjuvants modulate the immune response to different T-helper cell type (Th1 and Th2) (Golding 1991; Martin et al., 1991; Audibert and Lise, 1993; Cooper, 1994). The Th1 type response is accompanied by IL2 and IFNγ production (Shearer and Clerici, 1994) and is usually observed after viral, intracellular bacterial or parasitic infections as well as to antigens injected with live viruses (Coutelier et al., 1987). Stimulation of Th1 type response leads to a cell-mediated immune response (delayed type hypersensitivity) and production of relatively high levels of IgG2a antibodies in mice. In recent years several adjuvant formulations including Freund's complete adjuvant, Syntex adjuvant formulation-1, muramyl dipeptide, lipopolysaccharide, monophosphoryl lipid A, γ inulin, stearyl tyrosine, liposomes, QS21 have been shown to stimulate the Th1 type response in mice (Allison and Byars, 1990; Audibert and Lise, 1993; Kensil et al., 1993; Cooper, 1994; Gupta and Siber, 1994a; 1995a). Antigen delivered by *Salmonella typhimurium* for mucosal immunization also elicited Th1 type response in mice (Staats et al., 1994). The Th2 type response is modulated by IL-4 and IL-10 (Shearer and Clerici, 1994) and is stimulated by protein antigens or inactivated organisms. Stimulation of Th2 type response leads to production of IgG1 and IgE antibodies in mice (Golding, 1991). Th2 type response also results into eosinophilia and mucosal mastocytosis (Cooper, 1994) which are important components of the immune response to parasites (helminths). Aluminum adjuvants and cholera toxin as a mucosal adjuvants are known to stimulate a Th2 type response (Audibert and Lise, 1993; Cooper, 1994; Staats et al., 1994; Gupta and Siber, 1994a; 1995a; Gupta et al., 1995a).

We evaluated IgG subclass antibodies to tetanus toxoid and diphtheria toxoid in mice injected with these antigens given on various adjuvants (Table 2). Antigens adsorbed onto aluminum adjuvants or calcium phosphate or soluble antigens elicited lower levels of IgG2a and IgG2b antibodies than those given with stearyl tyrosine, γ inulin, algammulin and certain liposome formulations. Analysis of IgG subclass antibodies is an indirect way of determining the type of T helper cell stimulated (Gupta and Siber, 1994a).

Modulation to Th1 type response may not have a significant role for infections that can be prevented by induction of serum antibodies (for example, for routine childhood vaccines against tetanus and diphtheria). But Th1 type response seems to play an important role for diseases in which cell-mediated immune responses are important for prevention or cure, for example, parasitic infections and human immunodeficiency virus (HIV) infections (Salk et al., 1993; Clerici and Shearer, 1994).

4. MODULATION OF MHC CLASSES

As T-cells recognize antigens on antigen presenting cells along with MHC molecules (Neefjes et al., 1991), the form and processing of antigen affect its recognition by T-cells and the type of T-cells elicited. Antigen processing can be modulated with adjuvants (Golding, 1991; Martin et al., 1991) leading to vaccines which can elicit both T-helper cells and cytotoxic T lymphocytes (CTL).

With the use of adjuvants, the immune response can be modulated to MHC class I or MHC class II response (Cooper, 1994). An MHC class I response usually appears after infections with intracellular pathogens, such as viruses, leading to CTL (Paul, 1993). The response is observed to endogenously synthesized proteins but not to exogenous protein or peptide antigens. Adjuvants such as immunostimulating complexes (ISCOMS) and QS21 have been shown to elicit CTL to exogenous proteins, peptides or inactivated viruses (Takahashi et al., 1990; Wu et al., 1992; Audibert and Lise, 1993; Cooper, 1994). On the other hand MHC class II response is usually elicited against exogenous protein antigens or inactivated organisms (Paul, 1993; Gupta and Siber, 1995a). MHC class II response is associated with antibody production and most adjuvants are efficient in eliciting this response.

5. DUAL ADJUVANTICITY OF PROTEIN-POLYSACCHARIDE CONJUGATES

As new vaccines are being developed, combination vaccines have become a necessity in order to simplify immunization schedules, increase the immunization coverage and reduce the cost of immunization. Combining vaccine antigens faces a number of problems (Ellis and Douglas, 1994) including antigenic competition and carrier-specific epitope suppression (Gupta et al., 1995b). To make combination vaccines successful the amounts of various antigens need to be optimized and use of potent adjuvants, which could minimize amounts of antigens, may be desirable. One category of vaccines being developed and combined with the routine childhood vaccine diphtheria-tetanus-pertussis (DTP) is polysaccharide-protein conjugates (Robbins and Schneerson, 1990). Hib conjugate vaccine has already been licensed in the United States (Food and Drug Administration, 1993a,b) and efforts are underway to develop conjugate vaccines from capsular polysaccharides of pneumococci and meningococci. It would be desirable to prepare a polyvalent conjugate vaccine against at least seven types of pneumococcal capsular polysaccharides (Siber, 1994). As more conjugate vaccines are being developed, it would be advantageous to use carrier proteins with clinical significance in order to avoid the unnecessary load of large amounts of carrier proteins to the immune system.

The primary aim of conjugating polysaccharides to proteins has been to provide T-dependent characteristics to polysaccharides so that these are immunogenic in infants and produce an anamnestic response (Robbins and Schneerson, 1990). Little attention has been paid to the immunogenicity of protein antigens and virtually no efforts have been made to eliminate or reduce the amount of free protein antigens used in combination vaccines that contain the same protein as a carrier coupled to Hib polysaccharide and as a component of DTP vaccine (Food and Drug Administration, 1993a,b). On the basis of our findings that large polysaccharides enhance immunogenicity of covalently-linked protein antigens (Gupta et al., 1994b,c), we developed a strategy to utilize existing protein antigens such as tetanus toxoid, diphtheria toxoid, pertussis toxoid and filamentous haemagglutinin (components of DTP vaccine containing acellular pertussis vaccine) for covalently coupling these proteins to each of 2 capsular polysaccharides from Hib and Pneumococci (7 types). We observed that the carrier proteins, tetanus toxoid, diphtheria toxoid and pertussis toxoid provided T-dependent characteristics to polysaccharides such as dextran and Hib capsular polysaccharide and the polysaccharides enhanced immunogenicity of the protein antigens (Gupta et al., 1994b,c). By this approach, it may be possible to eliminate the need for free proteins from combination vaccines, thereby reducing the antigen burden on the immune system and complications due to carrier specific epitope suppression (Herzenberg et al., 1983; Barington et al., 1993). This strategy would be useful for developing an economical, safe and potent combined diphtheria-tetanus-acellular pertussis-Hib-Pneumococcal vaccine.

6. SUMMARY AND CONCLUSIONS

In recent years much progress has been made in understanding the molecular basis for action of adjuvants, the role of cytokines and different types of cells involved in immune response and the correlates of immunity to various diseases. This has led to selective modulation of immune response to vaccine antigens by adjuvants. The immune response can be selectively modulated to different antibody isotypes, IgG subclasses, MHC classes and T helper cell types. The basic knowledge of modulation of immune response is very important for developing suitable vaccines for newly emerging diseases such as HIV infections or for diseases against which no effective vaccines are available. Modulation of immune response to appropriate type and level would also be useful for development of combination vaccines and for the development of vaccines requiring fewer injections to achieve protection (ideally single dose vaccines). For infections that can be prevented by induction of serum antibodies, aluminum adjuvants formulated under optimal conditions are the adjuvants of choice. But for the purified, subunit or synthetic vaccines and combination vaccines comprising of purified vaccine antigens, potent adjuvants may be necessary. Due to limitations of aluminum adjuvants, especially their inability to elicit cell-mediated immune responses such as cytotoxic T-cell responses, there is a need for alternative adjuvants, particularly for diseases in which cell-mediated immune responses are important for prevention or cure. Based on pre-clinical and preliminary clinical observations, it appears that the range of adjuvants accepted for human vaccines will expand in coming years.

7. ACKNOWLEDGMENTS

We are thankful to Peter Cooper from Australian National University, Canberra, Australia for collaboration on γ inulin project. We apologize for not quoting original contributions of many workers in order to restrict the length of the article. Our recent review articles (Gupta et al., 1993a; 1995a; Gupta and Siber, 1995a) provide these citations to the interested reader. The work described in this paper was supported by grants from National Institutes of Health (AI 33575) and World Health Organization.

8. REFERENCES

Allison, A.C., and Byars, N.E., 1990, Adjuvants for a new generation of vaccines, in: *New Generation Vaccines* (G.C. Woodrow, and M.M. Levine, eds.), Marcel Dekker, New York, pp. 129-140.

Alonso, M.J., Gupta, R.K., Min, C., Siber, G.R., and Langer, R., 1994, Biodegradable microspheres as controlled-release tetanus toxoid delivery systems, *Vaccine* 12:299-306.

Aprile, M.A., and Wardlaw, A.C., 1966, Aluminum compounds as adjuvants for vaccine and toxoids in man: A review, *Can. J. Publ. Health* 57:343-354.

Audibert, F.M., and Lise, L.D., 1993, Adjuvants: current status, clinical perspectives and future prospects, *Immunology Today* 14:281-284.

Barington, T., Skettrup, M., Juul, L., and Heilman, C., 1993, Non-epitope-specific suppression of the antibody response to *Haemophilus influenzae* type b conjugate vaccines by preimmunization with vaccine components, *Infect. Immun.* 61:432-438.

Cooper, P.D., 1994, The selective induction of different immune responses by vaccine adjuvants, in: *Strategies in Vaccine Design* (G.L. Ada ed.), R.G. Landes Company, Austin, pp. 125-158.

Coutelier, J.P., van der Logt, J.T., Heessen, F.W.A., Warnier, G., and van Snick, J., 1987, IgG2a restriction of murine antibodies elicited by viral infections, *J. Exp. Med.* 165:64-69.

Dahlback, M., Bergstr, H., Pauwels, R., and Bazin, H., 1983, The non-specific enhancement of allergy III. Precipitation of bronchial anaphylactic reactivity in primed rats by injection of alum or *B. pertussis* vaccine: Relation of response capacity to IgE and IgG2a antibody levels, *Allergy* 38:261-271.

Eldridge, J.H., Gilley, R.M., Staats, J.K., Moldoveanu, Z., Meulbroek, J.A., and Tice, T.R., 1989, Biodegradable microspheres: vaccine delivery system for oral immunization, *Curr. Topics Microbiol. Immunol.* 146:59-66.

Eldridge, J.H., Staas, J.K., Meulbroek, J.A., Tice, T.R., and Gilley R.M., 1991, Biodegradable and biocompatible poly(DL-lactide-co-glycolide) microspheres as an adjuvant for Staphylococcal enterotoxin B toxoid which enhances the level of toxin-neutralizing antibodies, *Infect. Immun.* 59:2978-2986.

Ellis, R.W., and Douglas, R.G., Jr., 1994, Combination vaccines, *Int. J. Technol. Assess. Hlth care* 10:185-192.

Food and Drug Administration, 1993a, Approval of a new *Haemophilus influenzae* type b conjugate vaccine and a combined diphtheria-tetanus-pertussis and *Haemophilus influenzae* type b conjugate vaccine for infants and children, *MMWR* 42:296-298.

Food and Drug Administration, 1993b, Approval of use of *Haemophilus influenzae* type b conjugate vaccine reconstituted with diphtheria-tetanus-pertussis vaccine for infants and children. *MMWR* 42:964-966.

Glenny, A.T., Pope, C.G., Waddington, H., and Wallace, U., 1926, The antigenic value of toxoid precipitated by potassium alum, *J. Pathol. Bacteriol.* 29:38-45.

Golding, B., 1991, Cytokine regulation of humoral immune responses, in: *Topics in Vaccine Adjuvant Research* (D.R. Spriggs, and W.C. Koff, eds.), CRC, Boca Raton, pp. 25-37.

Gupta, R.K., and Siber, G.R., 1994a, Comparison of adjuvant activities of aluminum phosphate, calcium phosphate and stearyl tyrosine for tetanus toxoid, *Biologicals* 22:53-63.

Gupta, R.K., and Siber, G.R., 1994b, Comparative analysis of tetanus antitoxin titers of sera from immunized mice and guinea pigs determined by toxin neutralization test and enzyme-linked immunosorbent assay, *Biologicals* 22:215-219.

Gupta, R.K., and Siber, G.R., 1995a, Adjuvants for human use: current status, problems and future prospects, *Vaccine* 13:1263-1276.

Gupta, R.K., and Siber, G.R., 1995b, Method for quantitation of IgG subclass antibodies in mouse serum by enzyme-linked immunosorbent assay, *J. Immunol. Methods* 181:75-81.

Gupta, R.K., Relyveld, E.H., Lindblad, E.B., Bizzini, B., Ben-Efraim, S., and Gupta C.K., 1993a, Adjuvants - a balance between toxicity and adjuvanticity, *Vaccine* 11:293-306.

Gupta, R.K., Siber, G.R., Alonso, M.J., and Langer, R., 1993b, Development of a single-dose tetanus toxoid based on controlled release from biodegradable and biocompatible polyester microspheres, in: *Vaccines 93* (F. Brown, R. Chanock, H. Ginsberg, and R. Lerner, eds.), Cold Spring Harbor Laboratory Press, Cold Spring Harbor, pp. 391-396.

Gupta, R.K., Higham, S., Gupta, C.K., Rost, B., and Siber, G.R., 1994a, Suitability of the Vero cell method for titration of diphtheria antitoxin in the United States potency test for diphtheria toxoid, *Biologicals* 22:65-72.

Gupta, R., Griffin, P., Lees, A., Mond, J., Varanelli, C., Wallach, D., Cooper, P., Alonso, M., Langer, R. and Siber, G., 1994b, Comparative evaluation of aluminum phosphate, calcium phosphate, stearyl tyrosine, γ inulin, conjugation to dextran, liposomes and poly lactide/glycolide microspheres as adjuvant delivery systems for tetanus and diphtheria toxoids. Paper presented at the 94th General Meeting of the American Society for Microbiology, May 23-27, 1994, at Las Vegas, NV. American Society for Microbiology, Washington, DC, p. 147.

Gupta, R.K., Siber, G.R., Lees, A. and Mond, J.J., 1994c, Conjugation of multiple copies of T-cell dependent antigens on a large molecular weight polysaccharide carrier enhances antibody response to both components. Paper presented at the Second International Conference on Vaccines: New Technologies & Applications, March 21-23, 1994, Alexandria, VA. Waltham: Cambridge Healthtech Institute.

Gupta, R.K., Rost, B.E., Relyveld, E., and Siber, G.R., 1995a, Adjuvant Properties of aluminum and calcium compounds, in: *Vaccine Design: The Subunit Approach* (M.F. Powell, and M.J. Newman, eds.), Plenum Publishing Corporation, New York, pp 229- 248.

Gupta, R.K., Anderson, R., Cecchini, D., Rost, B., Griffin, P., Benscoter, K., Xu, J., Montanez-Ortiz, L., and Siber, G.R., 1995b, Development of a guinea-pig model for potency/immunogenicity evaluation of diphtheria, tetanus, acellular pertussis (DTaP) and *Haemophilus influenzae* type b polysaccharide conjugate vaccines, *Dev. Biol. Stand.* 86:281-294.

Gupta, R.K., Varanelli, C.L., Griffin, P., Wallach, D.F.H. and Siber, G.R., 1995c, Adjuvant properties of non-phospholipid liposomes (Novasomes®) in experimental animals for human vaccine antigens. *Vaccine* (in press).

Herzenberg, L.A., Tokuhisa, T. and Hayakawa, K, 1983, Epitope-specific regulations, *Ann. Rev. Immunol.* 1:609-632.

Kensil, C.R., Newman, M.J., Coughlin, R.T., Soltysik, S., Bedore, D., Recchia, J., Wu, J.- Y., and Marciani, D.J., 1993, The use of Stimulon adjuvant to boost vaccine response, *Vacc. Res.* 2:273-282.

Martin, S., Daniel, S.L., and Rouse, B.T., 1991, Cytokines and regulation of cellular immune responses to viruses, in: *Topics in Vaccine Adjuvant Research* (D.R. Spriggs, and W.C. Koff, eds.), CRC, Boca Raton, pp. 39-50.

Morris, W., Steinhoff, M.C., and Russell, P.K., 1994, Potential of polymer microencapsulation technology for vaccine innovation, *Vaccine* 12:5-11.

Neefjes, J.J., Schumacher. T.N.M., and Ploegh, H.L., 1991, Assembly and intracellular transport of major histocompatibility complex molecules. *Curr. Opin. Cell. Biol.* 3:601- 609.

O'Hagan, D.T., Jeffery, H., and Davis, S.S., 1993, Long-term antibody responses in mice following subcutaneous immunization with ovalbumin entrapped in biodegradable microparticles, *Vaccine* 11:965-969.

Paul, W.E., 1993, The immune system, in: *Fundamental Immunology* (W.E. Paul, ed.) Third Edition, Raven Press, New York, pp. 1-20.

Ramon, G., 1925, Sur l'augmentation anormale de l'antitoxine chez les chevaux producteurs de serum antidiphterique, *Bull. Soc. Centr. Med. Vet.* 101:227-234.

Ramon, G., 1926, Procedres pour acroitre la production des antitoxines, *Ann. Institut Pasteur* 40:1-10.

Robbins, J.B., and Schneerson, R., 1990, Polysaccharide-protein conjugates: a new generation of vaccines. *J. Infect. Dis.* 161:821-832.

Salk, J., Bretscher, P.A., Salk, P.L., Clerici, M., and Shearer, G.M., 1993, A strategy for prophylactic vaccination against HIV, *Science* 260:1269-1271.

Shearer, G.M., and Clerici, M., 1994, CD4$^+$ functional T cell subsets: their roles in infection and vaccine development, in: *Strategies in Vaccine Design* (G.L. Ada ed.), R.G. Landes Company, Austin, pp. 113-124.

Siber, G.R., 1994, Pneumococcal disease: Prospects for a new generation of vaccines, *Science* 265:1385-1387.

Singh, M., Singh, O., Singh, A., and Talwar, G.P., 1992, Immunogenicity studies on diphtheria toxoid loaded biodegradable microspheres, *Int. J. Pharmaceutics* 85:R5-R8.

Staats, H.F., Jackson, R.J., Marinaro, M., Takahashi, I., Kiyono, H., and McGhee, J.R., 1994, Mucosal immunity to infection with implications for vaccine development, *Curr. Biol.* 6:572-583.

Takahashi, H., Takeshita, T., Morein, B., Putney, S., Germain, R.N., and Berzofsky, J.A., 1990, Induction of CD8+ cytotoxic T-cells by immunization with purified HIV-1 envelope protein in ISCOMs, *Nature (London)* 344:873-875.

Wu, J.-Y., Gardner, B.H., Murphy, C.I., Seals, J.R., Kensil, C.R., Recchia, J., Beltz, G.A., Newman, G.W., and Newman, M.J., 1992, Saponin adjuvant enhancement of antigen specific immune responses to an experimental HIV-1 vaccine, *J. Immunol.* 148:1519-1525.

16

UNIQUE IMMUNOMODULATING PROPERTIES OF DIMETHYL DIOCTADECYL AMMONIUM BROMIDE (DDA) IN EXPERIMENTAL VIRAL VACCINES[*]

D. Katz,[1] S. Lehrer,[1] O. Galan,[1] B. Lachmi,[1] S. Cohen,[1] I. Inbar,[1]
I. Samina,[2] B. Peleg,[2] D. Heller,[3] H. Yadin,[2] D. Chai,[2] E. Freeman,[1]
H. Schupper,[1] and P. Fuchs[1]

[1] Department of Virology, Israel Institute for Biological Research
P.O.B. 19, 74100, Ness-Ziona, Israel
[2] Kimron Veterinary Institute
Bet Dagan, Israel
[3] Faculty of Agriculture, The Hebrew University
Rehovot, Israel

1. INTRODUCTION

The adjuvant activity of dimethyl dioctadecyl ammonium bromide (DDA), a low molecular weight (631) lipoid amine composed of two 18 carbon long alkyl chains and two methyl groups, all bound to a positively charged quaternary ammonium molecule, was discovered by Gall in a survey of more than 100 chemicals (Gall, 1966). Since 1966 many papers were published showing the efficacy of DDA as an adjuvant for protein antigens (Veronesi et al, 1970; Stanfield et al, 1973), haptens (Dailey and Hunter, 1974; Snippe et al, 1977; Snippe et al 1977), tumors (Prager and Gordon ,1978), viruses (Kraaijeveld et al, 1980; Katz et al, 1991; Kraaijeveld et al, 1983; Smith and Ziola, 1986; Molitor et al, 1984/85; Rijke et al, 1988; Katz et al, 1992; Katz et al, 1993; Katz et al, 1994), protozoa (Lilleloch et al, 1993; Desowitz and Barnwell, 1980) and bacteria (Andersen, 1994).

It is presumed that for obtaining an optimal adjuvant response, a direct interaction of DDA and the antigen is needed. This interaction is possible either through electrostatic or hydrophobic bonds, enabled by the amphiphilic nature of DDA. However, there are some studies that indicate that the immunomodulatory properties of DDA are independent of its binding to the antigen (Hilgers et al, 1989; Katz et al, 1995; Gordon et al, 1980; Smith and Ziola, 1986).

---

[*] In commemoration of our colleague the late Dr. Haim Schupper.

Novel Strategies in Design and Production of Vaccines
Edited by S. Cohen and A. Shafferman, Plenum Press, New York, 1996

This presentation is a summary of our studies with DDA as an adjuvant in experimental viral vaccines in which the immunomodulating properties of DDA are demonstrated. Some of the results were already published elsewhere and some were either presented at meetings or are shown here for the first time.

2. EXPERIMENTAL DESIGN

We have studied the adjuvant effect of DDA in three animal species with four inactivated viral vaccines: In mice, with two vaccines prepared from enveloped viruses: Semliki Forest virus (SFV) (Katz et al, 1991) and rabies virus (RV) (Katz et al, 1994); in chickens with another enveloped virus, Newcastle disease virus (NDV) (Katz et al, 1993) and in calves with a nonenveloped virus, foot and mouth disease virus (FMDV) (Katz et al, 1992). Experimental details will be described for each individual experiment in the "RESULTS" section.

3. RESULTS

3.1. the Adjuvant Effect of DDA in Mice Vaccinated with Inactivated SFV on Total ELISA Antibodies and Antibody-Isotypes in Groups of Vaccinated Mice - Comparison to Other Adjuvants

Groups of 6 random bred, 5-7 weeks old, ICR female mice (Charles River, UK) were inoculated subcutaneously with β–propiolactone inactivated SFV (V), in saline (SAL) and the following adjuvants: Complete Freund's adjuvant - Difco, USA (CFA), Aluminum hydroxide - Alhydrogel, Superfos, Denmark (Al) and DDA (100 μg/dose) - Eastman-Kodak, USA (Figure 1). A fifth (negative control) group was inoculated with saline. A second injection, containing virus only, was given 14 days later. Blood was drawn on days 10, 17, and 27 afterwards. Total antibody and antibody-isotypes were determined by ELISA and expressed as positive to negative ratios (P/N). Since no marked differences within the groups were observed in these samples, the results summarized in Figure 1, represent the average responses in each group on days 10, 17 and 24 days after booster. The antibody-isotype response of convalescent mice that recovered from a live SFV (LIVE V) infection is also shown in Figure 1 for comparison.

A relatively high total antibody response was induced by Al and DDA but not by CFA. Alhydrogel and inactivated SFV induced mainly IgG1 isotypes while DDA and CFA

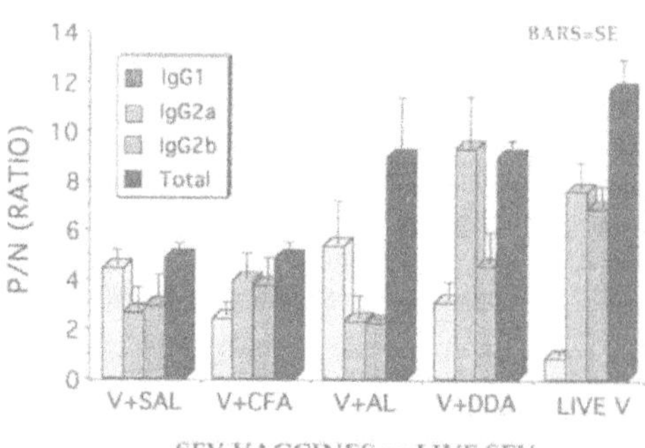

Figure 1. Total ELISA antibodies and antibody-isotypes in groups of mice vaccinated with inactivated SFV vaccines; Comparison of responses to convalescent mice.

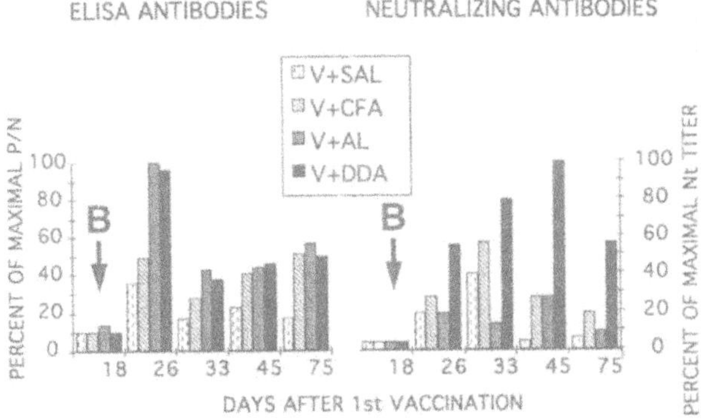

Figure 2. Effect of adjuvants on the induction of ELISA and neutralizing antibodies.

induced more of the IgG2a antibodies and IgG2b antibodies. Convalescent mice did not produce IgG1 antibodies at all but did produce a high proportion of IgG2a and IgG2b antibodies.

3.2. Induction of ELISA-Antibodies and Neutralizing Antibodies to SFV by Different Adjuvants

In another experiment , depicted in Figure 2, we examined the effect of adjuvants on the induction of antibodies by the micro-Nt test in comparison to ELISA. Groups of mice were vaccinated with inactivated SFV with adjuvants and boosted 18 days later with inactivated virus without adjuvants. Sera were drawn at different times after vaccination, pooled and tested. Results are expressed as percentage of the maximal antibody response in this experiment, which was P/N=15.5 for ELISA and neutralization titer of 1000 for the micro-Nt.

Results indicate that DDA induced a relatively strong neutralizing antibody response which lasted longer than those induced by other adjuvants. The difference between the adjuvants in the induction of ELISA antibodies was less prominent for most of the samples, except for the 26th day after vaccination where Al and DDA induced relatively more antibodies than CFA.

3.3. DTH in Mice Vaccinated with SFV Vaccines

In order to see whether the mixing of antigen and DDA is necessary for the demonstration of an optimal cell mediated immunity (CMI) as evaluated by an assay for DTH (delayed type hypersensitivity), we inoculated one group of mice with a mixture of DDA and inactivated SFV antigen (DDA+SFV), a second group with DDA first and antigen one day later (-1 DDA, SFV) and a third group with DDA and antigen inoculated at the same time but at two separate sites (DDA, SFV). In addition, for comparison, one group of mice was inoculated with SFV without adjuvants (SFV), another group with buffer (PBS) and three other with mixtures containing the viral antigens and CFA (CFA+SFV), TiterMax (nonionic block copolymers emulsified in squalene) - CytRx, USA (T/M+SFV) and Optivant (micron sized particles of β glucan polymer) - Transgenic Sciences Inc. USA (OPT+SFV). Six days later the mice were tested for induction of DTH (Katz et al, 1991). Results are summarized in Figure 3.

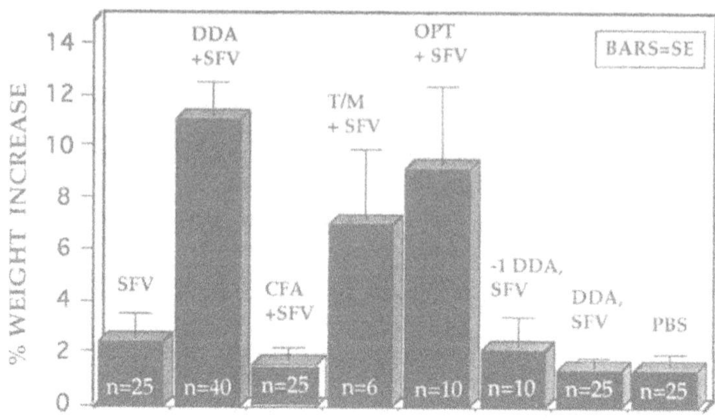

Figure 3. Effect of adjuvants (DDA, CFA, Optivant and TiterMax) on the DTH responses in SFV vaccinated mice.

DDA induced a high DTH response to SFV but only when administered mixed with the antigen. Injection of DDA 1 day earlier or at a separate site did not induce any response. High DTH responses were also induced by Optivant and by TiterMax. Unlike previously shown (Katz et al, 1991), in this experiment , CFA did not induce a DTH response.

3.4. the Adjuvant Effect of DDA in Mice Vaccinated with Inactivated Rabies Virus

The rabies antigen used in this experiment was prepared from the commercial human diploid cell culture, β-propiolactone inactivated, rabies vaccine (RV), (Merieux, France). Five groups, of 18 female mice per group were injected subcutaneously at the age of 5 weeks with 0.2 ml of the following preparations: RV in PBS (RV(PBS)); RV containing 1% aluminum hydroxide (RV(Al)); RV containing 100 μg DDA per dose (RV(DDA)); RV emulsified in 50% CFA (RV(CFA)); RV mixed with Optivant (RV(OPT)). Each preparation contained one tenth of the original concentration of the vaccine. An additional control group was inoculated with PBS. For determination of DTH, 12 mice of each group where inoculated on the 6th day after vaccination, into the right footpad with a 1:2.5 dilution of RV(PBS) and into the left footpad with PBS. The weight difference between the footpads was measured 24 hours later. Two weeks after vaccination, blood was drawn from the tail vein of the remaining 6 mice and a booster injection containing RV(PBS) was given. Blood samples were further drawn on days 29 and 74 after first injection. Sera were tested for ELISA antibodies utilizing a CVS 21 rabies strain as capture antigen. Positive to negative ratios (P/N) were calculated relatively to the PBS control group. Neutralizing antibodies were determined by NTCEIA. Results are summarized in Table 1.

Primary ELISA-antibody responses at 14 days after immunization were low in all vaccinated groups of mice. Primary neutralizing antibodies could not be detected in the RV(Al) and RV(DDA) groups and were low in all other groups. All mice responded in a typical secondary antibody response after the booster injection. There was no clear-cut correlation between the ELISA and NTCEIA. CFA and Al induced an enhanced ELISA-antibody response (compared to the RV(PBS) group). An enhanced neutralizing antibody

Table 1. Immunomodulative properties of adjuvants (DDA, CFA, Al and Optivant) in experimental inactivated rabies virus (RV) vaccines in mice

Vaccine	ELISA antibodies (P/N)			Neutralizing antibodies (titer[•])			DTH (%) weight increase
	14*	29*	74*	14*	29*	74*	
RV (PBS)	3.5	3.6	7.7	30	559	1135	1.5±1.2
RV (OPT)	3.4	3.5	4.8	50	143	170	3.8±1.7
RV (Al)	3.5	6.8	9.5	NEG	1679	5390	3.9±0.9
RV (DDA)	2.0	5.4	6.1	NEG	226	652	9.6±1.5
RV (CFA)	3.8	8.2	15.4	67	733	280	9.3±1.5

*Days after first vaccination (booster injection with RV was given on day 15.
[•]Reciprocal of dilution resulting in 50% neutralization; NEG=less than 50% neutralization.

response was induced only by Al (and none by DDA and CFA). The RV(OPT) group produced the lowest amount of antibodies by the two tests.

The highest DTH responses to rabies antigen stimulation were induced by DDA and CFA. Al and Optivant induced intermediate responses which were only slightly higher than the response in the RV(PBS) group.

3.5. the Adjuvant Effect of DDA in Chickens Vaccinated with Inactivated NDV Vaccines

Chickens (White Leghorn, 5 weeks old, roosters) were inoculated subcutaneously with 0.5 ml of 500 HA units of β-propiolactone inactivated NDV vaccines in combination with different adjuvants: DDA, CFA and commercial mineral oil vaccine (MABAT, Israel). Antibodies were assayed by the hemagglutination inhibition test (HI) and by the hemadsorption inhibition (HAdI) (an *in vitro* microneutralization test). CMI was tested by the wattle inoculation test for the determination of DTH and by an *in vitro* peripheral blood lymphocyte proliferation (LP) assay. Resistance of chickens was tested by a high challenge dose containing 2×10^5 LD$_{50}$ of a velogenic, locally isolated, NDV strain (Katz et al, 1993).

3.5.1. the Effect of DDA and Mineral Oil Emulsion on the Induction of HI-Antibodies, HADI Antibodies and Resistance to NDV in Vaccinated Chickens. The results at three weeks after one single inoculation of chickens with different vaccine preparations are summarized in Table 2.

Vaccines containing 8 mg of DDA induced similar amounts of HI antibodies to the mineral oil based vaccines. Significantly lower amounts were induced by 4 mg and 0.5 mg of DDA. The amount induced by 0.5 mg of DDA was not statistically different from the amount induced by the non-adjuvanted NDV vaccines. Eight mg of DDA induced higher titers of neutralizing (HAdI) antibodies than the commercial mineral oil based vaccine. Post-challenge, survival values, ranging from 66% to 93%, obtained with all 3 doses of DDA and with the mineral oil based commercial vaccine, were statistically similar. DDA-vaccines containing, crude NDV antigen, derived from NDV infected and inactivated allantoic fluid preparations (NDV(AL FL)) or a semi-purified NDV preparations ((NDV(PUR), induced similar results.

3.5.2. DTH in Chickens Vaccinated with NDV Vaccines. The DTH response to stimulation with an inactivated NDV antigen preparation was tested in NDV vaccinated roosters by the wattle inoculation test (Katz et al, 1993). Three groups of chickens were

Table 2. Effect of DDA containing NDV-vaccines on antibody production and resistance to challenge in comparison to the commercial mineral oil adjuvanted vaccine

Material injected (0.5 ml/chicken)	Number of chickens per group	Antibodies HI ± se [a] ($\log_2$)	Antibodies HAdi [b] ($\log_2$)	% survival (challenged with 2×10^5 LD$_{50}$)
NDV(AL FL)[c] + 8 mg DDA	14	4.1 ± 0.6	5.2	71
NDV(PUR)[d] + 8 mg DDA	15	5.0 ± 0.6	5.8	73
NDV(AL FL) + 2 mg DDA	15	3.0 ± 0.4	Not done	84
NDV(PUR) + 2 mg DDA	15	2.8 ± 0.5	Not done	93
NDV(AL FL) + 0.5 mg DDA	15	2.0 ± 0.4	Not done	66
NDV(PUR) + 0.5 mg DDA	15	2.5 ± 0.5	Not done	73
NDV+OIL (MABAT)	30	4.5 ± 0.6	2.1	80
NDV(AL FL)	15	1.0 ± 0.3	1.0	13
NDV(PUR)	13	2.1 ± 0.7	1.5	23
AL FL [e]	10	0.8 ± 0.3	0.5	0
UNTREATED	25	0.3 ± 0.2	0.5	8

[a] Hemagglutination inhibition geometric mean titer ± standard error; [b] Hemadsorption inhibition test performed on pooled serum samples; [c] Crude NDV preparations derived from clarified infected allantoic fluids; [d] Semipurified (by ultracentrifugation) NDV preparations; [e] Uninfected allantoic fluid.

inoculated with mixtures of NDV and adjuvants: NDV+CFA, NDV+DDA (2 mg DDA per dose), and NDV in mineral oil (MABAT (OIL) as shown in Figure 4. Three other groups which served as controls were inoculated with DDA alone, with NDV antigen in saline and with saline. The number of chickens in the group (n) is indicated in the figure. Eight days post vaccination, chickens were tested for specific DTH responses to NDV by inoculation of the right wattle with antigen and the left wattle with saline. DTH responses are expressed as the width difference in mm of the right and left wattles ± standard error (SE).

The results (Figure 4) indicate that all adjuvants induced DTH responses which were higher than those induced by the virus alone. DDA induced the highest DTH response, CFA an intermediate response and mineral oil induced the lowest response.

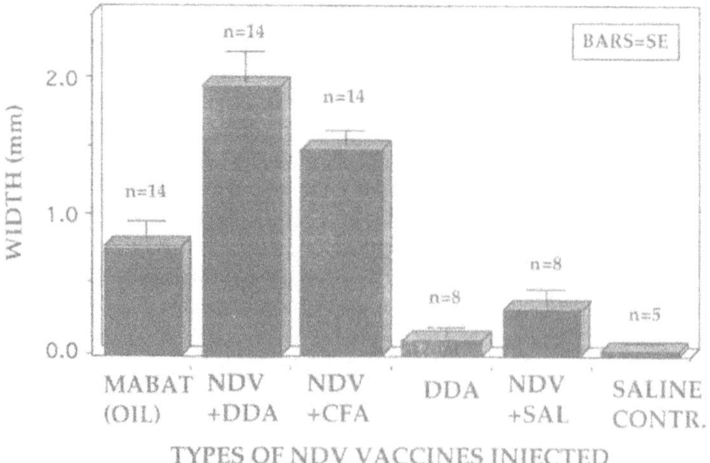

Figure 4. Effect of adjuvants (DDA, CFA and mineral oil) on the DTH responses in NDV vaccinated chickens.

In another experiment (results not shown) significant stimulation indices (SI) in the LP assay, were obtained after a booster injection with the antigen alone at 10 days after the first inoculation. Blood lymphocytes were obtained 8 days later and stimulated in vivo by the NDV antigen. DDA induced significantly higher stimulation indices as compared to CFA and mineral oil, although the HI antibody titers in all adjuvanted groups were similar (Katz et al, 1993).

3.6 the Effect of DDA and AL/SAP Adjuvants on the Induction of Neutralizing Antibodies and DTH to FMDV in Vaccinated Calves

In preliminary experiments DDA had a very small adjuvant effect on the induction of antibodies to FMDV. Since FMDV does not possess a lipid envelope we assumed that the reason for this poor response was due to loss of antigenicity at the low pH (6.0-6.5) of the saline solution that we used or due to lack of interaction of the antigen with DDA under the regular working protocol that we used (Katz et al, 1991). For the experiments presented here, we have replaced the saline solution with buffer (PBS, pH 7.2-7.4) to protect antigenicity and to facilitate electrostatic interaction between the DDA and FMDV antigen. DDA-FMDV mixtures were incubated for at least 1 hour at room temperature before injection. Six, 6 - months old calves, were inoculated with ethylene-diimide inactivated FMDV (FMDV) vaccines (O1 dalton, 3 µg/ dose) only, 8 calves were inoculated with FMDV + 4 mg of DDA/dose, 8 calves with FMDV + 16 mg DDA/dose, 7 calves with the commercial preparation of Al/Sap (Aluminum hydroxide-saponin - Sefic, Denmark) and another 7 calves with FMDV in a double oil emulsion (DOE) preparation. On day 32, 3 calves of each group, were tested for DTH by inoculating, intradermally, 0.2 ml containing 10 µg of the FMDV antigen. The skin width difference between the inoculated site and an uninoculated site was measured 24 to 72 hours later. The remaining calves were boosted subcutaneously with 2 ml containing 3 µg FMDV antigen. All animals were bled on day 0, 32 and 58 after first vaccination for determination of neutralizing antibodies. Results are summarized in Table 3.

Significant amounts of neutralizing antibodies were induced by all vaccines. On day 32, after one single injection, the FMDV(Al/Sap) and the FMDV(+16mg DDA) vaccines induced the highest antibody titers. After the booster injection the FMDV(DOE) induced the highest antibody titer but all other adjuvanted vaccines elicited relatively high titers as well. A dose effect of the DDA can be seen, 4 mg of DDA induced less antibodies than 16 mg of DDA.

Because of the small numbers of calves that were tested for DTH and the high standard deviations obtained, clear cut conclusions are not possible. However, while DDA

Table 3. Immunomodulative properties of adjuvants in experimental inactivated FMDV vaccines in calves

Vaccine	Neutralizing antibodies (GM±SD[*])			DTH (mm) skin width
	0*	32*	58*	
FMDV (PBS)	1.7±0.8	4.0±1.8	5.4±1.0	1.3±0.5
FMDV (+4 mg DDA)	2.7±0.5	3.2±1.3	6.3±1.3	1.3±1.5
FMDV(+16 mg DDA)	2.4±1.1	6.4±1.7	6.8±0.8	0.3±0.6
FMDV (Al/Sap)	2.4±0.9	7.1±1.6	7.7±1.1	5.0±3.7
FMDV (DOE)	2.1±0.7	4.9±0.9	8.9±1.7	3.5±3.6

*Days after first vaccination (booster injection with FMDV was given on day 32.
[*]Geometric mean titer ± standard deviation (Log_2).

vaccines did not induce a DTH response at all, some responses were obtained with the FMDV(Al/Sap) and the FMDV(DOE) vaccines. It is interesting to note that most of the calves (13/15) that were tested for DTH, including those that did not respond in the DTH assay, had significant amounts of antibodies in their blood.

In a similar experiment (Results not shown) we increased the incubation time of the DDA-FMDV mixtures to 24 hours in the cold room (4°C). This was done in order to enable a better interaction and binding of the antigen to the DDA. In general, antibody titers in this experiment were similar to the titers obtained in the previous experiment, indicating that the modified procedure for the preparation of the vaccine had no additive effect on antibody production.

3.7. DDA TOXICITY AND SIDE EFFECTS

To the best of our knowledge the toxicological properties of DDA have not yet been systematically studied. In the following experiment we have tried to determine the toxicity of DDA in mice.

Seven groups of ICR mice, 10 mice per group, were inoculated intraperitoneally with 0.2 ml of the following concentrations of DDA: 0, 2, 4, 8, 16, 32 and 100 mg/ml. Mice were weighed just before inoculation (day-0), and on days 2 and 7 . Results are summarized in Figure 5.

Statistically significant weight losses (relative to day-0) were observed on the second day after inoculation only in the groups that received high concentrations of DDA (16, 32 and 100 mg/ml). One mouse, of the group injected with 100 mg/ml, died on the 5th day after inoculation. On day 7, however, all mice showed a normal weight as compared to the control group.

4. DISCUSSION

In this presentation we have summarized our studies on the adjuvanticity of DDA in comparison to other adjuvants. Unlike previously believed (Snippe et al, 1977), it is now clear, from our and other studies, that DDA is capable of inducing not only CMI but also enhanced antibody responses to a variety of antigens (Hilgers et al, 1989; Katz et al, 1995). DDA induced enhanced humoral antibody responses to most of the inactivated viral antigens tested. In some experiments a single booster injection with antigen alone was necessary to

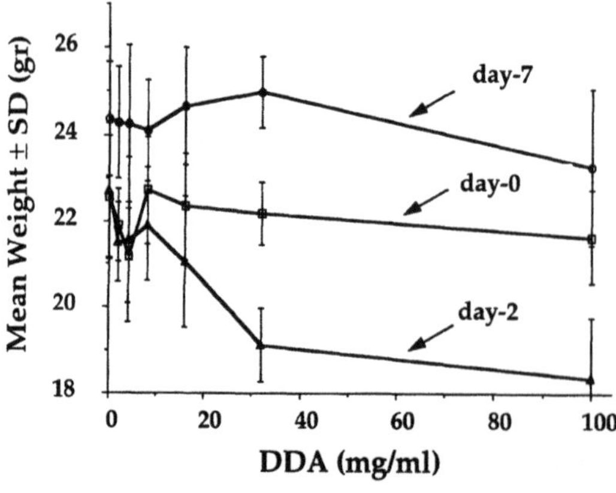

Figure 5. Toxicity of DDA in mice. (Standard deviation values (SD) are indicated by bars).

demonstrate the adjuvant effect of DDA in comparison to the non-adjuvanted vaccines. With the rabies antigen, DDA did not enhance the humoral antibody response, probably because of the high immunogenicity of the RV antigen by itself.

We have shown that different adjuvants may induce functionally different antibodies. In the SFV and NDV experimental systems, DDA induced higher titers of neutralizing antibodies than ELISA or HI antibodies, respectively. On the other hand, in the rabies experimental system higher titers of neutralizing antibodies were induced by aluminum hydroxide. The significance of this differential immunomodulation for the induction of protective immunity is not yet understood. In the NDV experimental system, where challenge experiments were performed, we could not demonstrate any direct correlation between the titers of HI or neutralizing (HAdI) antibodies and resistance to challenge. Moreover, protection did not correlate directly with CMI (DTH and LP) as well. Mineral oil containing vaccines that induced a low DTH response and no activity in LP assay, protected to the same extent as the DDA-vaccines which induced a very high CMI response. However, it seems that certain levels of antibodies and/or CMI are necessary for resistance since most of the susceptible chickens had no detectable immune response or very low levels of antibodies and CMI.

Adjuvants also influence the antibody isotype profile. In the SFV experiments in mice, we demonstrated that DDA induced a higher amount of IgG2a and IgG2b antibodies and a lower amount of the IgG1 antibodies as compared to the aluminum hydroxide based vaccines. This pattern was similar to the pattern of isotypes induced by CFA or by a non-lethal virus infection. IgG2a and IgG2b antibodies, which are complement binding antibodies in mice, are believed to correlate better with protection (Katz et al, 1991).

DDA induced an enhanced neutralizing antibody response to inactivated FMDV, a non-enveloped virus. The adjuvant activity seemed to be pH dependent, indicating that certain electrostatic conditions may be necessary for the interaction of the adjuvant and the antigen. However, these conditions were not sufficient for the induction of an enhanced DTH response, presumably because of the absence of a lipid-lipid interaction of the adjuvant with the antigen. Although no clear conclusion can be drawn from our preliminary, small scale, DTH-experiment, it seems to support other authors' findings who also obtained poor results with DDA and another non-enveloped virus (EMC) (Kraaijeveld et al, 1983).

DDA induced a high cell mediated immune response in combination with enveloped virus vaccines (SFV, RV and NDV). The response was equal to, or higher than, the response obtained with mineral oil based adjuvants and always higher than the response obtained with aluminum hydroxide. We have also shown, in the SFV experimental system that DDA had no adjuvant effect when administered separately from the antigen. This finding indicates, most probably, the need for a direct interaction of the DDA adjuvant with the antigen (Hilgers et al, 1989; Katz et al, 1995), contradict other authors' results (Gordon et al, 1980; Smith and Ziola, 1986).

In spite of being a surfactant, able to lyse red blood cells (Gall, 1966), it is believed that the toxicity of DDA is low (Katz, et al, 1995). No significant local reactions have been observed with any of our DDA vaccines, although mineral oil and CFA containing vaccines did occasionally induce local swelling and/or granuloma. This is probably true for most of the DDA studies that we are aware of, including the human trials (Veronesi et al, 1970: Stanfield et al, 1973). Our own toxicity study in mice (Figure 5) demonstrated indeed the very low toxicity of DDA.

In conclusion, DDA, a simple synthetic chemical, exhibited excellent adjuvanticity in several of our experimental systems. Although enhanced antibody responses were induced with most viruses, excellent CMI responses were obtained only with enveloped (lipid coated) viruses. Most convincing were the NDV studies in which a high degree of protection to a large velogenic-NDV challenge dose was achieved after one single inoculation of a DDA containing vaccine. For non-lipid antigens, it would be interesting to study the immuno-modulating properties of covalently bound DDA analogs. We hope that the unique immuno-modulating properties of DDA and of other lipoid amines with similar properties (Katz et al, 1995) as reflected in our and other studies, will finally be exploited for improving the efficacy of many of the veterinary and human vaccines.

5. REFERENCES

Andersen, P., 1994, Effective vaccination of mice against *Mycobacterium tuberculosis* infection with a soluble mixture of secreted mycobacterial proteins, *Infect. Immun.* 62:2536-2544.

Dailey, M. O., and Hunter, R. L., 1974, The role of lipid in the induction of hapten-specific delayed hypersensitivity and contact sensitivity, *J. Immunol.* 112:1526-1534.

Desowitz, R. S., and Barnwell, J. W., 1980, Effect of selenium and dimethyl dioctadecyl ammonium bromide on the vaccine-induced immunity of Swiss-Webster mice against Malaria (*Plasmodium berghei*), *Inf. Immun.* 27:87-89.

Gall, D., 1966, The adjuvant activity of aliphatic nitrogenous bases, *Immunol.* 11:369-386.

Gordon, W. C., Prager, M. D., and Carroll, M. C., 1980, The enhancement of humoral and cellular immune responses by dimethyldioctadecylammonium bromide, *Cell. Immunol.* 49:329-340.

Hilgers, L. A. T., Zigterman, G. J. W. J., and Snippe, H., 1989, Immunomodulating properties of amphiphilic agents, in: Autoimmunity and Toxicology, Kammuler, M. E., Bloksma, N., and Seinen, W. (Eds), Elsevier Science Publishers B. V. pp. 293-306.

Katz, D., Lehrer, S., Galan, O., Lachmi, B., and Cohen, S., 1991, Adjuvant effect of dimethyl dioctadecyl ammonium bromide, complete Freund's adjuvant and aluminum hydroxide on neutralizing antibody, antibody-isotype and delayed-hypersensitivity responses to Semliki Forest virus in mice, *FEMS Microbiol. Immunol.* 76:305-320.

Katz, D., Chai, D., Wasserman, A., Reshef, A., Davidson, M., and Yadin, H., 1992, The adjuvant activity of dimethyl dioctadecyl ammonium bromide (DDA)in foot and mouth disease vaccines, The first TAHRP workshop / April 10-16, 1992 (abstract).

Katz, D., Inbar, I., Samina, I., Peleg, B., and Heller, D., 1993, Comparison of dimethyl dioctadecyl ammonium bromide, Freund's complete adjuvant and mineral oil for induction of humoral antibodies, cellular immunity and resistance to Newcastle disease virus in chickens, *FEMS Immunol. Med. Microbiol.* 7:303-314.

Katz, D., Freeman, E., Schupper, H., Galan, O., and Fuchs, P., 1994, Immunomodulation in rabies postexposure prophylaxis, *Supplement to JAMA Southeast Asia (December 1994), Proceedings to 4th WPCCID,* pp. 235-239.

Katz, D., Kraaijeveld, C. A., and Snippe, H., 1995, Synthetic lipoid compounds as antigen-specific immu-nostimulators for improving the efficacy of killed-virus vaccines, in: *The Theory and Practical Application of Adjuvants, Stewart-Tull, D. E. S., (Eds), John Willey and Sons Ltd.* pp. 37-50.

Kraaijeveld, C. A., Snippe, H., Harmsen, M., and Boutahar-Trouw, K. B., 1980, Dimethyl dioctadecyl ammonium bromide as an adjuvant for delayed hypersensitivity and cellular immunity against Semliki Forest virus in mice, *Arch. Virol.* 65:211-217.

Kraaijeveld, C. A., Riviere, G., Boutahar-Trouw, K. B., Jansen, J., Harmsen, M., and Snippe, H., 1983, Effect of the adjuvant dimethyl dioctadecyl ammonium bromide on the humoral and cellular immune responses to encephalomyocarditis virus, *Antiviral Res.* 3:137-149.

Lilleloch, H. S., Lindblad, E. B., and Nichols, M., 1993, Adjuvanticity of dimethyl dioctadecyl ammonium bromide, complete Freund's adjuvant and corynebacterium parvum with respect to host immune response to coccidial antigens, *Avian Diseases,* 37:731-740.

Molitor, T. W., Joo, H. S., and Thacker, B. J., 1984/85, Potentiating effect of adjuvants on humoral immunity to porcine parvovirus vaccines in guinea pigs, *Vet. Microbiol.* 10:209-218.

Prager, M. D., and Gordon, W. C., 1978, Enhanced response to chemoimmunotherapy and immunoprophylaxis with the use of tumor-associated antigens with a lipopphilic agents, *Cancer Res.* 38:2052-2057.

Rijke, E. O., Loeffen, A. H. C., and Lutticken, D., 1988, The use of lipid amines as immunopotentiators for viral vaccines, in: *Advances of Immunomodulation, Bizzini, B., and Bonmassar, E. (Eds.), Pithagora Press, Rome-Milan,* pp. 433-443.

Smith, R. H., and Ziola, B., 1986, Cyclophosphamide and dimethyl dioctadecyl ammonium bromide immu-nopotentiate the delayed-type hypersensitivity response to inactivated enveloped viruses, *Immunology,* 58:245-250.

Snippe, H., Belder, M., and Willers, J. M. N., 1977, Dimethyl dioctadecyl ammonium bromide as adjuvant for delayed hypersensitivity in mice, *Immunology*, 33:931-933.

Snippe, H., de Reuver, M. J., Beunder, J. W., van der Meer, J. B., van Wichen, D. F., and Willers, J. M. N., 1982, Delayed type hypersensitivity in rabbits. Comparison of the adjuvants dioctadecyl ammonium bromide and Freund's complete adjuvant, *Int. Arch. Allergy Appl. Immun.* 67:139-144.

Stanfield, I. P., Gall, D., and Bracken, M., 1973, Single-dose antenatal tetanus immunization, *Lancet* i: *215-219*.

Veronesi, R., Correa, A., and Alterio D., 1970, Single dose immunization against tetanus: promising results in human trials, *Rev. Inst. Trop. Med. Sao. Paulo 12:46-54*.

17

CHALLENGES IN THE DEVELOPMENT OF COMBINATION VACCINES

Ronald W. Ellis

Department of Virus and Cell Biology
Merck Research laboratories
West Point, Pennsylvania 19486

There has been increased interest in the last decade in the development of new vaccines, especially for pediatric use. Newer vaccines that have been licensed and recommended for widespread pediatric immunization include those for *Haemophilus influenzae* type *b* (Hib), hepatitis B (HB), and most recently in some countries varicella and *Bordetella pertussis* (acellular pertussis). Clinical trials are ongoing in infants for vaccines for *Streptococcus pneumoniae* (pneumococcal), hepatitis A (HA), and *Neisseria meningitidis* (meningococcal), among others. As a consequence, there is a tremendous opportunity to prevent the morbidity and mortality associated with these infectious diseases and to do so with a significantly favorable cost:benefit. However, each new vaccine would require additional injections which may become so numerous as to discourage widespread immunization. As a consequence, medical practitioners, patients, parents and others are very interested in the development of combination vaccines, whereby individual vaccines are mixed before delivery for administration in a single injection. Such mixing can take place at the point of manufacturing or filling or within a syringe or vial at the time of immunization.

There are two combination vaccines which enjoy widespread pediatric usage in many countries. Diphtheria-tetanus-pertussis (DTP) is a mixture of inactivated, killed or nonreplicating vaccines (5). Measles-mumps-rubella (13) is a mixture of live attenuated vaccines which undergo limited replication in vaccinees. These two vaccines form the basis for future pediatric combination vaccines, since live and nonreplicating vaccines ordinarily are not expected to be compatible for combinations. Currently, *ca.* 12-16 injections are administered to each child in many countries by the age of six. If combination vaccines can be fully developed, there might be only 6-7 injections instead (Table 1). There also may be the opportunity for new combination vaccines for adults. A 23-valent pneumococcal (Pn) vaccine is indicated for older adults (8); also available is a combination of T and D vaccines. With frequent use in adults, a combination of HA and HB vaccines may become useful. Combinations of some of these four vaccines with acellular pertussis and polio also may be attractive and promote increased use of vaccines in adults.

In order for the tremendous promise of combinations vaccines to be fulfilled, there are numerous technical, clinical, manufacturing and marketing challenges to be addressed. The complexity of these challenges is such that the vaccine developer and regulatory

Novel Strategies in Design and Production of Vaccines
Edited by S. Cohen and A. Shafferman, Plenum Press, New York, 1996

Table 1. Potential future U.S. recommendation for pediatric vaccinations

		2 mo.	4 mo.	6 mo.	15 mo.	4-6 yr.
Diphtheria Tetanus Pertussis Haemophilus b Hepatitis B Polio (injected)	DTP-Hib-HepB-IPV	X	X	X	X	X
Measles Mumps Rubella Varicella	M-M-R®II M-M-R-V				X	4-15 yr. (X)

Total # injections = 6-7

agencies treat each combination vaccine as a new product. However, the first issue that must be addressed is that individual vaccines to be combined should be indicated for administration at the same ages as established through clinical trials of each vaccine. The three components of DTP vaccine each were developed as separate vaccines before being combined in the 1940s. A 3-dose primary series in infancy (2-4-6 months of age in some countries, 2-3-4 or 3-4-5 months or similar schedules in other countries) was shown to elicit immune responses that have been associated with protection against clinical disease. Subsequent booster doses are indicated at *ca.* 15-18 months and 4-6 years of age. Therefore, other new individual pediatric vaccines should be evaluated clinically at *ca.* 2, 4, 6 and 15 months of age by coadministration, then ultimate combination with DTP. A major direction in combination vaccine development is the anticipated widespread licensure of acellular pertussis (P_{ac}) vaccines in developed countries. These vaccines, of which at least 8 are in recently completed protective efficacy trials, show much improved tolerability profiles compared to the whole-cell pertussis (P_{wc}) vaccines which have been used for over 40 years. As a result, most new combination vaccines utilize P_{ac} as part of their DTP component. The degree of comparability in protective levels will influence the rate at which P_{ac} vaccines and their combinations replace P_{wc} vaccines in developed countries. However, due to cost and relative supply, it is anticipated that developing countries may continue to use P_{wc}-based vaccines.

The Hib conjugate vaccines are indicated for the prevention of invasive Hib disease in infants and young children. These vaccines consists of the Hib capsular polysaccharide (PRP) of different sizes conjugated to different carrier proteins (in order to make PRP immunogenic in infants): D toxoid (PRP-D), T toxoid (PRP-T), mutant D toxin (HbOC), and meningococcal outer membrane protein complex (PRP-OMPC). HbOC, PRP-OMPC and PRP-T have been licensed for infants in the United States and other countries at *ca.* 2, 4, 6, and 15 months (HbOC, PRP-T) or 2, 4, and 12-15 months of age (PRP-OMPC). Since all these vaccines are compatible with the DTP schedule, DTP_{wc}-Hib combination vaccines have undergone extensive evaluations and have been licensed on the basis of immunogenicity for all 4 component vaccines. DTP/HbOC is mixed at the time of manufacture and filled into vials (16). DTP_{wc} is used to rehydrate the lyophilized PRP-T vaccine at the time of administration (2).

The recombinant-derived HB vaccine is a second-generation product following the plasma-derived HB vaccine (9). Many countries worldwide are adopting policies of routine HB immunization of adolescents or infants as the most effective strategy for reducing the incidence of disease, depending on the country (3). There are two recommended immunization schedules in the United States: *ca.* 0, 1, 6 and 12 months of age to afford an earlier dosing regimen and faster protection and *ca.* 2, 4, 6 and 15 months of age, which is compatible with the DTP dosing schedule. DTP_{wc}/HB and Hib/HB vaccines have been developed and evaluated clinically, which also may serve as stepping-stones toward DTP/Hib/HB.

Both live and inactivated polio vaccines have been available for decades; polio vaccine is itself a combination of three poliovirus strains mixed at the time of manufacture. Developed countries use mostly the live oral polio vaccine (OPV) with use of the inactivated polio vaccine (IPV) increasing, while developing countries use OPV for reasons of relative cost and convenience (no injection). Use of OPV has successfully eradicated wild-type polio from the Western Hemisphere (14) and other developed countries; as a result the only cases of polio in these areas are vaccine-associated. This is stimulating public health officials to potentially recommend routine use of IPV for at least the first two or three doses, especially as part of a combination vaccine, to be followed by OPV. DTP_{wc}/IPV and $DTP_{wc}/IPV/Hib$ vaccines have been licensed in some countries on the way toward the potential $DTP_{wc/ac}/Hib/HB/IPV$ vaccine which would prevent 6 diseases.

The measles, mumps and rubella vaccines were each clinically tested and licensed in the 1960s, then were combined into a single vaccine which was licensed in the 1969 for immunization at 12-15 months of age (13). There have been subsequent recommendations in many countries in the 1980s for a booster dose upon entry to grade school or high school. Recently a live attenuated varicella vaccine (11) has been developed. It was licensed for use in young children in Japan and South Korea in the 1980s and most recently in the United States and Germany for routine immunization of children over 12 months of age. Given the same age indication for immunization, the combination measles-mumps-rubella-varicella vaccine has been tested clinically (4). However, since there are no other live attenuated vaccines which likely will be licensable for routine pediatric use in the foreseeable future, this quadrivalent vaccine represents the most complex cocktail of live vaccines at this time. Furthermore, the challenge of stabilizing these 4 vaccines mixed together has not been trivial.

The second issue for creating new combination vaccines is that the final combination product must be pharmaceutically acceptable in terms of physical interactions, adjuvants, preservatives and excipients and must be stable for a period of long-term storage.

Excipients in combination vaccines originate during the manufacture of an individual vaccine or are added at the point of combination of the vaccines; those derived from individual vaccines do not necessarily contribute to the stability of the final combination product. Buffers in the final mixture may ensure the stability of the component vaccines during long-term storage and may control physical interactions, such as aggregation. Bulking agents, *e.g.* lactose, confer a physical mass to a lyophilized vaccine that renders it visible at the time of reconstitution and administration. Preservatives are used in multidose vials to ensure that contaminating microorganisms inadvertently introduced into the vial by multiple needle punctures of the stopper cannot grow. Preservatives also may be needed in cases where the sterility of vaccines cannot be assured readily. To the extent possible, the concentration of excipients should be tabulated and justified, since a buffer constituent of one component vaccine may affect the stability of another component vaccine in the final combination.

A critically important excipient in most inactivated vaccines is the adjuvant, a nonantigenic component which increases the immune response to the vaccine antigen. The only currently licensed adjuvants are aluminum salts such as phosphate and hydroxide, although many new adjuvants are being evaluated clinically and preclinically (1). Aluminum salts bind noncovalently to inactivated vaccine antigens and influence their presentation to the immune system. There may be physical interactions among different aluminum-adsorbed antigens in a combination which may affect their immunogenicity and stability. This issue may be addressed through the use of appropriately selected aluminum salts for all components and by stably adsorbing each antigen to aluminum before final mixture into a combination. If a component vaccine that is not aluminum adsorbed is mixed with other adsorbed vaccines, the antigen may be adsorbed to aluminum in the course of mixing depending on the particular aluminum and buffer composition. While this adsorption may be desirable in some cases (6), it may be deleterious in other cases. Aluminum salts also can adjuvant any extraneous proteins carried along with an individual vaccine component, with the theoretical possibility of inappropriate immune responses to such proteins.

The chemical nature of all antigens and excipients in the combination vaccine contributes to potential physical interactions among components, with the possibility for noncovalent binding or aggregation which may affect the consistency and stability of the final product. This may lead to the final combination product appearing clumpy, discolored, or otherwise nonuniform in nature, thereby requiring vigorous mixing to ensure uptake into a syringe and delivery. In order to ensure uniformity of the final suspension for ease of administration by the medical practitioner, the formulation of individual component antigens or buffers should be optimized. This becomes an increasing challenge as the number of individual vaccines to be combined increases. Furthermore, since each component antigen (with aluminum) must occupy a certain minimum volume to retain stability, there is a yet-to-be-determined limitation to the total number of component vaccines that can be combined while retaining stability and physical uniformity of the mixture.

It is desirable from a marketing perspective that a vaccine be stable for a minimum of 18 months to 2 years to assure full use of inventory in the field. Hence, the vaccine developer must define the expiration date, *i.e.*, the end of dating period, of the final filled product. The dating period is established by a program of stability studies of each of the component vaccines in combination by analytical assays that measure stability. In this regard, the most important assays measure properties of the vaccine which correlate with immunogenicity. The dating period must be independently established for each presentation, *e.g.*, a prefilled syringe or a vial, whether single, 5-dose, 15-doses, *etc.*, at the intended temperature of storage (typically 2-8°C, sometimes frozen). Furthermore, the dating period within the production facility for each individual bulk component vaccine before mixing into combination must be determined.

There are instances where there is inherent incompatibility among vaccines or their associated stabilizers or preservatives. For example, many DTP_{wc} vaccines contain thimerosal as preservative, which cannot readily be removed from the production process. For making a combination vaccine, it has been shown that thimerosal gradually destroys the immunogenic potency of IPV (7). To circumvent this incompatibility, DTP_{wc} and IPV are filled into separate chambers of a two-chambered syringe, such that instantaneous mixing occurs only at the time of injection.

The third issue for combination vaccines is clinical evaluation with proper controls. Important elements of evaluation include study design, tolerability, immunogenicity and efficacy.

Combination vaccines ordinarily are constituted of vaccines which either individually (*e.g.*, HB, Hib) or in combination (*e.g.*, DTP) have been licensed previously. In order to afford the best comparison with its component vaccines, clinical studies of combination vaccines should be well controlled. Separate study arms would compare the new combination with its licensed components, *e.g.*, Hib/HB would be compared with concomitant administration into separate sites of Hib and HB and each injected separately and DTP/Hib with

DTP and Hib (not each of D, T, P and Hib). Controlled studies which are prospective, randomized and multicentered would provide the opportunity to detect safety-related and immunological interactions among the vaccines.

As revealed in well-controlled safety studies, the adverse-experience profile of a combination vaccine may be expected to be no worse than that of the component vaccine which is least well tolerated. Generally a certain minimum number of subjects (*e.g.*, >1000) should have received the combination vaccine in order to be able to tabulate its relatively safety. There also may be new rare adverse experiences, *e.g.*, 1 per 10,000 vaccinees, that cannot be observed in the limited number of subjects tested prelicensure. Hence, postmarketing safety studies and national reporting through routine vaccine usage (*e.g.*, the Vaccine Adverse Experience Reporting System in the United States) may enable such rare events to be documented.

The immune response to a particular vaccine generally should not be significantly lower in a combination than when administered separately. If lower, the issue would be whether there is clinical significance in terms of actual increased risk of disease in the combination. For instance, in a trial in which Hib and DTP_{wc} were mixed and coadministered in the same syringe, the anti-pertussis antibody responses were significantly lower in the DTP_{wc}/Hib group than in the DTP_{wc}-only group (12). The immunological basis for such lower responses, termed immunological interference, is not well understood. On the other hand, immunological enhancement has been observed; the DTP_{wc}/HbOC combination vaccine elicits higher immune responses against most of the vaccine antigens than do DTP_{wc} and HbOC administered concomitantly in different arms (16). Neither immunological enhancement nor interference is routinely observed in preclinical evaluations in animals, which means that the results of clinical evaluations can be empirical.

It is ordinarily not possible for ethical reasons to evaluate the efficacy of a combination vaccine in a placebo-controlled clinical trial, given that its component vaccines have been proven or accepted as efficacious. Thus, efficacy of component vaccines in combination is judged from a surrogate assay for efficacy, a serological assay whose results have been shown to correlate with protection from disease. One of the best known surrogate assays is the anti-HBs assay for antibodies to HB surface antigen, in which an anti-HBs response ≥ 10 mIU/mL has been shown to correlate with protection against hepatitis B (10). Thus, the percent of vaccinees with anti-HBs ≥ 10 mIU/mL becomes the key readout for the efficacy of HB vaccine in a combination.

The fourth issue for combination vaccines is manufacturing and associated regulatory affairs. There are many quality-control assays which are performed on each bulk component vaccine before mixing and on both the bulk combination vaccine and final filled vials or syringes. All assays on all components and on the combination must give satisfactory results for the vaccine to be released for clinical evaluation or to the market. In addition, 3-5 consecutive manufacturing batches must be produced during development as consistency lots, which prove the consistency of manufacture of the combination product. Consistency is judged by the results of all quality-control assays as well as by the results of clinical trials on the consistency lots. Furthermore, consistency lots are put into stability studies as described above in order to validate the dating period for the final filled vaccine. The number of quality-control assays on a combination vaccine is much higher than for a single-component vaccine; hence, combination products are more complex from both a manufacturing and regulatory perspective.

The final issue for combination vaccines relates to marketing. Combination products offer a significant opportunity to simplify immunization schedules by decreasing the number of injections per visit. However, there are many related combinations available or being developed (DTP/Hib, DTP/IPV, Hib/HB, DTP/HB, DTP/HB/Hib, DTP/HB/Hib/IPV) which may create confusion for medical practitioners in both the private and public sectors. Hence, companies will need to present these products in simple form to these groups, assuring clear labeling with respect to identity of component vaccines, compatibility/incompatibility with other vaccines, and flexibility of age of administration. Different medical practitioners will prefer different presentations, single- or multi-dose vial or prefilled syringe. The most widely used combination products likely will be those which incorporate the largest number of vaccines in presentations preferred by the medical community in a particular country and labelled as clearly as possible.

REFERENCES

1. Allison, A.C., and Byars, N.E., 1992, Immunological adjuvants and their mode of action. In R.W. Ellis (ed.), Vaccines: New approaches to immunological problems. Stoneham, MA. Butterworth Publishers, 431-449.

2. Avendana, A., Ferreccia, C., Lagos, R., *et al. Haemophilus influenzae* type *b* polysaccharide-tetanus protein conjugate vaccine does not depress serologic responses to diphtheria, tetanus or pertussis antigens when coadministered in the same syringe with diphtheria-tetanus-pertussis vaccine at two, four and six months of age, *Pediatr Infect Dis J,* 1993, 12: 638-643.

3. Calandra, G.B., and West, D.J. Recommendations for prevention of hepatitis B with vaccine. In R.W. Ellis (ed.), Hepatitis B vaccines in clinical practice. New York: Marcel Dekker, 1993, 1-16.

4. Dennehy, P.H., Saracen, C.L., and Peter, G. Seroconversion rates to combined measles-mumps-rubella-varicella vaccine of children with upper respiratory tract infection, *Pediatrics,* 1994, 94: 514-516.

5. Giebing, P.G., Hall, C.B., and Plotkin, S.A. (eds.). Reports of the Committee on Infectious Diseases, 20th ed. Elk Grove Village, IL: American Academy of Pediatrics, 1986.

6. Paradiso, P.R., Hogerman, D. A., Madore, D.V., *et al.* Safety and immunogenicity of a combined diphtheria, tetanus, pertussis and *Haemophilus influenzae* type *b* vaccine in young infants, *Pediatrics,* 1993, 92: 827-832.

7. Sawyer, L.A., McInnis, J., Patel, A., *et al.* Deleterious effect of thimerosal on the potency of inactivated poliovirus vaccine, *Vaccine ,* 1994, 12: 851-856.

8. Shapiro, E.D., Berg, A.T., Austrian, R., *et al.* The protective efficacy of polyvalent pneumococcal polysaccharide vaccine, *New Eng J Med,* 1991, 325, 1453-1460.

9. Stevens, C.E., Taylor, P.E., Tong, M.J., *et al.* Yeast-recombinant hepatitis B vaccine: Efficacy with hepatitis B immune globulin in prevention of perinatal hepatitis B virus transmission, *JAMA,* 1987, 257, 2612-2616.

10. Szmuness, W., Stevens, C.E., Zang, E.A., *et al.* Controlled clinical trial of the efficacy of the hepatitis B vaccine (Heptavax B): A final report, *Hepatology,* 1981, 1, 377-385.

11. Takahashi, M., Okuno, Y., Otsuka, T., *et al.* , Development of a live attenuated varicella vaccine. *Biken,* 1975, 18, 25-33.

12. Watemberg, N., Dagan, R., Arbelli, Y., *et al.* Safety and immunogenicity of *Haemophilus influenzae* type *b*-tetanus protein conjugate vaccine, mixed in the same syringe with diphtheria-tetanus-pertussis vaccine in young infants, *Pediatr Infect Dis J,* 1991, 10, 758-763.

13. Weibel, R.E., Buynak, E.B., McLean, A.A., *et al.* Follow-up surveillance for antibody in human subjects following live attenuated measles, mumps and rubella virus vaccines. *Proc Soc Exp Biol Med,* 1979, 162: 328.

14. World Health Organization, Weekly Epidemiological Record, April 7, 1995, pp. 97-101.

18

POLYSACCHARIDE CONJUGATE VACCINES FOR THE PREVENTION OF GRAM-POSITIVE BACTERIAL INFECTIONS

Robert Naso and Ali Fattom

W. W. Karakawa Microbial Pathogenesis Laboratory
Univax Biologics, Inc.
12280 Wilkins Avenue, Rockville, Maryland, 20852

Among the most problematic Gram-positive bacteria with regard to human pathology are Staphylococcal species including *S. aureus* and *S. epidermidis*, Enterococcal species including *E. faecalis* and *E. faecium*, and Streptococcus species including *S. pneumoniae* and Group B Streptococcus, among others.

1. INTRODUCTION

Infections by most, if not all of these Gram-positive bacteria, have been of growing medical concern due to an increased incidence of infection observed especially in hospitals and other health care institutions world-wide. As an example, over the last 10 years, the number of combined staphylococcal blood stream infections in the U.S. has increased from just over 0.5 infections per 1000 discharges in 1980 to more than 3.0 such infections in 1990[2]. This is in comparison to the relatively stable number of blood stream infections with Gram-negative bacteria, which has remained between 1.5-2.0 infections per 1000 discharges over this same period. Today, *S. aureus* is the most common organism causing bacteremia, accounting for about 25% of blood isolates[3].

Even more disturbing is the increasing trend toward antibiotic resistance shown by these and other Gram-positive bacteria. There has been an inexorable increase in antibiotic resistance among staphylococci over the last several decades until today when 30-50 percent of *S. aureus* infections are resistant to most antibiotics, leaving these isolates sensitive only to Vancomycin[15]. The alarming appearance of Vancomycin resistance among enterococci, the incidence of which is 15-20% or more[4], raises the specter that soon both staphylococci and enterococci will be untreatable with antibiotics. Many investigators are fearful that this trend will lead us to a return to the days before antibiotics when staphylococci killed tens of thousands of people each year.

Those at highest risk of infection by Gram-positive bacteria are those who are hospitalized. Patients undergoing major surgery, victims of severe trauma, patients in

Novel Strategies in Design and Production of Vaccines
Edited by S. Cohen and A. Shafferman, Plenum Press, New York, 1996

intensive care units, those receiving transplants and very low birth weight neonates are at major risk of infection, as are cancer and AIDS patients and those on dialysis for end-stage kidney disease. Infections include bacteremia, surgical wound and deep tissue infections, pneumonia and peritonitis, and these infections often progress to sepsis and septic shock. Mortality rates from hospital acquired infections with these bacteria can be as high as 40% and the morbidity associated with these infections greatly increases the cost of medical care not to mention the increase in pain and suffering associated with these infections.

2. RESULTS AND DISCUSSION

With this backdrop, it should be clear that the development of alternative methods to prevent and treat Gram-positive bacterial infections in at-risk populations is of great importance. Scientists at Univax Biologics, Inc., in collaboration with many investigators including Drs. Robbins and Schneerson at the NIH, are developing vaccines which have great promise as effective antimicrobials to combat Gram-positive bacterial infections. Our strategy is being applied to both Gram-positive and Gram-negative bacteria but in this article we will limit our consideration to the Gram-positive bacteria and concentrate primarily on staphylococci, especially *S. aureus*. We are developing a core immunization technology that will result in vaccines that can prevent bacterial infections in immunocompetent individuals who are at long term risk for infection. Such individuals include, for example, peritoneal and hemodialysis patients and individuals with prosthetic devices such as hip replacements.

There remains, however, a population of patients who are at very high and very immediate risk for infection - who either don't have time to respond to a vaccine, or because they are immunocompromised, cannot respond adequately to a vaccine. These individuals include shock trauma patients, neonates, emergency surgery patients and cancer and AIDS patients.

An example of the problem can be seen in an evaluation of *S. aureus* infections in shock trauma patients. A recent study at the University of Maryland at Baltimore Hospital shows that there is a biphasic trend in *S. aureus* infections. The overall incidence of *S. aureus* infections in those admitted to the shock-trauma unit was approximately 8%. A high incidence of *S. aureus* pneumonia and bacteremia (30/57) can be seen within ten days of admission to the trauma unit, followed by a second period of increased infections (7/57) 20-30 days later (Fattom, manuscript in preparation). While it is possible that the second period of risk could be addressed by a vaccine, clearly the first could not. Another way of protecting these individuals must be found. For these individuals, we are developing specific human polyclonal antibodies for use to passively immunize against disease. In this scenario, the vaccine, now called an immunizing agent, is used to immunize normal, healthy people who then donate their plasma. From the pooled, donated plasma is generated purified polyclonal antibodies that contain a high titer of antibody to the vaccine components. These purified antibodies are then administered to patients who are otherwise at immediate risk for infection. The circulating half-life of such antibodies is usually in the order of 14-21 days - so passive immunization such as this can be expected to provide protection for perhaps as long as a month, although additional dosing at monthly intervals is possible, if needed, to extend protection even longer.

As with any strategy to approach a complex biological issue, the devil is in the details.

First and foremost, is the question of selection of the appropriate target antigen as the vaccine and immunizing agent. What component of Gram-positive bacteria will induce antibodies that will be protective? Ideally, a highly immunogenic surface component shared by clinically significant isolates and integrally involved in *S. aureus* pathogenicity would be the best target. In a search for such a vaccine candidate and to better understand the

Type 5:   →4)-βD-Man*p*NAcA(1→4)-αL-Fuc*p*NAc(1→3)-βD-Fuc*p*NAc(1-
                         3
                         ↑
                        *O*Ac

Type 8:   →3)-βD-Man*p*NAcA(1→3)-αL-Fuc*p*NAc(1→3)-βD-Fuc*p*NAc(1-
                         4
                         ↑
                        *O*Ac

Figure 1. Structures of Type 5 and Type 8 *S. aureus* capsular polysaccharides[8,14].

pathogenicity of *S. aureus*, a number of investigators including Karakawa, Vann, Fournier, Robbins, Arbeit and Fattom used a series of antibodies to whole cell vaccines and later a series of monoclonal antibodies to evaluate different *S. aureus* clinical isolates[1,9,22] (Fattom, unpublished results). They showed that all clinical *S. aureus* isolates possess capsular polysaccharides, and they determined that there were at least 8 such capsular types. Initially, it was feared that any vaccine composed of *S. aureus* capsular polysaccharides must contain all 8 polysaccharides. Of all the clinical isolates examined, however, two capsular types, type 5 and type 8, were the predominant types causing infections. In fact, it is now known that approximately 90% of all clinical isolates of *S. aureus* fall into these two capsular types.

Karakawa also showed that production of polysaccharides was significantly reduced in the presence of phosphorus at levels that might be used in common growth media. It has also been shown that when *S. aureus* is grown to stationary phase in low phosphate media, visible capsules could be observed by microscopy[9]. Subsequently, Fattom and his colleagues at the NIH, showed that significant amounts of polysaccharide could be purified from bacteria grown *in vitro* [5-8].

The structures of the repeating units in the type 5 and type 8 capsular polysaccharides have now been determined (Figure 1).

Notice that the structures of these two capsular polysaccharides are similar in that both are linear copolymers composed of repeat units containing one mole of *O*-acetylated mannoseamineuronic acid and two moles of fucosamine. Differences between these two capsular polysaccharides regarding glycosidic linkages and O-acetylation sites, however, make these two structurally related capsular polysaccharides immunologically distinct; antibodies to one do not recognize the other[10]. The implication of these observations is clearly that a vaccine composed of *S. aureus* capsular polysaccharide may be effective but in order to be effective it must contain both type 5 and type 8 capsular polysaccharides.

In addition, true to their title as capsular polysaccharides, *S. aureus* types 5 and 8 capsular polysaccharides have two other properties that qualify them as true capsular polysaccharides - that is, *S. aureus* capsular polysaccharides promote both bacterial virulence and bacterial survival in blood[11,12,13].

The ability of capsular polysaccharide to promote bacterial survival and an early hint of the protective value of antibodies to capsular polysaccharides can be shown in a rather simple experiment in which encapsulated bacteria (grown to stationary phase) and non-encapsulated bacteria (grown to early log phase) are incubated in human whole blood. The unencapsulated bacteria are quickly killed while the encapsulated bacteria survive incubation in whole blood. However, addition of antibodies to *S. aureus* capsular polysaccharides facilitate the killing of the encapsulated bacteria (Figure 2).

Proving that *S. aureus* capsular polysaccharides are virulence promoting factors took more effort but it has now been clearly shown that encapsulated *S. aureus* is more potent than unencapsulated *S. aureus* in a mouse mortality model. In an experiment in which mice were injected intraperitoneally with 10^5 CFU of encapsulated *S. aureus* (grown to stationary

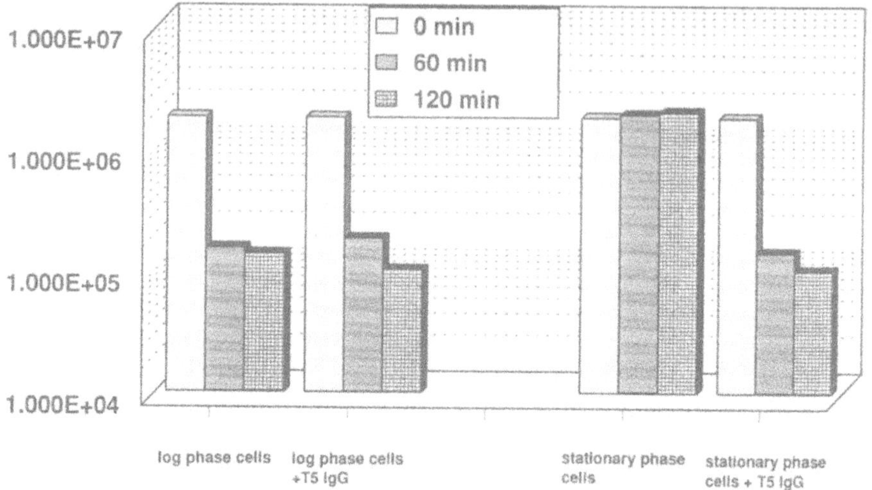

Figure 2. Viability of *S. aureus* in whole blood and the effect of specific antibodies (IgG).

phase) or the same number of unencapsulated *S. aureus* (grown to log phase), the mortality after 24 hours was 40 % for the unencapsulated bacteria and 80% for the encapsulated bacteria. After 48 hours, the mortality was 50% for the unencapsulated bacteria and 90% for the encapsulated bacteria (Fattom, *et al.*, manuscript in preparation).

Other studies have shown that the type 5 and type 8 *S. aureus* capsular polysaccharides are non-immunogenic in mice and this property has been shown for other polysaccharides to be predictive of immunogenicity in immunocompromised individuals[16,17]. In order to increase their immunogenicity, the polysaccharides have been conjugated to carrier proteins and the immunogenicity of the conjugates have been evaluated in mice where they have been shown to be highly immunogenic raising significant levels of capsular polysaccharide specific antibodies[5,6,7]. Two such conjugate polysaccharide vaccines composed of capsular polysaccharide conjugated either to *P. aeruginosa* exotoxin A or to recombinant exoprotein A (rEPA), a non-toxic form of exotoxin A, have been further evaluated for safety and immunogenicity in humans[7] (Welch et al., manuscript in preparation; Fattom, et al., manuscript in preparation).

The bivalent form of the capsular polysaccharides, which contains both type 5 and type 8 polysaccharides conjugated to rEPA, is called StaphVAX. StaphVAX has now been evaluated for safety and immunogenicity in over 80 volunteers including 40 healthy volunteers and 40 individuals with end-stage renal disease (ESRD).

The safety profile of StaphVAX has been excellent. There was some mild, local reactogenicity in about 30% of the vaccine recipients and very mild systemic symptoms in a few patients.

The immunogenicity of the bivalent conjugate vaccine in healthy volunteers has also been excellent. Response rates to the vaccine were in the >90% range. Geometric mean titers of capsular polysaccharide specific antibodies as measured by ELISA reached 50-100 ug/ml in the responders (those responding to both capsular polysaccharides with >25 µg/ml specific antibody levels and levels 4-times pre-immunization levels) two weeks after a single dose of the vaccine. The peak levels of antibodies were in the 70-170 ug/ml range six weeks after the immunization and levels in the 50-100 ug/ml range remained in the circulation for more than a year.

In other studies, antibodies from rabbits and normal healthy human donors immunized with StaphVAX were tested in opsonophagocytosis assays[6]. In this assay, bacteria are mixed with complement and with human polymorphonuclear cells either in the presence or absence of antibodies from immunized or control individuals. If the antibodies opsonize or coat the bacteria, they are capable of enhancing the ability of the PMN cells to phagocytose the bacteria. The results showed that both sera and purified IgG from either rabbits or humans immunized with StaphVAX has the ability to stimulate the phagocytosis of homologous *S. aureus* by human PMN cells *in vitro* (results not shown).

In ESRD patients, the response rates to StaphVAX were about 60%, lower than that seen in healthy volunteers. Peak geometric mean antibody titers in ESRD patients were in the 50-120 ug/ml range in the responders, with titers in the 40-70 ug/ml range persisting for greater than 26 weeks post-immunization. While the response rates to the vaccine are lower than desired in the ESRD study, preliminary data indicate that an improvement in response rates may be achievable by increasing the dose of vaccine and/or by giving a booster injection of vaccine. Additional dosing studies are underway.

It is also important to note that, to date, StaphVAX has only been tested in humans in a saline formulation. Results in animals (not shown) indicate that increased immune responses to the vaccine can be achieved if the vaccine is formulated in adjuvants such as monophosphoryl Lipid A (Ribi ImmunoChem Research, Inc., Hampton, Montana), Stimulon™ (Cambridge Biotech, Worcester, Massachusetts) and in Novasomes™ (Novasome, Inc., Rockville, Maryland), a non-phospholipid liposome-like delivery system (Fattom, *et al.*, manuscript in preparation). Additional animal studies are underway evaluating these adjuvants and human studies with one or more of these adjuvants may be initiated later this year.

Supported by these results, a Phase II clinical study of StaphVAX in 100 vaccinated chronic ambulatory peritoneal dialysis (CAPD) patients is also now underway. These patients are reportedly at high risk for staphylococcal infections. Results relating to immunogenicity and infection rates are expected from this study around the end of this summer.

Also underway are Phase 1 donor stimulation studies which are clinical studies in potential plasma donors to determine safety, immunogenicity and the parameters of antibody production in plasma donors during and after repeated plasmapheresis. These studies are expected to be expanded toward the end of this year so that we may begin collecting larger amounts of stimulated plasma from vaccinated donors. Antibody will be purified from these plasma pools for passive immunization studies. The IgG antibody generated in this fashion is referred to as StaphGAM. Research pools of plasma from vaccinated donors have already been made, as have been research lots of StaphGAM.

While we await data relating to efficacy from human studies, we are encouraged by the relatively good immunogenicity of the conjugate *S. aureus* vaccine in normal healthy volunteers. The high titers of antibody and the longevity of the antibody response in healthy volunteers bodes well for our interest in using this vaccine in plasma donors to raise antibodies for passive immunization of at risk patients.

As a surrogate for data on efficacy in humans (which will come from subsequent studies) we do have promising results for both active and passive immunization in animal models.

In the active immunization model, mice are immunized subcutaneously (SQ) with three injections of StaphVAX at 2.5 ug/mouse administered at two week intervals. Control mice are sham immunized with saline. Mice are then challenged intraperitoneally (IP) with 2×10^5 CFU *S. aureus* in the presence of 5-6% hog mucin, a reagent which has been shown to potentiate killing by the bacteria. The results four days after challenge show 80% survival in the vaccinated group and only 30% survival in the saline control group. The protective

Table 1. Passive immunity against *S. aureus* type 5 challenge in mice

Group	3 Hrs post-challenge mortality	24 Hrs post-challenge mortality	48 Hrs post challenge mortality
648 µg StaphGAM	0/5	0/5	0/5 (0%)
342 µg StaphGAM	0/5	1/5	1/5 (20%)
162 µg StaphGAM	0/5	1/5	1/5 (20%)
72 µg StaphGAM	0/5	2/5	2/5 (40%)
Standard IgG	0/5	4/5	4/5 (80%)
Saline	0/5	5/5	5/5 (100%)
Saline; challenged with 5% mucin only	0/5	0/5	0/5 (0%)

value of active vaccination is statistically significant with a P value of 0.04 (Fattom, *et al.*, manuscript in preparation).

In order to test efficacy of passive immunization using antibodies generated to StaphVAX, we injected mice IP with various levels of StaphGAM. This antibody was generated in normal, healthy volunteers which had been vaccinated with StaphVAX. The IgG antibody was purified from the pooled plasma from the vaccinated individuals by Cohn fractionation. Twenty four hours after receiving the antibodies, the mice were challenged IP with 2×10^5 CFU *S. aureus* in hog mucin. The results (Table 1) show that StaphGAM is able to provide protection from mortality in a dose dependent fashion; with 40% mortality in mice receiving the low 72 ug dose of StaphGAM to 0% mortality in mice receiving the high 648 ug dose of StaphGAM (P<0.05). Standard IgG given at the high dose was not able to afford any protection to the mice.

In an attempt to determine if passive immunization given sub-cutaneously to the mice would protect against IP challenge, we injected mice sub-cutaneously with 400 ug of StaphGAM IgG (Table 2). Forty-eight hours later, the mice were challenged IP with 2×10^5 CFU of *S. aureus* in hog mucin. While control standard IgG provided no significant protection (10/15 mice died), the mice receiving StaphGAM were protected from mortality associated with the challenge (P<0.05).

3. SUMMARY AND CONCLUSIONS

In summary, the type 5 and type 8 capsular polysaccharides of *S. aureus* are characterized as having properties conducive to their use as vaccines to prevent and/or treat *S. aureus* infections or for use as immunizing agents to raise specific polyclonal antibodies

Table 2. Subcutaneous passive immunization against *S. aureus* challenge in mice: Mortality between 16 hr and 6 days post-challenge

Group	Mortality between 16 Hr and 6 Days Post-Challenge							
	16h	18hr	20hr	24hr	42hr	4day	5day	6day
StaphGAM SQ	0/15	0/15	0/15	0/15	0/15	0/15	0/15	1/15
Control IgG SQ	2/15	2/15	3/15	3/15	6/15	9/15	10/15	10/15
Saline SQ	1/6	1/6	3/6	4/6	4/6	4/6	4/6	5/6
Saline SQ; challenged with 5 % mucin only	0/6	0/6	0/6	0/6	0/6	0/6	0/6	0/6

for passive immunization of those at risk for *S. aureus* infections. These properties of the type 5 and type 8 *S. aureus* capsular polysaccharides are summarized as follows. Compared to proteins, *S. aureus* capsular polysaccharides have a simple structure - they are polymers of repeating units and the polymers vary in length. The repeat units of the polysaccharides contain one mole of mannoseamineuronic acid and two moles of fucosamine. The immunodeterminants on the capsular polysaccharide are directed primarily to glycosidic bonds and antigenic side groups such as *O*-acetylation sites. The capsular polysaccharides are surface components, they are available exposed on the bacterial surface, and they are formed preferentially under growth conditions of low phosphate and in late log and stationary phase of growth. Capsular polysaccharides are virulence promoting factors and they protect *S. aureus* against phagocytosis and complement mediated killing. Type 5 and type 8 capsular polysaccharides make up approximately 90% of all clinical *S. aureus* isolates. Low titers of antibodies to type 5 and type 8 capsular polysaccharides are present in many healthy humans, but capsular polysaccharides alone are poor, T-cell independent immunogens. The capsular polysaccharides can be made immunogenic by conjugation to carrier proteins and the immunogenicity of the conjugates can be increased through the use of adjuvants. Capsular polysaccharide conjugate vaccines are safe and immunogenic in humans, and antibodies to capsular polysaccharides are opsonic and induce opsonophagocytosis *in vitro*. Active immunization with a capsular polysaccharide conjugate vaccine (StaphVAX) and passive immunization with antibodies to StaphVAX (StaphGAM) can provide protection against *S. aureus* challenge in animal models

While the impressive results in animal models, may or may not be predictive of the value of active and passive immunization in humans, we are optimistic that vaccines to Gram-positive bacteria, such as *S. aureus* can be made and will be effective. Results in the next few years from clinical trials of StaphVAX and StaphGAM should be forthcoming and will determine the true promise of this approach to preventing serious bacterial infections. Univax is also well along in developing similar vaccines for *S. epidermidis* and for enterococci. A combination vaccine and a combination specific polyclonal antibody addressing these three Gram-positive pathogens may be extremely important armaments in the war against nosocomial bacterial infections.

4. REFERENCES

1. Arbeit, R. D., W. W. Karakawa, Vann, W. F. and Robbins, J.B., 1984, Predominance of two newly described capsular polysaccharide types among clincial isolates of *Staphylococcus aureus*. Diagn. Microbiol. Infect. Dis. 2:85-91.
2. Banerjee, S. N., Emori, T. G., Culver, D. H., Gaynes, R. P., Jarvis, W. R., Horan, T. J., Edwards, J. R., Tolson, J., Henderson, T., Martone, W. J , Secular Trends in Nosocomial Primary Bloodstream Infections in the United States, 1980-1989, Am. J. Med., 1991, 91:865-895.
3. Centers for Disease Control, 1991, Mortality patterns - United States, 1988, Morbid. Mortal. Weekly Rep., 40:493-502.
4. Centers for Disease Control, 1993, Nosocomial Enterococci Resistant to Vancomycin - United States, 1989-1993, Morbid. Mortal. Weekly Rep., 42:597-599.
5. Fattom, A., Schneerson, R., Szu, S. C., Vann, W. F., Shiloach, J., Karakawa, W. W., and Robbins, J. B., 1990, Synthesis and immunologic properties in mice of vaccines composed of *Staphylococcus aureus* type 5 and type 8 capsular polysaccharides conjugated to *Pseudomonas aeruginosa* exotoxin A, Infect. and Immun. 58:2367-2374.
6. Fattom, A., Schneerson, R., Watson, D. C., Karakawa, W. W., Fitzgerald, D., Pastan, I., Li, X., Shiloach, J., Bryla, D. A., and Robbins, J. B., 1993, Laboratory and clinical evaluation of conjugate vaccines composed of *Staphylococcus aureus* type 5 and type 8 capsular polysaccharides bound to *Pseudomonas aeruginosa* recombinant exoprotein A, Infect. and Immun. 61:1023-1032.

7. Fattom, A., Shiloach, J., Bryla, D., Fitzgerald, D., Pastan, I., Karakawa, W. W., Robbins, J. B., and Schneerson, R., 1992, Comparitive immunogenicity of conjugates composed of the *Staphylococcus aureus* type 8 capsular polysaccharide bound to carrier proteins by adipic acid dihydrazide or N-succinimidyl-3-(2- pyridyldithio)propionate, Infect. and Immun. 60:584-589.

8. Fournier, J.M., Vann, W. F. and Karakawa, W. W., 1984, Purification and characterization of *Staphylococcus aureus* type 8 capsular polysaccaride, Infect. Immun. 45:87-93.

9. Hochkeppel, H. K., Braun, D. G., Vischer, W., Imm, A., Sutter, S., Staebubli, U., Genheim, R., Kaplan, E. L., Boutonnier, A. and Fournier, J. M., 1987, Serotyping and electorn microscopy studies of *Staphylococcus aureus* clinical isolates with monoclonal antobodies to capsular polysaccharides types 5 and 8, J. Clin. Microbiol. 25:526-530.

10. Karakawa, W. W. and Vann, W. F., 1982, Capsular polysaccharides of *Staphyloccus aureus*, Semin. Infect. Dis. 4:285-293.

11. Karakawa, W. W., Sutton, A., Schneerson, R., Karpas, A., and Vann, W. F., 1988, Capsular antibodies induce type-specific phagocytosis of *Staphylococcus aureus* by human polymorphonuclear leukocytes, Infect. Immun. 56:1090-1095.

12. Karakawa, W. W., Fournier, J.-M., Vann, W. F., Arbeit, Schneerson, R., and Robbins, J.B, 1986, Methods for the serological typing of the capsular polysaccharides of *Staphylococcus aureus*, J. Clin. Microbiol. 22:445-447.

13. Karakawa, W. W., 1992, Editorial. The role of capsular polysaccharide antigens in *Staphylococcus aureus*. Int. J. Med. Microbiol. 277:415-418.

14. Moreau, M., Richards, J. C., Fournier, J-M., Byrd, R. A., Karakawa, W. W., and Vann, W. F., 1990, The structure of the type 5 capsular polysaccharide of *Staphylococcus aureus*. Carbohydr. Res. 201:285-297.

15. Panililio, A. L., Culver, D. H., Gaynes, R. P., Banerjee, S., Henderson, T. S., Tolson, J. S., and Martone, W. J., Methicillin-resistant Staphylococcus aureus in U.S. hospitals, 1975-1991, Infec. Control and Hosp. Epidemiol., 1992, 13:582-586.

16. Robbins, J. B., and Schneerson, R., 1990, Polysaccharide-protein conjugates. A new generation of vaccines. J. Infect., Dis. 161:821-832.

17. Robbins, J. B., Schneerson, R., Vann, W. F., Bryla, D. A., and Fattom, A., 1995, Prevention of systemic infections caused by Group B Streptococcus and *Staphylococcus aureus* by multivalent polysaccharide-protein conjugate vaccines. NYAS: Combined Vaccines, New York Acadamy of Science Annals, In Press.

19

PRODUCTION OF INFLUENZA VIRUS IN CELL CULTURES FOR VACCINE PREPARATION

O.-W. Merten,[1] C. Hannoun,[2] J.-C. Manuguerra,[2] F. Ventre,[2] and S. Petres[1]

Institut Pasteur
[1] Laboratoire de Technologie Cellulaire
[2] Unité d'Ecologie Virale
25, rue du Docteur Roux, F-75015 Paris, France

ABSTRACT

Influenza virus strains of different types for use as an inactivated vaccine have been successfully grown in different cell lines. Increasing titres were obtained with BHK-21/BRS, VERO and MDCK cells. Cultures in stationary flasks, in spinner cultures or in large bioreactor systems were tested and the optimal conditions were studied. MDCK cells grown in serum-free medium before and during the virus production phase were found to yield high titres in the presence of trypsin. Satisfactory results were obtained with egg-adapted strains of human and equine origin as well as with strains just isolated from human patients without any further passages in eggs or cell culture.

INTRODUCTION

Virus for influenza vaccine is massively produced in chick embryos and it is necessary to obtain and to process large numbers of embryonated eggs for a routine production. In case of the emergency of a new virus strain, production of a large number of vaccine doses would be difficult and a simpler method would be necessary. In addition, recent data show that passage in chick embryos induces or facilitates changes in the structure of the hemagglutinin and of other genes of the virus, making it different from the wild form (Oxford et al., 1987, 1991, Robertson et al., 1987, Wang et al., 1989). There is more concern about the sequence changes in the hemagglutinin since the antibodies elicited by the vaccine will not correspond exactly to the constitution of the epidemic virus (Wood et al., 1989).

Early attempts to grow the virus in cell cultures have been only poorly successful, except in primary monkey kidney cell cultures, and even so, the titres obtained were not satisfactory. The introduction of trypsine into the culture media changed the situation and several cell types were then used for virus isolation or culture. However, the amount of virus produced was not always high enough to reach production requirements (Pyhala et al., 1987).

In our experiments, the first attempts were made using Vero cells (monkey) because these cells have already been accepted for the production of other inactivated vaccines. Then, other cells such as BHK-21/BRS (hamster) and MDCK (dog) were also used in further experiments for the sake of comparison.

Experiments were first conducted in small scale microcarrier cultures in order to study the effects of medium changes. Here, cell growth as well as virus production were compared when serum-containing (SCM) or serum-free (SFM) media were used for cell growth. Virus inoculation and production was always done in SFM. In a second step, large amounts of cells were used in agitated cultures using microcarriers. Finally, the conditions for bioreactor systems have been developed for the production of larger volumes of virus suspension.

MATERIALS AND METHODS

Cells and cell culture: The following three cell lines were used: Vero cells (WHO-1878) were obtained from Dr. F. Horaud (Institut Pasteur, Unité de Virologie Médicale), BHK-21 C13 were adapted at the Institut Pasteur to growth in suspension in SFM, this so adapted clone was named BHK-21/BRS (Merten et al., 1994, Perrin et al., 1995), MDCK were originally obtained from NIH, (Bethesda, USA). The cells were grown in SFM: Vero and BHK-21/BRS in MDSS2 (Merten et al., 1994) (Axcell Biotechnologies, n° 34601), and MDCK in a slightly modified version of MDSS2. In the case of Vero cells, a part of the routine cultures were kept in SCM (DMEM (Axcell Biotechnologies, n° 35213SP) + 2% new born calf serum (NCS), Gibco). In general, the cells were passed once (Vero, MDCK) or twice (BHK-21/BRS) a week. The cells have been tested for absence of mycoplasmas.

All cells used for the study are coming from stocks in liquid nitrogen, frozen in the culture medium to which 10% dimethylsulfoxid and in the case of the SFM methylcellulose (0.1%) have been added (Merten et al., 1995).

Small scale microcarrier batch cultures for media comparison: Cells were washed once with PBS, trypsinized with trypsine/versene (0.25%/0.01% final concentrations), and washed twice with the medium to be used. The cultures were started with $2*10^5$ c/ml in the presence of the microcarriers (Dormacell 2.6, Pfeifer & Langen) by using a culture volume of 25ml. After onset, the tubes were agitated at 8rpm at 37° C (Thermolyne agitator). 50% of the media were changed at the following time points: 145h, 240h, 313h, and 597.75h after sedimentation of the microcarriers. For cell counting, samples of 0.5ml were taken from each culture and were treated with 0.5ml 0.1M citric acid containing 0.1% crystal violet. After incubation at 37 °C for at least one hour, the released cell nuclei were counted.

At 409.25h the cells were infected with influenza virus (A/Shanghai) already passed on Vero cells for several times: The cells/microcarriers were washed twice with Hank's solution, the cells were infected with 1ml (SCM-culture) or with 0.4ml (SFM-culture) of a diluted virus suspension (1/10) in 10 ml SFM. After an incubation of 0.5 hour at 25 °C without agitation, the tubes were filled up to 25 ml with SFM to which trypsine (Worthington, USA) and gentamycine have been added (final concentrations: 5 µg/ml and 50 µg/ml, respectively). The cultures were agitated again.

Virus production was determined by hemagglutination (Dowdle et al., 1979). The results of the hemagglutination tests or HA test carried out on samples are given in HA units or HAU. In order to evaluate the cumulative production of virus or the specific productivity, the amounts of virus are given as if the total volume of the infected fluid was concentrated into 1 ml.

Small scale T-flask cultures for comparing the production of different virus strains: The cultures were started as described for the small scale microcarrier cultures by inoculating 25cm2 T-flasks (Costar) with $2*10^6$ cells in 10ml of SFM. One week later the cultures were inoculated as described previously by using the A/Shanghai, 12 times passed on Vero cells, as reference, and 10 other strains and recent isolates (see Fig. 5). Virus production was determined by hemagglutination.

Reactor Cultures

The following general conditions were employed: pH = 7.20, regulation by injecting CO_2 or $NaHCO_3$ (75g/l), pO_2: 20% air saturation, regulation by injecting air, O_2, or N_2, temperature: 37°C.

Vero and MDCK cells were grown on microcarriers: Superbead-Flow (cat. n° : 60-085-12), concentration: 5g/l (NewBrunswick Scientific Celligen reactor) [NSB], 6.25g/l (Biolafitte ICC 1L) [ICC 1L]. The cells were prepared as for the Vero batch cultures in tubes. The microcarriers were prepared as recommended by Pfeifer and Langen.

For starting the microcarrier cultures, the cells were incubated in the bioreactor in the presence of the microcarriers, and this suspension was discontinuously agitated for 5 minutes with an interruption of 10 minutes. After 12 hours, agitation was set continuously. BHK-21/BRS cells were grown in suspension culture (Perrin et al., 1995).

Reactors: NSB: Working volume: 2 l, cell retention by a sedimentation device (NewBrunswick), perfused culture, agitation: 40 rpm.

ICC 1L: Working volume: 1.6 l, cell retention by a spinfiltre (pore diameter of 20 μm (Biolafitte)), perfused culture, agitation: 50rpm.

Virus inoculation: The reactor cultures were inoculated with 3 ml of a virus suspension (12th passage of A/Shanghai/11/87 on Vero for infecting Vero and MDCK cultures: 7th passage of A/equine/Miami E2 on BHK-21 for BHK-21/BRS cultures) after having stopped the continuous alimentation. After an incubation phase of at least 45 minutes, trypsine (final concentration: 2 μg/ml) and gentamycine (final concentration: 50 μg/ml) were added to the culture and the continuous alimentation was restarted by using SFM containing trypsine and gentamycine. The perfusion rate was chosen with respect to the cell density. Samples were taken once or twice a day for cell counting and the determination of virus production.

Cell counting: Vero and MDCK cells were counted after treatment of an aliquot with crystal violet/citric acid. Vero and BHK-21/BRS cells were counted after trypsinisation. An aliquot of 0.5ml of the culture was incubated with 0.5ml of trypsine/versene (final concentration: 0.25%/0.01%) at 37°C for 10 minutes and then counted after treatment with trypane blue in a Mallassez chamber.

The virus titres were determined by hemagglutination using chicken red blood cells.

Virus Purification

Crude medium from infected cultures was clarified by centrifugation at 1500g for 30 minutes. The clarified supernatant was then centrifuged at 15000g for 3 hours after a dilution with 2 volumes of cold distilled water. The pellet was reconstituted in STE buffer (TRIS-HCl 0.01 M; NaCl 0.15 M; EDTA 0.001; pH = 7.4) and left over night. After resuspension in 1/10th of initial volume in the same buffer, the preconcentrated virus was deposited on the top of a prepared continuous gradient of potassium tartrate (50% - 10%) in centrifugation tubes. These tubes were then centrifuged at 20000 rpm (80000 g) for 18h. The visible opaque bands containing the virus were carefully separated into fractions, which were separately titred after dilution at 1/500 in TRIS-NaCl by the standard hemagglutination technique using chicken or guinea pig red blood cells according to the virus.

RESULTS

Vero

The first step of the development of an industrial process for the production of an influenza vaccine, was the choice of the cell line and the medium for cell growth. As Vero cells have been used for the production of viral vaccines for more than 10 years (Montagnon et al., 1984), we have chosen this cell line for influenza virus production. The use of the SCM (DMEM+2%NCS) and the SFM (MDSS2), previously developed for the production of rabies virus on BHK-21/BRS cells (Merten et al., 1994, Perrin et al., 1995) had to be tested because for virus production, generally trypsine containing media are used, and trypsine is inactivated by serum proteins. Agitated tube cultures of Vero cells grown on DEAE- dextrane microcarriers revealed that cell growth was about twice as fast in SCM (μ = 0.0047 ± 0 /h) than in SFM (μ = 0.0021 ± 0.0006 /h). Four-hundred hours after start,

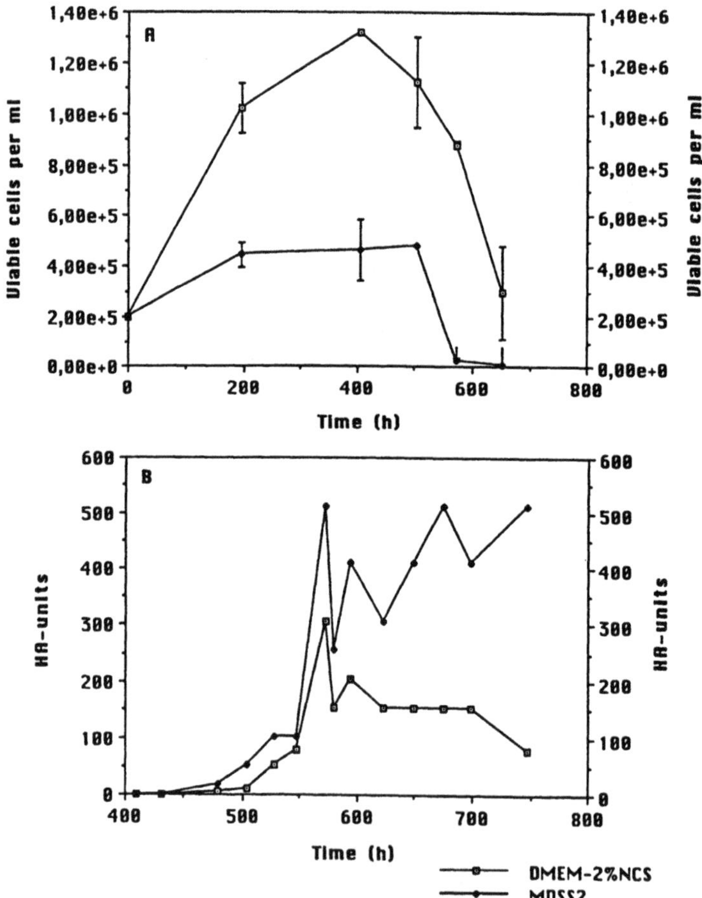

Figure 1. Comparison of cell growth of Vero cells (A) in SCM (DMEM+2%NCS, square) and SFM (MDSS2, diamond) and influenza virus (A/Shanghai/11/87) production (B) in SFM after two washings in Hank's solution.

$1.3*10^6$ c/ml and $0.45*10^6$ c/ml were obtained in SCM and SFM, respectively (Fig. 1A), and were infected with influenza virus (A/Shanghai/11/87 (H3N2)) by using the SFM MDSS2 in all cases. Despite the important differences in cell density, the virus production was inverse, and 256-512 and 160-320 HAU were obtained for the cultures derived from SFM and SCM for cell growth, respectively (Fig. 1B). Not only the SFM derived cultures were superior for the virus titres obtained, but the virus production was also accelerated for at least 24 hours in comparison to the SCM-derived cultures. The specific productivities were 320.9 ± 67.5 and 9.8 ± 0.2 HAU/10^6 cells and hour (values calculated between day 6 and day 7 "post-infection") for SFM and SCM-derived cultures, respectively. By using Fibracel as carrier, where the cells grow in a sponge-like structure, cell growth was equal in SCM and SFM, however, virus production was only possible when cells were grown in SFM. Certainly due to problems of infection of cells too far away from the free circulating medium, only low titres of maximally 64-128 HAU were obtained (not shown). These results led us to the conclusion that a serum-free medium for cell growth as well as for the virus production phase is necessary for an optimal virus production rate. In addition, technical systems allowing a rather easy contact between cells and medium are necessary in order to facilitate the homogeneous infection of cells. Finally, the cell density itself is a very important factor, wherefore high cell density cultures have to be chosen in order to maximise virus production. For the process development we have chosen a perfusion reactor based process where the cells are grown on classical DEAE-dextrane based carriers by using the SFM MDSS2.

Under these conditions $2.5*10^6$ c/ml of Vero cells can be obtained after 200 h. The infection of virus done at a cell density of about $1.5*10^6$ c/ml (at 148h) led to a correct virus production (Fig. 2A). Virus titres of 128-256 HAU were obtained four days after inoculation (Fig. 2B). Because a residual viable cell density of about $8*10^5$ c/ml could be maintained at a perfusion rate of about 0.01 /h, the virus production phase could be prolonged for up to 14 days post infection. The virus production rate varied between 0 and 15 HAU/10^6 cells and hour (average: 4 ± 2.5 HA- units/10^6c.h). During the production phase (4-15 days post infection) altogether $1.7*10^6$ HAU (110000 per day) were produced by using 7.7 l of medium.

BHK-21/BRS

BHK-21/BRS cells originally adapted to growth in serum-free suspension cultures for the production of rabies virus (Perrin et al., 1995) were used to replace Vero cells. Because BHK-21/BRS cells can grow in MDSS2 in a perfusion reactor in suspension a more cost-effective production of influenza virus than by using Vero cells should be possible. However, as for Vero cells, titres do not exceed 128 HAU because the virus kills the cells rather rapidly, leading to a short virus production phase (not shown). Using a 1.6 l perfusion reactor, altogether $5.91*10^5$ HAU (148500 per day) were produced by using 3.5 l of medium.

MDCK

The relatively low titres obtained with Vero and BHK-21/BRS cells and in the case of the use of Vero cells the relatively long delays between virus inoculation and virus production led to the use of MDCK-cells generally used for establishing new virus strains.

These cells showed a relatively fast growth and it was possible to obtain about $3.5*10^6$ c/ml 4 days after onset of the culture (Fig. 3A). On day 6 the culture was infected with the influenza virus strain A/Shanghai-11/87 and cell growth was still detected up to 3 days post infection ($6.2*10^6$ c/ml). During the whole culture duration during which the cell density was beyond 10^6 c/ml a perfusion rate of at least 0.0312 /h was used.

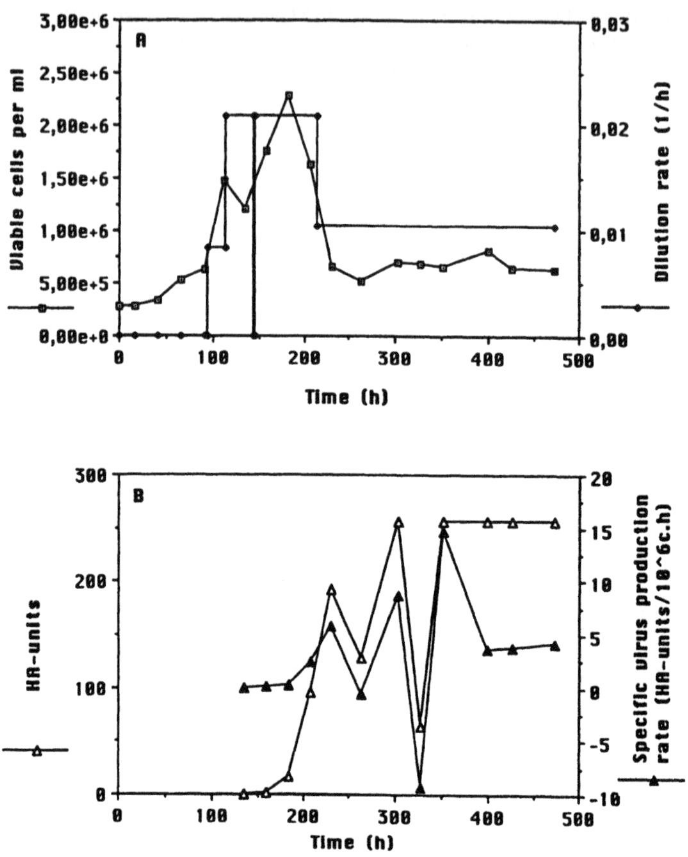

Figure 2. Vero grown on Superbead-microcarriers in a 2 l Celligen bioreactor, presented are cell number per ml (squares) and perfusion rate (diamonds) in A, and titre (HAU, open triangles) and the specific virus production rate (HAU/10⁶ c.h, full triangles) in B. The culture was infected at 144.25 h with influenza virus (A/Shanghai/11/87).

Already two days after virus inoculation a titre of 1280 HAU was obtained which increased to 1920 HAU one day later (Fig. 3B). With the continuation of the perfusion and the reduction of the cell density the titres fell to values of 256-512 HAU. The specific virus production rate ranged from 0 to 15 HAU/10⁶c.h (average: 9.3 ± 4.5, between day 2 and day 4 post virus inoculation). Using this 1.6 l perfusion reactor, altogether 7.28*10⁶ HAU (1.23*10⁶ per day) were produced by using 8.7 l of medium.

Comparison of the Three Cell Lines for Virus Production

The above mentioned results make it evident that MDCK is the best choice for an industrial production of an influenza vaccine. However, for giving a more comprehensive view of the production capacities of these cell lines, the cumulative virus productions were compared (Fig. 4). MDCK cells produced much more rapidly than Vero or BHK-21/BRS cells. When normalised values are compared (normalised for 5*10⁶ c/ml using a perfusion reactor of 2 l), MDCK cells produce about twice as fast as Vero cells and almost 7 times faster than BHK-21/BRS cells (Table 1). Comparing Vero and BHK- 21/BRS cells, the factor

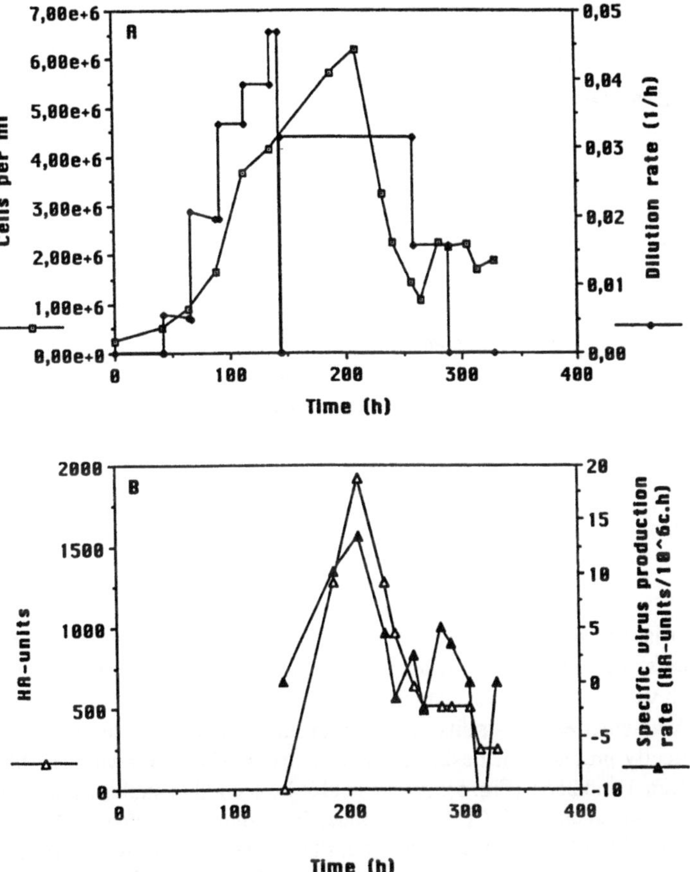

Figure 3. MDCK grown on Superbead-microcarriers in a 1.6 l Biolafitte ICC11 bioreactor, presented are cell number per ml (squares) and perfusion rate (diamonds) in A, and titre (HAU, open triangles) and the specific virus production rate (HAU/10^6c.h, full triangles) in B. The culture was infected at 143.75 h with influenza virus (A/Shanghai/11/87).

is about 3.2. The differences are due to the specific production rates and to the duration of the virus production phase. Whereas MDCK showed a maximum daily specific production rate of 14.8 ±4.8 between day 2 and day 4 post infection, BHK-21/BRS and Vero showed a maximal specific virus productivity of 5.3 and 5.8, respectively. However, BHK-21/BRS produced at this rate only for 2 to 3 days, whereas Vero cells produced at a quite constant rate starting two days after virus inoculation. So, important quantities of virus can be produced by using Vero cells, which are equivalent to those produced by MDCK. The main difference is that by using MDCK cells 6 days are sufficient for getting 4.1 ± 2.6 *10^6 HAU, whereas 14 days are necessary for getting 5.1*10^6 HAU by using Vero cells. BHK-21/BRS is following with a tenth of the mentioned values (0.566*10^6 HAU in about 5 days).

Production of Other Virus Strains

The interest of cell culture based virus production is not only the industrial production of viral vaccine after having adapted the virus during several passages on cells cultivated in

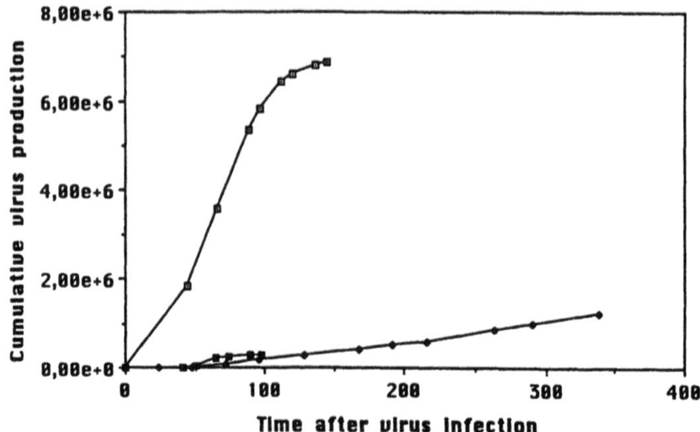

Figure 4. Comparison of the cumulative influenza virus production for the following cell lines: MDCK (culture shown in Fig. 3, open squares), Vero (culture shown in Fig. 2, diamonds), and BHK-21/BRS (culture grown in a 1.6 l Biolafitte ICC11 bioreactor, 5.96*10^6 c/ml were infected with influenza virus (A/equine/Miami E2), full squares).

flasks, but it is very important to test if newly established strains can be produced in cell cultures (flasks, reactors) directly without adaptation. So, confluent cultures in T-flasks were infected with various virus strains which have been established very recently or during the last years. Altogether eleven strains of human influenza virus were tested, of which seven could be directly produced in flasks cultures by using MDCK grown in SFM. The titres varied between 4 and 256+ (Fig. 5). As it can also be seen, that strains established recently which were passaged on MDCK cells only once, like A/Paris/457/95 or B/Paris/503/95, can be produced to high titres. On the other hand, titres obtained with A-strains and B-strains, are comparable. Finally, for the virus strains successfully produced, high titres were obtained already three days after virus inoculation.

Recently, we propagated the strains A/Paris/457/95 and B/Paris/503/95 on MDCK cells grown on microcarriers in bioreactors and titres of 512-1024 HAU could be obtained for both virus strains, indicating that even completely new strains (A and B) can be successfully produced in perfused serum-free microcarrier cultures of MDCK.

Table 1. Comparison of the cumulative virus production for three cell lines used for the production of influenza virus (normalised for a 2 l perfusion reactor, and 5*10^6 c/ml for first three days after virus inoculation)

Cell line	Virus strain	Maximum daily production HA-u/10^6c.h	Cumulative production + reactor content	Cumulative production per day
BHK-21/BRS (n = 7)	Miami	5.291 (J3 ± J1) ± 4.3998	566132 (J5 ± J0.82) ± 224187	113226
Vero (average)	Shanghai	5.804 (J4) 4.001 ±2 .464 (J2-J14)	5093349 (J14)	363810
MDCK (n = 6)	Shanghai	14.79 ± 4.780 (J3.3 ± J0.7)	4141548 (J5.8 ± J0.75) ± 2578052	714060

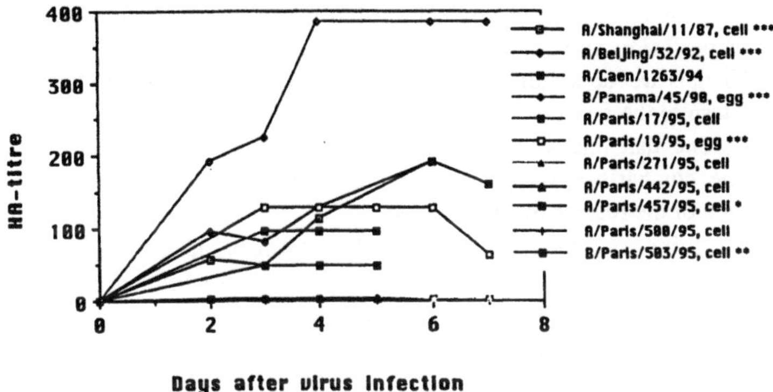

Figure 5. Production of various influenza virus strains by MDCK grown in SFM in T-flasks. Notation: *** maximum HA-titre: equal or higher than 128, ** maximum HA-titre: 64-128, * maximum HA-titre: 32-64.

Virus Purification

The virus produced in MDCK cells was found to be identical to the egg grown preparations of the same strain in terms of sedimentation characteristics, migration in the density gradient and morphology.

DISCUSSION

Today, the influenza vaccine production process is still based on embryonated eggs. This method of production conveys many major drawbacks such as inflexibility of the production process, modification of the hemagglutinin molecule due to successive egg passages, contamination of the final product by egg derived substances with the possibility of allergic reactions. In order to solve these problems we undertook the present development to replace the ancient production process by a modern cell culture based reactor production process.

The starting point was the development of a production process for rabies vaccine which is based on the BHK-21 C13 derived clone BHK-21/BRS growing in suspension in SFM (Merten et al., 1994, Perrin et al., 1995). The medium developed for this process and commercialised under the name MDSS2, supports growth of Vero cells (Merten et al., 1994) and, after a slight modification of the composition, also growth of MDCK cells. The use of SFM for this purpose has two advantages. First, the production of influenza virus has to be done in the presence of trypsine and the use of a SCM would inactivate the trypsine rather rapidly. Even the use of a SCM only for cell growth followed by a vigorous washing step and a virus production phase in SFM is not a viable approach because virus production is retarded and, in general, lower than in a complete serum-free process. Second, the problem of BSE and other contaminants originated from serum or serum-based products can be avoided when SFM are used for the production of biotechnological products for human and veterinary use.

The choice of the cell line used is obvious. Vero cells have been used for the production of viral vaccines for humans for more than ten years (Montagnon et al., 1984), whereas BHK-21 C13 cells are used for the production of veterinary vaccines (e.g. Capstick et al., 1962, Radlett 1987) and rather recently also for the production of recombined proteins for human therapy (Bödeker et al., 1994). Although both cell lines grow well in the SFM, they are not very interesting for the production of influenza virus, because the maximal titres obtainable in perfusion cultures ranged only between 256 and 512 HAU. In addition, BHK-21/BRS cells are too rapidly killed by the virus leading generally to low overall virus production. Despite the fact that Vero cells are able to produce the virus over a time of at least 14 days, and that relatively large quantities of virus can be produced under these conditions, the comparison with a MDCK-based process is negative due to the long occupation time of the reactor by the process.

By comparing the three cell lines tested the MDCK based serum-free process shows many advantages. MDCK does not only produce rather rapidly influenza virus after infection, but this cell line produces very high titres of up to 2000 HAU in a very short time during perfusion. This fast virus production combined with a rather rapid cell growth for biomass production allows an overall process duration of 11 to 14 days. The process presented here, is based on a 1.6 l perfusion reactor, used altogether 12.3 l of SFM of which only 3.6 l (about 30%) were used for cell growth and the rest for virus production. This signifies that a large quantity of the medium is used for the production of virus.

Other aspects of this new process was to show that the so produced virus can be purified by the same methods developed for the egg-based process and that new non-adapted virus strains can be produced without difficulties. The production of other virus strains was possible without major difficulties, however, some strains were not produced very probably due to a non-viable inoculum. The titres obtained with these strains ranged from 4 to 512 in T-flask cultures. These titres are already rather high. However, when perfusion cultures are used instead of T-flask cultures, titres of up to 2000 HAU can be obtained. Whereas the A/Shanghai/11/87 strain was produced up to 190 HAU in T-flasks, almost 2000 HAU were obtained in the perfusion culture. Similar results were found with the strains B/Paris/503/95 and A/Paris/457/95 for which 96 HAU and 48 HAU, respectively, were obtained in T-flasks whereas perfusion cultures produced titres of 512 to 1024 HAU. This signifies that the perfusion reactor based process is much more efficient than a classical batch process. These results are comparable with those presented for the production of rabies virus by using a serum- free perfusion process of BHK-21/BRS cells (Merten et al., 1994, Perrin et al., 1995). Here again, the perfusion process produced much more virus than the batch process. The increase in the efficiency of perfusion processes can be explained with the fact that the processes are based on rather high cell densities, that the cells are fed regularly, and that almost "steady state" conditions can be maintained during the virus production phase.

REFERENCES

Bödeker, B.G.D., Newcomb, R., Yuan, P., Braufman, A., and Kelsey, W., 1994, Production of recombinant factor VIII from perfusion cultures: I. Large- scale fermentation. In: Spier, R.E., Griffiths, J.B., and Berthold, W. (eds.): Animal Cell Technology: Products of Today, Prospects for Tomorrow, pp. 580-583,Butterworth-Heinemann, Oxford.

Capstick P.B., Telling, R.C., Chapman, W.G., and Stewart, D.L., 1962, Growth of a cloned strain of hamster kidney cells in suspended cultures and their suceptibility to the virus of foot-and-mouth disease. Nature 195: 1163-1164.

Merten, O.-W., Kierulff, J.V., Castignolles, N., and Perrin, P., 1994, Evaluation of the new serum-free medium (MDSS2) for the production of different biologicals: Use of various cell lines. Cytotechnology 14: 47-59.

Merten, O.-W., Petres, S., and Couvé , E., 1995, A simple serum-free freezing medium for serum free cultured cells. Biologicals 23: 185-189.

Montagnon, B., Vincent-Falquet, J.C., and Fanget, B., 1984, Thousand litre scale microcarrier culture of Vero cells for killed polio virus vaccine. Promising results. Develop. biol. Standard. 55: 37-42.

Oxford J.S., Corcoran T., Knott R., Bates J., Bartolomei O., Major D., Newman R.W., Yates P., Robertson J.S., Webster R.G. et al., 1987, Serological studies with influenza A(H1N1) viruses cultivated in eggs or in a canine kidney cell line (MDCK), Bull. WHO 65: 181-187.

Oxford J.S., Corcoran T., Bootman J., Major D., Yates P., Robertson J.S. and Schild G.C., 1991, Direct isolation in eggs of influenza A(H1N1) and B viruses with hemagglutinins of different antigenic and amino-acid composition. J. Gen. Virol. 72: 185-189.

Perrin, P, Madhusudana, S., Gontier-Jallet, C., Petres, S., Tordo, N., and Merten, O.-W., 1995 An experimental rabies vaccine produced with a new BHK-21 suspension cell culture process: use of serum-free medium and perfusion-reactor system. Vaccine 13: 1244-1250.

Pyhala R., Pyhala L., Valle M. and Aho K., 1987, Egg-grown and tissue culture grown variants of influenza A(H3N2) virus with special attention to their use as antigens in seroepidemiology. Epidem. Inf. 99: 745-753.

Radlett, P.J., 1987, The use of BHK suspension cells for the production of foot and mouth disease vaccines. In: Fiechter, A. (ed.): Advances in Biochemical Engineering/Biotechnology, Vol. 34, pp. 129-146, Springer- Verlag, Berlin-Heidelberg.

Robertson J.S., Bootman J.S., Newman R., Oxford J.S., Danoels R.S., Webster R.G. and Schild G.C., 1987, Structural changes in the hemagglutinin which accompany egg adaptation of an influenza A(H1N1) virus. Virology 160: 31- 37.

Rocha, E.P., Xo, X., Hau, H.E., Allen, J.R., Regnery, H., and Cox, N., 1993, Comparison of 10 influenza A(H1N1 and H3N2) hemagglutinin sequences obtained directly from clinical specimens to those of MDCK-cell and egg- grown viruses. J. Gen. Virol. 74: 2513-2518.

Wang M.L., Katz J.M. and Webster R.G., 1989, Extensive heterogeneity in the hemagglutinin of egg-grown influenza viruses from different patients. Virology 171: 275-279.

Wood J.M., Oxford J.S., Dunleavy U., Newman R.W., Major D. and Robertson J.S., 1989, Influenza A(H1N1) vaccine efficacy in animal models is influenced by two amino-acid substitutions in the hemaglutinin molecule. Virology 171: 214-221.

20

ANALYSIS OF *BORDETELLA PERTUSSIS* SUSPENSIONS BY ELISA AND FLOW CYTOMETRY

W. Jiskoot,[1] J. Westdijk,[1] C. H. K. Reubsaet,[2] and E. C. Beuvery[1]

[1] Laboratory for Product and Process Development
[2] Laboratory for the Control of Biological Products
National Institute of Public Health and Environmental Protection (RIVM)
P.O. Box 1, 3720 BA Bilthoven, The Netherlands

1. INTRODUCTION

In our institute the production of whole-cell pertussis vaccine is being upgraded. This requires fast, reliable *in-process* controls, the results of which should correlate with the protective activity *in vivo*. For routine vaccine production, *Bordetella pertussis* suspensions are diluted to a final strength on the basis of their opacity, expressed as International Opacity Units (IOU), and the potency is evaluated on the basis of the mouse protection test (MPT) according to Kendrick et al.[1] These tests do not meet the above criteria for *in-process* controls. The opacity not only depends on biomass concentration but also on varying properties such as cell size, cell surface roughness and the amount of lysed and any other particulate material. Moreover, IOU values are not predictive for the antigen contents. On the other hand, the MPT is time-consuming and poorly reproducible.

Here we present three ELISAs for the quantification of Pertussis Toxin (PT), Filamentous Haemagglutinin (FHA), and 92-kD Outer Membrane Protein (92-kD OMP) on the bacterial cell wall. Furthermore, the use of the flow cytometer for determining the antigen content per cell and other cell properties is introduced. Both techniques are valuable for monitoring the quality of *B. pertussis* cell suspensions as a function of strain, cultivation conditions, and inactivation method.

2. EXPERIMENTAL PROCEDURES

2.1. Samples

B. pertussis cell suspensions were obtained from routine production batches and experimental batches of different strains, whether or not heat-inactivated, as indicated in Table I.

Novel Strategies in Design and Production of Vaccines
Edited by S. Cohen and A. Shafferman, Plenum Press, New York, 1996

Table I. Sample description

Cultivation number	Strain	Scale (Litres)	Inactivation[*]
1 (0)	134	350	no
1 (10)	134	350	yes
2 (0)	CS	350	no
2 (10)	CS	350	yes
3 (0)	134	800	no
3 (10)	134	800	yes
4	509	800	yes
5	134	800	yes
6	509	350	no
7	509	800	no

[*]Heating for 10 min at 56°C

2.2. ELISA

For determining PT, FHA, and 92-kD OMP contents, twofold dilution series of *B. pertussis* cell suspensions were preincubated with a fixed dilution of mouse monoclonal antibodies (Mabs) raised against PT, FHA, and 92-kD OMP, respectively. After incubation, the antibody excess was determined in an antigen-specific ELISA by transferring the mixtures to 96-well microtitration plates coated with the antigen (PT, FHA, or 92-kD OMP), and subsequent incubation with a fixed dilution of sheep anti-mouse immunoglobulin peroxidase conjugate. After the addition of substrate and colour development, the absorbances of the dilution series of samples and references (purified antigens) were read and titres were calculated.

2.3. Flow Cytometry

The Mabs that were used in the ELISA described above were also used for flow cytometric analysis. Diluted cell suspensions were incubated with Mab and subsequently, after washing and resuspending, with goat anti-mouse immunoglobulin fluorescein isothiocyanate conjugate. After washing and resuspending, the suspensions were analysed with a FACScan flow cytometer (Becton Dickinson).

For cell integrity studies, diluted cell suspensions were incubated with either fluorescein diacetate or propidium iodide and analysed by flow cytometry.

2.4. Mouse Protection Test (MPT)

Immunisation of mice with sample and intracerebral challenge with *B. pertussis* strain 18323 was performed as described by Kendrick et al.[1]

3. RESULTS AND DISCUSSION

The results of ELISA and MPT are summarised in Fig. 1. Large intra-strain (batch-to-batch) as well as inter-strain variations in antigen content per IOU and relative PT/FHA/92-kD OMP ratio were detected by ELISA. In general, the apparent PT content was relatively low as compared to the FHA and 92-kD OMP contents. The antigen contents were not substantially affected by heat inactivation. Furthermore, the 92-kD OMP content roughly correlated with the potency as determined with the MPT, a finding that was observed before

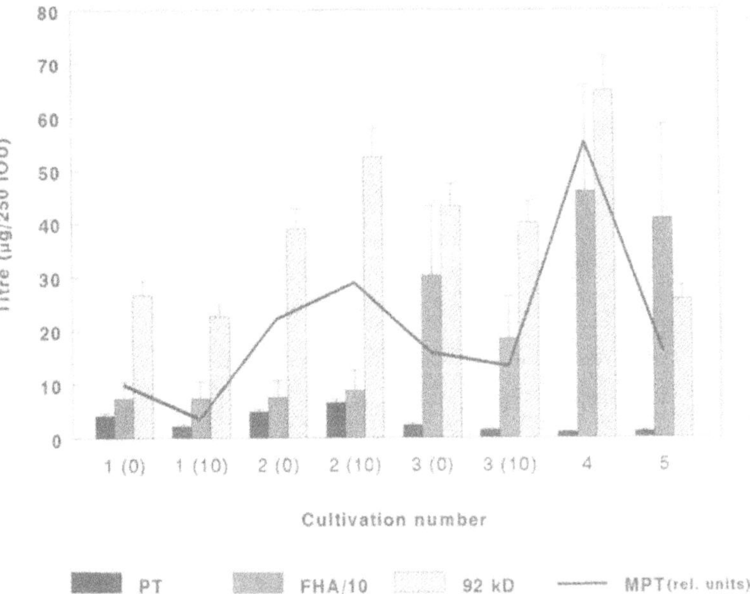

Figure 1. Antigen contents (ELISA) and potency (MPT) of *B. pertussis* suspensions. Samples are described in Table I. Error bars indicate upper limits of estimated standard deviations.

by Poolman et al.[2] The reproducibility of the ELISAs (see error bars in Fig. 1) is significantly better than that of the MPT (errors not shown). Therefore, ELISA is an attractive test not only for evaluating final products but also for aiding in the optimisation of cultivation and inactivation procedures.

Flow cytometry has proven to be a valuable tool in the analysis of eukaryotic cells[3] and is rapidly gaining importance in the characterisation of bacterial cells[3,4]. It is a powerful technique with regard to its ability to measure individual cells and, hence, to detect heterogeneity within a cell population. Dot plots (graphs of forward scatter against side scatter intensity) of *B. pertussis* cell populations typically show large "clouds" with a relatively broad distribution of forward scatter intensity and less variation in side scatter intensity, indicating large variations in cell size but fairly homogeneous cell morphology (results not shown).

The antigen contents of *B. pertussis* cells were analysed by flow cytometry and the results were compared with ELISA. Fig. 2 shows the plots of cell number versus fluorescence intensity (a direct measure for the FHA and 92-kD OMP contents) of samples 6 and 7. The average FHA content of the cells of sample 7 was considerably higher than that of sample 6. Furthermore, the plots suggest heterogeneity in the FHA content per cell withing each of the two cell suspensions, i.e., the presence of subpopulations with different FHA expression levels. In contrast, the 92-kD OMP contents were comparable and were more homogeneous for either sample. The PT content was hardly detectable by flow cytometry (results not shown). These results are in excellent agreement with the ELISA results presented in Table II: a relatively high FHA content of sample 7, similar 92-kD contents, and low PT titres.

Flow cytometry after incubation of *B. pertussis* cells with fluorescein diacetate and propidium iodide as markers was used to monitor the integrity of the bacterial cells. Fluorescein diacetate (non-fluorescent) is known for its active uptake and subsequent

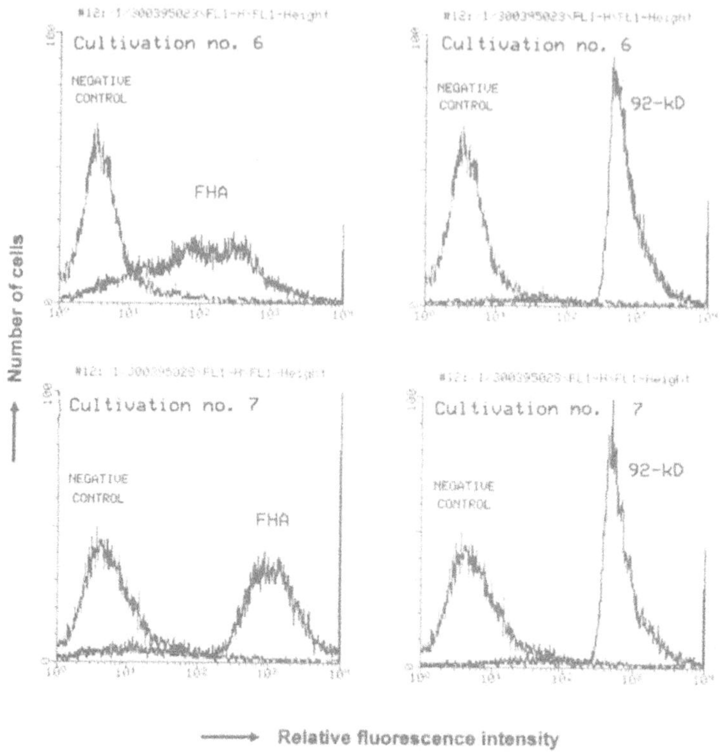

Figure 2. Relative fluorescence intensity (as a measure for FHA and 92-kD OMP contents) of *B. pertussis* cell samples 6 and 7 (see Table I) as determined by flow cytometry.

intracellular, enzymatical conversion to (fluorescent) fluorescein[3,4]. Propidium iodide is a fluorescent dye which intercalates with DNA[3,4].

The results of flow cytometric analysis of samples 6 and 7 with fluorescein diacetate and propidium iodide as markers are shown in Fig. 3. From the strong fluorescence signals it can be concluded that both markers pass the cell membranes and that fluorescein diacetate is hydrolysed to fluorescein. The fluorescein and propidium iodide contents per cell tend to be higher for sample 6 in comparison with sample 7. The applicability of flow cytometry in combination with fluorescent markers for the characterisation of *B. pertussis* and other bacterial cells is currently under investigation. The uptake rate and/or conversion rate, as well as the maximal fluorescence per cell may be indicative parameters for the integrity of bacterial cells.

Table II. ELISA titres of samples (cultivation numbers) 6 and 7

Cultivation number	PT (µg/250 IOU)	FHA (µg/250 IOU)	92-kD OMP (µg/250 IOU)
6	3.0	60	88
7	6.3	332	65

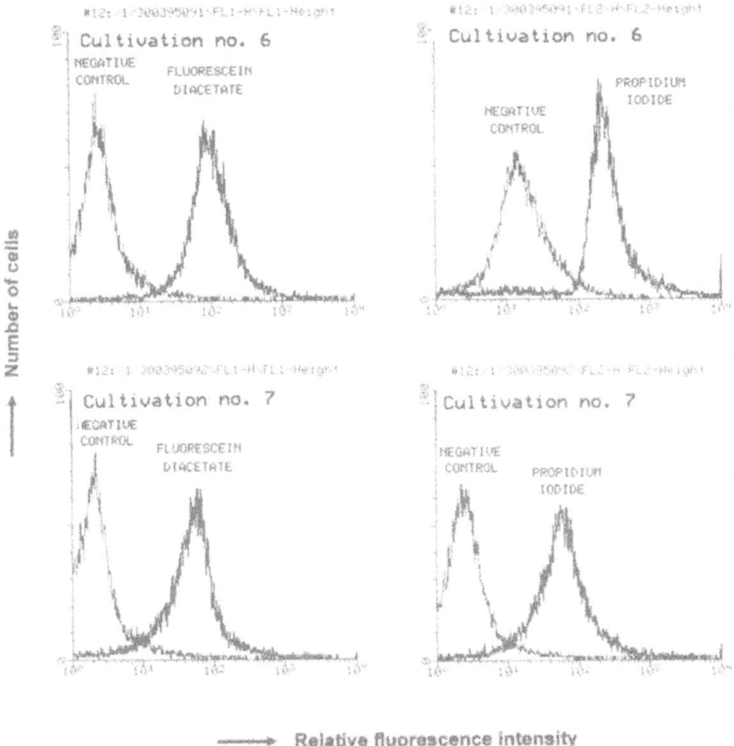

Figure 3. Relative fluorescence intensity of *B. pertussis* cell samples 6 and 7 (see Table I) after incubation with fluorescein diacetate and propidium iodide.

In conclusion, both ELISA and flow cytometry can be used as predictive techniques for the quality of *B. pertussis* cell suspensions. As such, they are of great value as *in-process*, final bulk, and final lot controls.

4. REFERENCES

1. Kendrick, P., Eldering, G., Dixon, M.K., and Mishner, J. (1947) Mouse protection tests in the study of pertussis vaccine, Am. J. Public Health 37, 803-810.
2. Poolman, J.T., Hamstra, H.-J., Barlow, A.K., Kuipers, B., Loggen, H., and Nagel, J. (1990) Outer membrane vesicles of *Bordetella pertussis* are protective antigens in the mouse intracerebral challenge model, in: Proceedings of the Sixth International Symposium on Pertussis, Department of Health and Human Services, Food and Drug Administration, Bethesda, MD, pp. 148-155.
3. Melamed, M., Mullaney, P., and Mendelsohn, M. (1990) Flow Cytometry and Sorting, Second Edition, Wiley-Liss, New York, NY.
4. Lloyd, D. (1993) Flow Cytometry in Microbiology, Springer-Verlag, London.

21

CLINICAL TRIALS OF *SHIGELLA* VACCINES IN ISRAEL

D. Cohen,[1] S. Ashkenazi,[1] M. Green,[1] M. Gdalevich,[1] M. Yavzori,[1]
N. Orr,[1] G. Robin,[1] R. Slepon,[1] Y. Lerman,[1] C. Block,[1] I. Ashkenazi,[1]
D. Taylor,[2] L. Hale,[2] J. Sadoff,[2] R. Schneerson,[3] J. Robbins,[3] M. Wiener,[1]
and J. Shemer[1]

[1] Israel Defence Force, Medical Corps
[2] Walter Reed Army Institute of Research
   Washington, DC.
[3] Laboratory of Developmental and Molecular Immunity, NICHD, NIH
   Bethesda, Maryland

1. INTRODUCTION

Shigellosis or bacillary dysentery is caused by organisms belonging to genus *Shigella*, divided into four species (*S. dysenteriae, S. boydii, S. flexneri* and *S. sonnei*). With the exception of *S. sonnei* which has a single serotype, each species is divided into several serotypes according to the O-polysaccharide antigen of the cell wall (*S. dysenteriae* has 12 serotypes, *S. flexneri* has 6 serotypes, and *S. boydii* has 18 serotypes). *Shigella* spp. are invasive organisms that penetrate into the enterocytes of the colon epithelium, escape very quickly from the phagocytic vacuole and multiplicate intracellularly. Although non-motile, shigellae can move on an actin skeleton and spread to adjacent cells. The inflammatory process is usually limited to the lamina propria and does not involve the spread of *Shigella* deeper, into the submucosa. Pathogenesis in *Shigella* spp. is associated with a constellation of genes encoded on both the chromosome and a large 140 MDa virulence plasmid. These genes can be divided into two groups: regulatory genes and structural genes. The 140 MDa plasmid encodes for all the genes essential for invasion of *Shigella* into the epithelium of the colon. Regulatory genes are located on the virulence plasmid or on the chromosome.

The initial manifestations of acute shigellosis are usually fever, malaise, abdominal pain and watery diarrhea. The disease may progress, with the appearance of tenesmus, and of blood and mucus in the stool. Infection caused by *S. dysenteriae* type 1 and sometimes by *S. flexneri* may cause severe protein-loss. Extra-intestinal complications may include reactive arthritis, toxic megacolon, bacteremia and hemolytic-uremic syndrome.

Shigellosis is endemic throughout the world. The disease is hyperendemic in developing countries. The annual global incidence of shigellosis is around 200 million cases, with more than 650,000 fatal cases of the disease (Institute,1986).

Novel Strategies in Design and Production of Vaccines
Edited by S. Cohen and A. Shafferman, Plenum Press, New York, 1996

Israel is highly endemic for shigellosis, having a reported incidence of disease about 20-30 times higher than that of the United States (Green, 1991). Young children, mainly of nursery school age appear to be particularly vulnerable to the disease, which accounts for approximately 600 pediatric admissions per year. The use of antibiotic treatment in shigellosis is becoming more and more problematic in Israel, since clinical isolates are becoming increasingly resistant to antimicrobial agents (Smollan, 1992; Ashkenazi, 1993). Shigellosis causes about five deaths in Israel each year, typically in the pediatric and geriatric age groups (Green, 1991). In addition to children, soldiers serving under field conditions constitute another risk group for shigellosis (Green, 1987; Cohen, 1991). Of 420 laboratory-investigated outbreaks of diarrhea occurring in the Israel Defence Force between 1985 and 1993, 181 (43%) were caused by *Shigella* organisms. The relative importance of *S. sonnei* and *S. flexneri* as etiologic agents of epidemic shigellosis in the IDF is similar, each of these species being responsible for about 45% of these outbreaks. *S. boydii* and *S. dysenteriae* are involved in the rest of the outbreaks. The very low infectious dose of *Shigella*, of about 10^2-10^3 organisms (DuPont, 1989), and difficult field conditions facilitate the transmission of the pathogen, explaining the partial failure of routine sanitary and hygienic measures to prevent the sporadic and epidemic occurrence of shigellosis among Israeli military populations (Green, 1987; Cohen, 1991). In such circumstances, effective vaccination appears to be the only reliable means of preventing outbreaks.

2. CURRENT STRATEGIES IN THE DEVELOPMENT OF *SHIGELLA* VACCINES

Candidate *Shigella* vaccines developed in the last five decades have not reached an acceptable level of safety and efficacy. There are neither licensed vaccines for it, nor consensus on the relative importance of the host components responsible for protective immunity to shigellosis. Since there is evidence that shigellosis confers protection against recurrent disease due to the homologous *Shigella* group (Cohen, 1988; Herrington, 1990), it has been assumed that an efficient *Shigella* vaccine should induce, to a comparable extent, the same immune mechanisms as natural infection does, without causing the symptoms of diarrhea or bacillary dysentery. New generations of live-attenuated or subunit vaccines are currently employed to deliver the O-polysaccharide, the protective antigen of *Shigella*.

Formal and co-workers constructed an *E. coli* K12-*S. flexneri* 2a hybrid vaccine by conjugal transfer of the 140 MDa *S. flexneri* invasion plasmid and genes encoding for the *S. flexneri* 2a LPS into an *E. coli* K12 recipient (Formal, 1984; Newland, 1992). Lindberg and his group in Sweden induced *aro* mutations in *Shigella* spp. wild strains and obtained auxotrophic live-attenuated *Shigella* vaccines which showed a good level of safety and immunogenicity in humans (Lindberg, 1990; Li, 1993). Sansonetti and coworkers reached attenuation of a *S. flexneri* 5 strain by a deletion in the plasmid *ics* (encoding for cell-to-cell spread) followed by an insertional mutation in the chromosomal *iuc* (encoding for aerobactin) (Sansonnetti, 1989). Recently, deletion mutations in the chromosomal gene *aro*A and plasmid gene *virG* were induced in a wild-type *S. flexneri* 2a by Noriega and coworkers to engineer an oral vaccine prototype capable of penetrating the intestinal epithelial cells but incapable of extensive intracellular replication (Noriega, 1994). In view of previous studies among Israeli recruits, showing a strong association between serum anti-LPS IgG antibodies and protection against shigellosis, Robbins, Schneerson and co-workers developed at NIH *Shigella* conjugate vaccines capable of inducing high levels of such antibodies when administered parenterally (Robbins, 1992; Chu, 1992; Taylor, 1993). A subunit *Shigella* vaccine composed of *S. sonnei* or *S. flexneri* 2a hydrophobically-complexed with proteosomes, meningococcal outer membrane proteins, has been developed in the Israel Defence Force Medical Corps by Orr and coworkers. Oral or intranasal immunization with one or two doses of this proteosome-LPS vaccine induced strong local and systemic immune responses in mice and showed a high level of protection against *Shigella* keratoconjunctivitis (Séreny test) in guinea pigs (Orr, 1993).

3. SAFETY, IMMUNOGENICITY AND PRELIMINARY EFFICACY STUDIES OF CANDIDATE *SHIGELLA* VACCINES IN THE ISRAEL DEFENCE FORCE

Double-blind, randomized, placebo-controlled studies of safety, immunogenicity and preliminary efficacy of the oral, attenuated *E. coli* K12-*S. flexneri* 2a (*EcSf2a-2*) vaccine and the parenteral *S. sonnei* and *S. flexneri* type 2a conjugate vaccines have been conducted in the Israel Defence Force (IDF).

3.1. Safety and Immunogenicity of the Oral, Attenuated *E. coli* K12-*S. flexneri* 2a (*EcSf2a-2*) Hybrid Vaccine

The vaccine was constructed at the Walter Reed Army Institute of Research (WRAIR) by conjugal transfer of the 140-MDa invasion plasmid of *S. flexneri* 5 (strain M90T) into an *E. coli* K12 recipient (strain 395-1, lactose-negative, streptomycin-resistant) (Formal, 1984). Subsequent conjugal transfer from the *S. flexneri* 2a Hfr donor (strain 256) of the *his*, *pro* and *arg* chromosomal markers in separate matings allowed the expression the *S. flexneri* 2a LPS surface antigen and stabilized the expression of the plasmid-encoded invasiveness phenotype. A further attenuation of the vaccine strain was obtained by P1 transduction of a tetracycline-resistance transposon (Tn10)-inactivated *aroD* gene followed by selection of a tetracycline-sensitive strain with a growth requirement for para-aminobenzoic acid, a precursor of folic acid not available in mammalian cells (Newland, 1992).

Sixty volunteers received the vaccine and 59 received placebo. Fifty three volunteers were given the full regimen of the vaccine (4 doses) on days 0, 3, 14 and 17. The vaccination doses ranged between 4.1×10^8 and 1.1×10^9 cfu. The *EcSf2a-2* vaccine was well tolerated by the volunteers. None of the volunteers lost any training time due to complaints occurring after vaccination (Cohen, 1994). No significant difference in the rate of any reported gastrointestinal or non-gastrointestinal symptom, following the 4 doses of vaccine or placebo, was detected between vaccinees and placebo recipients. Symptoms were most frequent after dose 1, and decreased at doses 2, 3 and 4 (Table 1).

Since no differences in the rate of these complaints were identified between vaccinees and placebos at any specific dose, it is possible that the sodium bicarbonate, which was given with the vaccine as well as with the placebo, could have been partly responsible. Recent data from a controlled study have shown a significant association between the concentration of the sodium bicarbonate solution administered prior to vaccination with the oral, whole cell/recombinant B subunit cholera vaccine and the extent of adverse reactions among volunteers (Sanchez, 1993). The decrease in the rate of these mild complaints following doses 2, 3, and 4 observed in our study may reflect physical and psychological accommodation of the volunteers to the vaccination regimen.

The vaccine strain was excreted by 69% and 67% of the vaccinees one day after receiving the second and the fourth dose, respectively. According to three parameters examined, namely antibiotic susceptibility, phage typing and restriction fragment length polymorphism (RFLP), the vaccine strain emerged genetically-stable after replication in

Table 1. Rate (%) of symptoms reported by 60 vaccinees and 59 placebo recipients within 3 days of each vaccine dose

	Dose 1		Dose 2		Dose 3		Dose 4	
	Vacc.	Plac.	Vacc.	Plac.	Vacc.	Plac.	Vacc.	Plac.
Loose stools	7	5	7	5	9	7	9	11
Diarrhea	5	2	5	2	2	4	4	2
Abdom. cramps or gurgling [a]	39	25	17	17	11	15	11	6
Vomiting	3	2	0	3	0	0	0	2
Malaise [b]	37	25	25	24	17	17	11	17
Loss of appetite [c]	25	24	14	19	7	19	9	11
Headache [d]	37	22	17	17	15	21	15	9
Fever (temp.$\geq$37.6°C)	5	0	2	0	2	2	2	0
Visits to Unit Clinic	13	5	0	0	0	2	0	0

[a]Mantel Haenszel Chi-Square for trend: p = 0.010 (Placebo); p<0.001 (Vaccine).
[b]Mantel Haenszel Chi-Square for trend: p = 0.205 (Placebo); p = 0.001 (Vaccine).
[c]Mantel Haenszel Chi-Square for trend: p = 0.109 (Placebo); p = 0.007 (Vaccine).
[d]Mantel Haenszel Chi-Square for trend: p = 0.131 (Placebo); p = 0.006 (Vaccine).
Statistical tests for differences between vaccine & placebo yielded p > 0.05 for all comparisons.

human gut and shedding. There was neither bacteriological nor serological evidence of transmission of the vaccine from vaccinees to placebo recipients throughout the follow-up. Eighteen of 26 (69.2%) and 11 of 30 (36.7%) vaccinees had a significant IgA secreting cell response 7 and 21 days after the first dose, respectively (Table 2). The rate and magnitude of the ASC response to the vaccine strain in this study (Cohen, 1994) were very similar to those observed among civilian and military volunteers in the United States (Kotloff, 1992; Taylor, 1994), but much lower than those detected among Israeli soldiers in the convalescent stage of shigellosis (91% response and mean of 1,432 spots per 10^6 cells) (Orr, 1992).

Significant IgA or IgG serum antibody response to *S. flexneri* 2a LPS was detected in 30% of the vaccinees (Table 3). The rate of IgG and IgA serum antibody responses to *S. flexneri* LPS among Israeli volunteers was slightly lower than that found in previous volunteer studies with the *EcSf* vaccine (Kotloff, 1992; Taylor, 1994) and much lower than the serum antibody response following *Shigella* natural infection (Cohen, 1989). A high systemic immune response to LPS was not anticipated since such a reaction had not been commonly observed in previous studies with live, oral attenuated *Shigella* and non-*Shigella* vaccines (Levine, 1972; Tramont, 1984)

Table 2. IgA antibody-secreting cell response (ASC) 7 and 21 days after vaccination

		No. tested	No. (%) with significant ASC response[a]	Arithmetic mean of positive results
Day 7	Vaccine	26	18 (69.2)	70.0
	Placebo	10	1 (10.0)	
Day 21	Vaccine	30	11 (36.7)	21.7
	Placebo	18	1 (5.6)	

[a]Significant ASC response - an ASC result equal to or higher than 9 spots/Mcells; this figure is based on the mean (1.58 spots/Mcells) ± 2SD (2 x 3.62 spots/Mcells) found among those receiving placebo.

Table 3. Number (%) of vaccinees with significant antibody response[a]

Time after vaccination	No. tested	IgA	IgG	IgA or IgG
Day 7	53	10 (18.9)	1 (1.9)	10 (18.9)
Day 14	53	4 (7.6)	2 (3.8)	4 (7.6)
Day 28	50	1 (2.0)	3 (6.0)	2 (4.0)
Total	53	15 (28.3)	6 (11.3)	16 (30.2)

[a]Based on Ratio=(Peak OD on days 7,14,28)/(OD on day 0) with Peak OD$\geq$0.15(IgA) or 0.25(IgG); Ratio>2.43(IgA) or 1.78(IgG) was used, based on mean+2SD found in placebo recipients.

ELISA results are based on adjusted OD calculated from a linear regression analysis of eight double dilutions.

3.2. Safety and Immunogenicity of the Parenteral, *S. sonnei*-rEPA and *S. flexneri* 2a-rEPA Conjugate Vaccines

The O-specific polysaccharides (O-SPs) of *P. shigelloides* type O17 (identical with the O-SP of *S. sonnei*) and of *S. flexneri* type 2a were prepared in pure form, free of significant amounts of LPS, protein or nucleic acid. Their structure was identified by ^{13}C N.M.R. and the serological identity verified by immunodiffusion. The O-SPs were then covalently bound to exoprotein A of *Pseudomonas aeruginosa* to form conjugates (Chu, 1992; Taylor, 1993). The O-SPs as conjugates had both increased immunogenicity and T-cell dependent properties in laboratory mice. The vaccines contained 25 µg of conjugate per human dose dissolved in saline with 0.01% thimerosal.

A phase 2 study of the *Shigella* conjugate vaccines was carried out among 192 Israeli soldiers. The volunteers were randomized to receive *S. flexneri* 2a-rEPA vaccine (n = 64), *S. sonnei*-rEPA (n = 66), or hepatitis B vaccine as control (n = 62). The last 33 (16 in *S. flexneri* 2a and 17 in *S. sonnei* vaccine groups) vaccinees received a second dose of the same vaccine 6 weeks later. The first injections of the conjugates and the hepatitis B vaccine elicited similar rates of minor local reactions. Tenderness was detected in 9.7% (6/62), 8.1% (5/62) and 5.0% (3/60), redness was observed in 1.7% (1/62), 3.2% (2/62) and 3.3% (2/60) of the volunteers, following vaccination with the *S. sonnei*, *S. flexneri* 2a and hepatitis B vaccines, respectively. The second injection of *S. sonnei*-*r*EPA induced pain at the injection site in 71.4% (10/14) of volunteers compared to 18.1% (2/11) who received hepatitis B vaccine (p = 0.01). These symptoms were considered mild and did not interfere with the activities of the volunteers. Two of 130 volunteers who received a conjugate vaccine had a slight increase in temperature (37.6°C and 37.7°C) within hours after vaccination, while one recipient of the hepatitis B vaccine had a temperature of 38.5°C, two hours after the first dose. One volunteer developed mild and self-limiting herpes zoster 48 hours following injection with *S. flexneri* 2a-*r*EPA. Slight transient increases in hepatic enzymes were recorded in two volunteers who received *S. flexneri* 2a-*r*EPA and in one who received *S. sonnei*-*r*EPA; these were not present any more upon a subsequent bleeding. All other volunteers had normal hepatic and renal function tests.

S. sonnei-*r*EPA elicited significant rises of IgG anti-LPS in 91% and of IgA in 88% of vaccinees 14 days after immunization. IgG and IgA GMT rose 41- and 141-fold, respectively, on day 14, and remained still significantly high 6 months later (23- and 26-fold, respectively). Only 17% of the volunteers showed a $\geq$4-fold rise in IgM anti-LPS, with levels after 6 months similar to those prior to vaccination. *S. flexneri* 2a-*r*EPA elicited lesser serum antibody responses than *S. sonnei*-*r*EPA. Fourteen days after immunization, 84% showed a $\geq$4-fold rise of IgG anti-LPS and 86% had a $\geq$4-fold rise of IgA. The preimmunization GMT

Table 4. Serum antibody responses to homologous LPS among recipients of *S. sonnei* and *S. flexneri* 2a conjugate vaccines

| | | *S. sonnei* | | | | | | | *S. flexneri 2* | | | | | |
| | | IgG | | IgA | | IgM | | | IgG | | IgA | | IgM | |
Weeks after Injection	No.	GMT	Percent $\geq$4-fold Response	GMT	Percent $\geq$4-fold Response	GMT	Percent $\geq$4-fold Response	No.	GMT	Percent $\geq$4-fold Response	GMT	Percent $\geq$4-fold Response	GMT	Percent $\geq$4-fold Response
0	49	151		16		497		48	90		40		410	
2	42	6260	91	2262	88	1058	17	44	1076	84	846	86	924	21
6	41	5937	88	930	83	784	5	44	850	86	253	52	883	11
24	40	3446	85	420	80	580	0	33	737	73	179	46	690	9

GMT = Geometric Mean Titer for an end-point of OD=0.3 calculated from slope based on 8 double dilutions.

IgG and IgA anti-LPS rose 12- and 21-fold on day 14 and was still 8-fold and 4-fold high, respectively, 6 months later. Only 21% of the volunteers showed a ≥4-fold rise in IgM antibodies on day 14. Six months later, the GMT was similar to the preimmunization level (Table 4). A second dose of either *S. sonnei-r*EPA or *S. flexneri* 2a-*r*EPA neither elicited a booster response nor increased the number of responders. IgG was the highest and most sustained Ig response elicited by the conjugates. There was only slight cross-reactivity of the two conjugates as only 2% of the volunteers produced a ≥4-fold rise to the heterologous LPS. None of the recipients of the hepatitis B vaccine developed a significant antibody response to either LPS.

S. sonnei-*r*EPA elicited significant IgA and IgG ASC responses in 78% and 83% of 23 vaccinees after the first dose. *S. flexneri* 2a-*r*EPA induced significant IgA ASC and IgG ASC rises in 68% and 58% of 19 volunteers similarly examined. The geometric mean ASCs elicited by *S. sonnei-r*EPA was $1159/10^6$ cells for IgA and 659 for IgG while *S. flexneri* 2a-*r*EPA elicited 242 for IgA and 121 for IgG. None of the vaccinees had a significant heterologous LPS response.

3.3. Preliminary Efficacy Studies

Following the phase 2 studies, a study of expanded safety, immunogenicity and preliminary efficacy of the oral *EcSf*2a-2 and the *S. sonnei* conjugate vaccines was performed in volunteers serving in areas with a high risk of exposure to *Shigella*. A five-month follow-up revealed enough cases of *S. sonnei* shigellosis to assess the efficacy of the *S. sonnei* conjugate. The recipients of *S. sonnei-r*EPA had a significantly lower rate of culture-proven *S. sonnei* shigellosis (p = 0.006) than the placebo group, yielding a level of 74% protective efficacy for this vaccine. These findings show that a single injection of *S. sonnei-r*EPA protects adults against homologous infection. We continue to study the conjugate vaccines in Israeli soldiers in order to confirm these promising findings as well as to elucidate the nature of the protective immunity exerted by this new type of enteric vaccine.

ACKNOWLEDGMENTS

These studies were supported by Grant Nos. DAMD 17-88-Z-8010 and DAMD17-93-V-3001 from U.S. Army Medical Research and Materiel Command, Fort Detrick, Frederick, Maryland; and in part by the National Institutes of Health, Bethesda, Maryland.

The authors are grateful to Ruhama Ambar, Ita Marcus, Tamar Sela, Rachel Heller-Mendelziss and Marcelo Low for very helpful technical assistance in the laboratory and field work.

4. REFERENCES

Ashkenazi S., May-Zahav M., Dinari G., Gabbay U., Zilberman A., and Samra Z. 1993. Recent trends in the epidemiology of *Shigella* infections. *Clin. Infect. Dis.* 17:897-899.

Chu C. Y., Liu B., Watson D., Szu S. C., Bryla D., Shiloach J., Schneerson R., and Robbins J. 1992. Preparation, characterization and immunogenicity of conjugates composed of the O-specific polysaccharide of *Shigella dysenteriae* type 1 (Shiga's bacillus) bound to tetanus toxoid. *Infect. Immun.* 59:4450-4458.

Cohen D., Green M. S., Block C., Rouach T., and Ofek I. 1988. Serum antibodies to lipopolysaccharide and natural immunity to shigellosis in an Israeli military population. *J. Infect. Dis.* 157:1068-1071.

Cohen D., Green M., Block C., Lowell G., and Ofek I. 1989. Immunoglobulin M, A, and G antibody response to lipopolysaccharide O antigen in symptomatic and asymptomatic *Shigella* infections. *J. Clin. Microbiol.* 27:162-167.

Cohen D., Green M., Block C., Slepon R., Ambar R., Wasserman S, and Levine M. M. 1991. Reduction of transmission of shigellosis by control of house flies (*Musca domestica*). *Lancet* 337:993-997.

Cohen D., Ashkenazi S., Green M. S., Yavzori M., Orr N., Slepon R., Lerman Y., Robin G., Ambar R., Block C., Taylor D. N., Hale T. L., Sadoff J. C., and Wiener M. 1994. Safety and immunogenicity of the oral *E. coli* K12-*S. flexneri* 2a vaccine (*EcSf2a-2*) among Israeli soldiers. *Vaccine* 12:1436-1442.

DuPont H. L., Levine M. M., Hornick R. B., and Formal S. B. 1989. Inoculum size in shigellosis and implications for expected mode of transmission. *J. Infect. Dis.* 159:1126-1128.

Formal S. B., Hale T. L., Kapfer C., Cogan J. P., Snoy P. J., Chung Y., Wingfield M. E., Elisberg B. L., and Baron L. S. 1984. Oral vaccination of monkeys with an invasive *Escherichia coli* K12 hybrid expressing *Shigella flexneri* 2a somatic antigen. *Infect. Immun.* 46:465-469.

Green M. S., Cohen D., Block C., Rouach T., and Dycian R. 1987. A prospective epidemiologic study of shigellosis. Implications for the new *Shigella* vaccines. *Isr. J. Med. Sci.* 23:811-815.

Green M. S., Block C., Cohen D., and Slater P. 1991. Four decades of shigellosis in Israel - the epidemiology of a growing public health problem. *Rev. Inf. Dis.* 13:248-253.

Herrington D. A., Van De Verg L., Formal S. B., Hale T. L., Tall B. D., Cryz S. J., Tramont E. C., and Levine M. M. 1990. Studies in volunteers to evaluate candidate *Shigella* vaccines. Further experience with a bivalent *Salmonella typhi-Shigella sonnei* vaccine and protection conferred by previous *Shigella sonnei* disease. *Vaccine* 8:353-357.

Institute of Medicine. Prospects for immunizing against *Shigella* spp. In: New Vaccine Development: Establishing Priorities; Diseases of Importance in Developing Countries, vol. 2; National Academic Press, Washington, D.C., 1986:329-337.

Kotloff L. K., Herrington D. A., Hale T. L., Newland J. W., Van De Verg L., Cogan J. P., Snoy P. J., Sadoff J. C., Formal S. B., and Levine M. M. 1992. Safety, immunogenicity, and efficacy in monkeys and humans of invasive *Escherichia coli* K12 hybrid vaccine candidates expressing *Shigella flexneri* 2a somatic antigen. *Infect. Immun.* 60:2218-2224.

Levine M. M., DuPont H. L., Gangarosa E. J., Hornick R. B., Snyder M. J., Libonati J. P., Glaser K., and Formal S. B. 1972. Shigellosis in custodial institutions. II. Clinical immunologic and bacteriologic response of institutionalized children to oral attenuated *Shigella* vaccines. *Am. J. Epidemiol.* 966:40-49.

Li A., Karnell A., Huan P. T., Cam P. D., Minh N. B., Tram L. N., et al. 1993. Safety and immunogenicity of the live oral auxotrophic *Shigella flexneri* SFL124 in adult Vietnamese volunteers. *Vaccine* 11:180-189.

Lindberg A. A., Karnell A., and Stocker B.A.D. Aromatic-dependent *Shigella* strains as oral live vaccines. In: Woodrow G. C., Levine M. M. (eds.), New Generation Vaccines. Vaccines against *Shigella* part II. Marcel Dekker, New York, 1990:677-687.

Newland J. W., Hale T. L., and Formal S. B. 1992. Genotypic and phenotypic characterization of an *aro*D deletion attenuated *Escherichia coli* K12-*Shigella flexneri* hybrid vaccine expressing *S. flexneri* 2a somatic antigen. *Vaccine* 10:766-776.

Noriega F. R., Wang J. Y., Losonsky G., Maneval D. R., Hone D. M., and Levine M. M. 1994. Construction and characterization of attenuated Δ*aro*A Δ*vir*G *Shigella flexneri* 2a strain CVD 1203, a prototype live oral vaccine. *Infect. Immun.* 62:5168-5172.

Orr N., Robin G., Lowell G., and Cohen D. 1992. Presence of specific immunoglobulin A secreting cells in peripheral blood following natural infection with *Shigella sonnei*. *J. Clin. Microbiol.* 30:2165-2168.

Orr N., Robin G., Cohen D., Arnon R., and Lowell G. H. 1993. Immunogenicity and efficacy of oral or intranasal *Shigella flexneri* 2a and *Shigella sonnei* proteosome-lipopolysaccharide vaccines in animal models. *Infect. Immun.* 61:2390-2395.

Robbins J. B., Chu C. Y., and Schneerson R. 1992. Hypothesis for vaccine development: serum IgG LPS antibodies confer protective immunity to non-typhoidal Salmonellae and Shigellae. *Clin. Infect. Dis.* 15:346-361.

Sanchez J. L., Trofa A. F., Taylor D. N., Kushner R. A., DeFraites R. F., Craig S. C., Rao M. R., Clemens J. D., Svennerholm A., Sadoff J. C., and Holmgren J. 1993. Safety and immunogenicity of the oral, whole cell/recombinant B subunit cholera vaccine in North American volunteers. *J. Infect. Dis.* 167:1446-1449.

Sansonnetti P. J. and Arondel J. 1989. Construction and evaluation of a double mutant of *Shigella flexneri* as a candidate for oral vaccination against shigellosis. *Vaccine* 7:443-450.

Smollan G. and Block C. 1992. Development of antimicrobial drug resistance among Shigellas isolated at an Israeli hospital from 1977 through 1990. *Publ. Health Rev.* 18:319-327.

Taylor D. N., Trofa A. C., Sadoff J., Chu C. Y., Bryla D. A., Shiloach J., Cohen D., Ashkenazi S., Lerman Y., Egan M., Schneerson R., and Robbins J. 1993. Synthesis, characterization, and clinical evaluation of conjugate vaccines composed of the O-specific polysaccharides of *Shigella dysenteriae* type 1,

Shigella flexneri type 2, *Shigella sonnei* (*Plesiomonas shigelloides*) bound to bacterial toxoids. *Infect. Immun.* 61:3678-3687.

Taylor D., Phillip D. F., Zapor M., Trofa A., Van de Verg L., Hartman A., Bendiuk N., Newland J. W., Formal S. B., and Sadoff J. C. 1994. Outpatient studies of the safety and immunogenicity of the auxotrophic *Escherichia coli-Shigella flexneri* hybrid vaccine candidate *EcSf*2a-2. *Vaccine* 12:565-568.

Tramont E. C., Chung R., Berman S., Keren D., Kapfer C., and Formal S. B. 1984. Safety and antigenicity of Typhoid-*Shigella sonnei* vaccine (Strain 5076-IC). *J. Infect. Dis.* 149:133-136.

22

HYPOTHESIS: HOW LICENSED VACCINES CONFER PROTECTIVE IMMUNITY

John B. Robbins, Rachel Schneerson, and Shousun C. Szu

Laboratory of Developmental and Molecular Immunity
National Institute of Child Health and Human Development, NIH
Bethesda, Maryland 20892

ABSTRACT

By examining experience with evaluation of licensed vaccines we theorize that a critical level of serum IgG confers protection against infectious diseases by killing or inactivating the inoculum. We found that efficacy is reliably predicted by measurement of serum antibodies elicited by vaccines, that serum IgG antibodies alone account for the protection conferred by passive immunization, that vaccine-induced "herd" immunity is best explained by inactivation of the inoculum on epithelial surfaces by serum antibodies and that serum antibodies induced by active immunization will neither treat disease symptoms nor eliminate the pathogen. If valid, this theory should facilitate research because knowledge of the pathogenesis of the disease symptoms may not be essential for vaccine development.

INTRODUCTION

Our theory about the mechanism of vaccines' protective action is based mostly upon indirect evidence from re-examination of epidemiologic, clinical and laboratory data. We considered the FDA requirements for vaccines as well as data about individual pathogens [19]. BCG and adenovirus vaccines were not considered because there is limited information about protective immunity to these organisms.

Licensed vaccines confer protective immunity by eliciting serum IgG antibodies which eliminate the inoculum by either killing bacteria, "inactivating" viruses or neutralizing toxins. For many of the diseases, vaccine-induced serum IgG inactivates the inoculum on mucous membranes. This explains how serum IgG anti-polysaccharide may prevent diseases caused by respiratory and enteric bacterial pathogens [81,99,109].

Other mechanisms may also be protective, such as serum IgM and IgA, secretory antibodies or T-cell mediated immunity which may be induced by licensed vaccines, disease with the homologous organism or by interaction with cross-reacting organisms.

Novel Strategies in Design and Production of Vaccines
Edited by S. Cohen and A. Shafferman, Plenum Press, New York, 1996

STANDARDIZATION OF VACCINES

Despite their heterogeneity, different routes of administration, the wide spectrum of diseases they prevent, and although they may induce more than one immune mechanism, regulatory agencies standardize vaccines only by their ability to elicit a protective level of serum antibodies in order to predict their effectiveness [Table 1].

The bioassays for some vaccines were developed for standardization when only incomplete knowledge was available about their mode of action. For example, cellular pertussis vaccines are assayed by survival of mice following intraperitoneal immunization and intracerebral challenge with *Bordetella pertussis* [83,87]. Now, there is convincing evidence for the *essential* role of serum neutralizing antibodies (antitoxin) in mediating the vaccine-induced protection of mice [21,75]. The newly licensed acellular vaccines must elicit antitoxin in mice by primary immunization and by a booster injection in children [21]. There is evidence now that serum antitoxin is both necessary and sufficient to prevent pertussis [51,75,87,91].

Diphtheria: Diphtheria toxoid is assayed by its ability to elicit ≥ 2 IU/mL serum antitoxin in guinea pigs and in humans.

Typhoid vaccines: There are three types of typhoid vaccines.Inactivated *Salmonella typhi* (cellular vaccines) are assayed by intraperitoneal immunization of mice followed by challenge with *S. typhi*: protection is related to the immunogenicity of the Vi capsular polysaccharide (Vi) [88] and there is evidence from animal and human studies that serum antibodies to this antigen alone confer protection [114]. The efficacy of Vi polysaccharide typhoid vaccine [114] is predicted by its ability to elicit serum antibodies. Neither the protective antigen(s) nor the host immune mechanism(s) responsible for protection elicited by Ty21a, an orally-administered attenuated strain of *S. typhi*,are yet known [57].

Cholera vaccines: There are two cholera vaccines. One, composed of inactivated strains of *V. cholerae* 01, serotypes Ogawa and Inaba, is evaluated in mice similarly to the cellular typhoid vaccines [64,99]. The efficacy of the cellular and LPS vaccines was related to their ability to elicit serum vibriocidal antibodies [11,99]. The second is an orally administered attenuated strain of *V. cholerae* 01 (CVD 103-HgR) [59]. The FDA required demonstration of a rise in serum vibriocidal antibodies for its licensure.

Capsular Polysaccharides: The 4-valent vaccine for *meningococci*, 23-valent vaccine for pneumococci, *H. influenzae* type b vaccine, Vi typhoid vaccine, are standardized by gel filtration to measure their molecular "size" which predicts their ability to elicit serum antibodies [113]. The FDA requires that a newly developed polysaccharide vaccine elicit a ≥ 4-fold rise of antibodies with antibacterial properties in $\geq 80\%$ of the recipients [113].

***Haemophilus* type b Conjugates:** WHO and the FDA specify that each new product shall elicit serum *H. influenzae* type b antibodies with bactericidal activity in infants [115].

Influenza virus: Prior to licensure of a new strain of influenza, demonstration that serum hemagglutinin-inhibiting antibodies are elicited by several consecutively manufactured lots is required.

Rubeola (measles): FDA required clinical studies of consecutively manufactured lots of the attenuated strain of measles virus for their ability to elicit serum neutralizing antibodies [110].

Rubella: Requirements for the new strain, RA 27/3, which replaced the original attenuated rubella virus included that 90% of recipients respond with a protective level of serum neutralizing antibodies [22].

Mumps: Mumps virus vaccine must elicit neutralizing antibodies in $\geq 5,000$ recipients.

Table 1. U.S. licensed vaccines

Vaccine	Type	Route
Adenovirus*	Live virus	Oral
Anthrax	Inactivated bacteria	S.C.
BCG	Attenuated live bacteria	I.D.
Cholera	Inactivated bacteria	S.C.
	Attenuated live bacteria	Oral
DTP	Toxoids, inactivated bacteria	I.M.
Hib conjugate	Polysaccharide-protein	I.M.
Influenza	Inactivated virus, components	S.C.
Japanese encephalitis	Inactivated virus	S.C.
Measles-mumps-rubella	Attenuated virus	
Meningococcus	A,C,Y,W135 polysaccharides	S.C.
Plague	Inactivated bacteria	I.M.
Pneumococcus	23-valent polysaccharide	S.C.
Polio (OPV)	Attenuated 3 types	Oral
(IPV)	Inactivated 3 virus types	S.C.
Rabies	Inactivated virus	I.M.
Typhoid	Inactivated bacteria	S.C.
(Ty21a)	Attenuated bacteria	Oral
Varicella	Attenuated virus	S.C.
Yellow fever	Attenuated virus	S.C.

*Recommended only for use in U.S. Armed Forces.
After: CDC. 1994. *MMWR*, Volume 43 [1].

Poliovirus: Both the inactivated and attenuated strains of poliovirus elicit serum neutralizing antibodies in monkeys and humans to the three virus serotypes in the vaccine.

Japanese Encephalitis Virus: The formalin-inactivated virus vaccine must elicit a serum neutralizing titer $\geq 1/10$ in mice. This level of serum antibody is also used to evaluate vaccine-induced protective immunity in humans [20].

In summary, the only immune response required by the FDA and other regulatory agencies for standardization of newly manufactured vaccine lots is their ability to stimulate protective levels of serum antibodies.

PASSIVELY ADMINISTERED SERUM IgG CONFERS IMMUNITY

Table 2 lists licensed immunoglobulins. Whether placentally transmitted or by injection of immunoglobulin, passively acquired antibodies confer protection to diseases covered by the above vaccines. Only serum IgG is transmitted from the mother to the human newborn. IgG comprises $\geq 90\%$ of the immunoglobulin used for passive immunization [52,108]. Accordingly, only serum IgG mediates passively-acquired protective immunity.

Passively acquired antibodies are effective in preventing systemic infections caused by respiratory capsulated pathogens [38,43,54] and the toxin-mediated diseases of diphtheria [71], pertussis [83] and tetanus [79]. Passive immunization with hyperimmune globulin, from adults injected with polysaccharide vaccines, prevents pneumococcal otitis media [94] considered as a "mucosal" disease. This finding provides evidence that serum IgG exerts antibacterial actions on the epithelial surfaces. A likely explanation is that specific serum

Table 2. U.S. Licensed Products For Passive Immunization

Disease	Biologic	Indication
Botulism	Specific equine Ig	Treatment
CMV	Hyperimmune human IV Ig	Prophylaxis
Diphtheria	Specific equine Ig	Treatment
Ig	Pooled human Ig	Hepatitis A, measles
Ig IV	Pooled human Ig	Ig deficiency, ITP, Kawasaki disease
Hepatitis B Ig	Immune human Ig	Hepatitis B
Rabies (HRIG)	Immune human Ig	Prophylaxis
Tetanus Ig (TIG)	Immune human Ig	Treatment
Vaccinia	Immune human Ig	Treatment
Varicella-zoster	Immune human Ig	Prophylaxis

After: CDC. 1994. *MMWR*, Volume 43 [1]

IgG inhibits colonization as was shown for immunization with polysaccharide vaccines for pneumococci [61], meningococci [44] and for *Haemophilus influenzae* type b [101].

Although the evidence is indirect placentally-transmitted antibody confers protection against cholera [26] and shigellosis (also considered as "mucosal" diseases), based on the rarity of cases up to ~6 months of age [26,35,37]. Although there are no clinical data, passively injected serum IgG anti-Vi confers protection to mice against challenge with *S. typhi* [40] and serum antibodies against the protective antigen protect mice against challenge with *Bacillus anthracis* [50].

Passively acquired antibodies prevent measles, rubella, mumps, poliomyelitis, varicella, hepatitis A and B, rabies, CMV and RSV [8,47,52,78,98]. With the exceptions of rabies and hepatitis B, these viral pathogens contact the host on the surface of mucous membranes. It is not known whether passive immunization also prevents colonization with or transmission of viral pathogens from a treated host.

High titered human antitoxin exerts therapeutic activity against pertussis [16,45] but whether this new product prevents infection with *B. pertussis* has not been reported. In mice, passive immunization with antitoxin prevents *B. pertussis* infection [83,87,90,91].

The successful experience with passive immunization in preventing bacterial and viral infections in patients with X-linked hypogammaglobulinemia provides evidence for our theory [17,38,91].

In summary, these data show that a critical level of serum IgG antibodies *alone* can prevent infectious diseases.

POLYSACCHARIDE *VS* PROTEIN ANTIGENS

The protective antigens of viral vaccines, tetanus, diphtheria and pertussis are proteins which are specific and T-cell dependent. The presence of serum antibodies to these proteins in an adult either follows disease caused by that pathogen or immunization with a specific vaccine.

Capsular polysaccharides are considered T-cell independent antigens and O-specific polysaccharides of LPS as haptens [81]. Acquisition of serum antibodies to these surface polysaccharides is age-related [38,43,54,81,85,86] and may occur without interaction the homologous organism [91]. The following illustrate this point: 1) isohemagglutinins are present in adults depending upon their blood group antigens [96]. Their ubiquitous presence is due to the terminal disaccharide structures of blood group antigens among the enteric flora and some parasites [3,85]; 2) despite the absence of Group A meningococci from the United States for about 50 years, most adults have antibodies to this capsular polysaccharide [43]. The stimuli for these Group A antibodies are likely several Gram-positive and Gram-negative enteric bacteria [48,104]; and 3) adults in Sweden and the United State have antibodies to the LPS of *Shigella dysenteriae* type 1 despite the absence of this pathogen [60,102]. The stimulus for "natural" antibodies is probably by identical or cross-reacting polysaccharides of the enteric and respiratory tract flora [53].

In summary, "natural" serum antibodies explain the age-related incidence of diseases whose protective antigens are surface polysaccharides. Antibodies to proteins, in contrast, are elicited either by infection or by immunization.

SERUM IgG ANTIBODIES ARE ON THE SURFACES OF MUCOUS MEMBRANES

Serum IgG is found on the mucosal surfaces of respiratory [76,80] and intestinal tracts [7,74,111] and on the cervix [15,24] probably by transudation [107]. In animals, serum antibodies to bovine serum albumin and *E. coli* and colostral antibodies to strain G206 of *E. coli* (O8:K87[B]K88ac[L]) induce rapid emigration of neutrophils onto the intestinal lumen without accompanying inflammation of the mucous membranes [9,93].

SERUM IgG-MEDIATED PREVENTION *VS* THERAPY

We infer that vaccine-induced serum antibodies must inactivate the inoculum to confer protection based upon comparison of the quantity required for prevention *vs* that required for therapy of *H. influenzae* type b meningitis [2,82]. The difference between the preventative dose of antibody (~1 mg) and the therapeutic dose (0.6 grams) is explained by the few organisms in the inoculum compared to the large number in the CSF of meningitis patients. Similar differences exist between the preventative *vs* the therapeutic doses for meningococcal and pneumococcal infections.

Passive immunization with immunoglobulin taken from adults prevents viral diseases [52]. But administration of immunoglobulin has no *therapeutic* effect upon infections caused by these viruses [52]. Recently, high-titered immunoglobulin or monoclonal anti-viral antibodies have shown therapeutic effects in animal models and in clinical diseases [23].

In summary, passively acquired serum IgG antibodies prevent systemic diseases and otitis media as an example of a mucosal disease. The preventative dose of antibody is low compared to the therapeutic level probably due to the number of organisms involved and serum IgG antibodies are found on mucous membrane surfaces.

EPIDEMIOLOGIC, CLINICAL AND IMMUNOLOGICAL DATA

Capsulated Bacterial Pathogens

The first randomized, placebo-controlled study of capsular polysaccharide vaccines was in a U.S. Army Technical School in 1940 [61]. The recruits received either pneumococcal types 1, 2, 5 and 7 (n=5239) or saline (n=5105). Participants were examined for pneumonia and for pharyngeal carriage of pneumococci over the next six-months. There was type-specific reduction of pneumonia in the vaccinees and 6 months later there was also a statistically significant reduction of pneumonia as well as carriage of *only* the vaccine types in both the vaccinees and in the controls. Similar effects of vaccine-induced capsular polysaccharide antibodies have been reported for meningococci and have been characterized as"herd" immunity [44,73].

"Infant" pneumococcal types are poor immunogens in children and failed to inhibit carriage in that age group [5,31,62]. Similarly, *H. influenzae* type b polysaccharide failed to stimulate protective antibody levels in children up to ~2-years of age [85,86,95] as well as affect pharyngeal carriage of this pathogen. But the improved *H. influenzae* type b conjugates [4,25,86,92] have virtually eliminated meningitis and other systemic infections, as well as pharyngeal carriage of this pathogen [12,101] despite incomplete rates of immunization. This "herd immunity" likely results from vaccine-induced serum antibodies eliminating the inocula on pharyngeal surfaces thereby preventing carriage and reducing their transmission. Protection conferred by Vi vaccines was presumed to be bacteriolysis of *S. typhi* in the bloodstream [88,114]. It is also possible that the inoculum (most often $\leq 10^3$ organisms [13] is killed on the intestinal surface by serum IgG anti-Vi. In order to increase its immunogenicity, conjugate technology has been adapted to Vi [100]. There is indirect evidence that a critical level of type-specific IgG antibodies will confer protective immunity to neonates against Group B streptococci [6].

Widespread immunization with conjugate vaccines could, theoretically, eliminate meningococci, *H. influenzae* type b and *S. typhi* because these organisms are inhabitants of and pathogens of humans only.

Lipopolysaccharides

Cholera. The symptoms of cholera are mediated largely by the actions of cholera toxin upon the small intestine [81,99]: systemic infection is rarely encountered. But neither serum nor secretory antitoxin confer protection against cholera in humans.

Resistance to cholera has been correlated only with a serum vibriocidal antibody titer of $\geq 1/160$ [11,64,99]. Parenterally administered inactivated cellular and LPS vaccines induced statistically significant protection against cholera in adults for ~6 months. These vaccines elicited mostly serum LPS antibodies with vibriocidal activity but did not induce antitoxin. Serum LPS antibodies are the main component that exerts this vibriocidal activity [64,67,99]. Age-related immunogenicity and effectiveness were also obtained with orally administered inactivated *V. cholerae* 01 [27]: addition of the B subunit of cholera toxin did not provide an increase in protection. An explanation for how serum vibriocidal (LPS) antibodies prevent a disease in which the pathogen is confined to the lumen of the intestine and the symptoms are caused by an exotoxin is as follows: 1) the inoculum of *V. cholerae* is low ($\leq 10^3$) [58]; 2) serum antibodies (and likely complement) are in intestinal fluid [7,74,81,99,111]; 3) the intestinal walls are in contact because of peristalsis; 4) *V. cholerae* are susceptible to lysis induced by antibodies and complement. Serum vibriocidal antibodies prevent cholera by inducing complement-mediated lysis of the inoculum of *V. cholerae* in the jejunum [81,99].

Shigellae, Enteroinvasive Escherichia Coli and Non-Typhoidal Salmonellae.
There is no consensus about what are the host protective immune moiety(ies) and there are no valid experimental models for most of these enteric pathogens. Based upon the *similarities* between their pathogenesis and upon limited information about protective immunity, we proposed that vaccine-induced serum IgG to the O-specific polysaccharides of non-typhoidal salmonellae and shigellae could confer protective immunity by killing the inoculum in the intestine [81]: 1) as with *V. cholerae* [122], a low inoculum of shigellae and of non-typhoidal

salmonellae ($\sim 10^3$) is sufficient to cause disease [32]; 2) the age-related susceptibility to these diseases may be explained by acquisition of serum antibodies to their surface polysaccharides: newborns by placental transmission and adults by either infection with the homologous organism or with cross-reacting antigens [3,48,53,60,81,85,86,96,102,104]; 3) full expression of their LPS is required for these pathogens to be virulent; 4) of the four major groups of pathogenic non-typhoidal salmonellae, only *S. typhimurium* (Group B) is a pathogen for animals: both actively induced or passively acquired serum O-specific antibodies confer protection in mice [18,109]; 5) convalescence from shigellosis confers only LPS-specific protective immunity [29,35,81]; 6) there is a correlation between pre-existing serum IgG-anti LPS and resistance to shigellosis [55]; 6) both shigellae and salmonellae are intracellular when the disease is manifest and it is improbable that serum antibodies will then be effective. Because shigellae and *E. coli* should be considered as one genus, our approach may be applied to vaccine development for pathogenic *E. coli* such as the O111 and O157 serotypes [28,49,81].

Preliminary data indicate that a *S. sonnei* O-specific polysaccharide conjugate elicits protective immunity in Israel Defense Forces recruits [28]. If substantiated by more extensive clinical trials, this finding provides evidence for our hypothesis that serum antibodies inactivate the inoculum of shigellae.

Serum Antitoxin (IgG) Exerts Anti-bacterial Immunity Against Diphtheria and Pertussis. *Corynebacterium diphtheriae* and *Bordetella pertussis* are not invasive and reside on the respiratory membranes. Both diseases can be prevented by vaccine-induced serum antitoxin [21,52,63,79,83,87,91]. Our explanation is that the toxin of each confers a selective advantage for each by providing a phagocyte-free milieu on the respiratory mucosa [1,83,87] and the antitoxin eliminates this advantage. Widespread usage of diphtheria toxoid vaccines has virtually eliminated toxigenic *C. diphtheriae* [63]. Pertussis antitoxin prevents colonization by this pathogen in mice and inhibits colonization and pertussis in children [1,83,90,91,103].

VIRAL DISEASES

Poliovirus: Poliovirus causes a mild and self-limited enteritis in most individuals: myelitis is not required for its transmission. The protective antigen ("D") is conformationally determined by the association of its four outer capsid polypeptides. Passively-acquired serum IgG prevents poliomyelitis [52,78] but its effect upon the viability of poliovirus in the intestine however, has not been studied. In The Netherlands and in Sweden, infants have been immunized with an improved Formalin-inactivated poliovirus vaccine (EIPV or Salk-type) [14,105] for ~30 years: compliance is almost 100%. The injected vaccine elicits mostly serum antibodies in infants [69,97] and its widespread use has eliminated poliovirus and poliomyelitis in these two countries [14]. The best explanation for this disappearance is that vaccine-induced serum antibodies inactivate intestinal poliovirus [34,42,89].

Measles: Its stormy development has led many to consider that the attenuated measles virus vaccine confers protection by eliciting both secretory antibodies and T-cell mediated immunity. Three factors: high rate of contagion, spread by patients only and a high rate and long duration of protective immunity following disease [56], accounted for the triennial cycle of measles in children prior to widespread immunization [36].

Passively acquired serum antibodies prevent measles [52]. There are no experimentally-based data that other immune components *prevent* measles in humans. Development of the Formalin-treated virus vaccine considered that the hemagglutinin (H) was the protective antigen and antibodies that inhibited virus-induced hemagglutination were presumed to mediate immunity. In some recipients of the formalin-inactivated vaccine, an unusual disease with wild-type measles resulted presumed to be caused by deposition of virus-antibody complexes [10,39]. Later, it was shown that another surface protein, the fusion (F) protein, was an important protective antigen and that the Formalin-treatment had abrogated the immunogenicity of this component [68].

Currently, the live virus vaccine is standardized and sero-epidemiologic studies measure the levels of serum neutralizing antibodies (anti-F) and antibodies to the F and H proteins. The attenuated strain has limitations: 1) maternally-derived antibodies persist in some infants up to 15 months and may inactivate the attenuated vaccine and; 2) antibody levels may wane after two decades in a sizable fraction of individuals vaccinated during infancy. Both limitations are probably due to the small amount and reduced level of replication of the virus ($\sim 10^5$) in the vaccine. If the hypothesis about the protective action of the F and possibly H proteins [106] is correct, these antigens, in amounts comparable to diphtheria and tetanus toxoids, could be incorporated into DTP and administered to infants.

Hepatitis A virus (HAV): HAV is acquired by ingestion of the pathogen. Passive immunization prevents HAV disease [52]. The development of Formalin-inactivated HAV has provided an important new vaccine [77,112]: It is likely that the ability of HAV vaccines to elicit neutralizing antibodies will be required by the FDA.

Varicella: Varicella is highly contagious and spread by aerosol. Following its establishment in the lungs, the virus spreads throughout the body: visible signs of disease are limited largely to the epidermis. FDA requires demonstration of serum neutralizing antibodies elicited by the vaccine in sero-negative recipients [41].

Rotavirus: Vaccine development for this important cause of infantile diarrhea has been complicated. Four serotypes cause the majority of diarrhea and vaccine-induced protection is largely serotype-specific. To-date, the best correlation with protective immunity to diarrhea caused by rotavirus is the level of serum serotype-specific antibodies [46].

In summary, serum IgG antibodies alone prevent viral diseases. Usage of inactivated poliovirus vaccine in infants provides evidence that serum antibodies eliminate the inoculum in the intestine.

INACTIVATED *VS* ATTENUATED ORGANISMS AS VACCINES

There is no evidence, to-date, that any vaccine-induced component other than serum antibodies *prevent* infectious diseases. Accordingly, an optimal vaccine would be one that elicits protective levels of serum IgG antibodies in all recipients for the longest duration.

SUMMARY

We propose that vaccine-induced serum IgG kills or inactivates the inoculum of the pathogen. For many infections, this inactivation is mediated by serum IgG that exudes onto epithelial surfaces. Although they may induce more than one immune component, vaccines are standardized by measurement of serum antibodies only. Serum IgG antibodies, whether passively-acquired or actively induced, *prevent* both bacterial and viral diseases. The difference in the amount of antibody required for prevention *vs* therapy is explained by the size of the inoculum which is several logarithms lower than the number of organisms in an established infection. Serum IgG is the only immunoglobulin provided by passive immunization and this Ig class will induce secondary biologic activities, such as complement-dependent lysis, opsonophagocytosis of bacteria or neutralization of viruses, required for inactivation of the inoculum. Vaccine-induced serum IgG to surface polysaccharides prevent carriage of bacterial pathogens by killing the inoculum on the pharyngeal mucosa. In order to confer protection, IgG antibodies must be present when the host encounters the pathogen. Because a single organism that enters the bloodstream may multiply and cause a systemic infection [66], vaccine-induced serum antibodies may also provide a second line of resistance. The study of enteric pathogens provides evidence that serum IgG kills the inoculum as the pathogen enters the jejunum.

If this theory is correct, serum IgG will inhibit the development of active immunity because these antibodies will eliminate the pathogen and there will be no immunogenic stimulus because the inoculum is small and short-lived. An immune individual will not transmit the pathogen because it is inactivated so quickly which accounts for the vaccine-induced "herd" immunity. Vaccine development should be directed towards initial contact with the pathogen because the levels of vaccine-induced serum antibodies will neither treat the symptoms of the disease nor eliminate the pathogen once a systemic infection is established. Based upon experience with licensed vaccines, we predict that a vaccine that induces serum neutralizing (inactivating) antibodies to all strains of HIV-1 would prevent AIDS [30]. This subject, reviewed from another perspective, is referred to the readers [84].

ACKNOWLEDGMENTS

We are grateful to Robert Austrian, Robert A. Chanock, Rajesh A. Gupta, Lars Å. Hanson, Birger Trollfors, David Towne and Joan D. Robbins for their comments and suggestions.

It is not possible to acknowledge all the contributions in the REFERENCES that formed the basis for our hypothesis.

REFERENCES

1. Ad Hoc Group for the study of pertussis vaccines. Placebo-controlled trial of two acellular pertussis vaccines in Sweden - protective efficacy and adverse events. Lancet i:955-960.

2. Alexander H.E. Experimental basis for treatment of *Haemophilus influenzae* infections. Amer. J. Dis. Child. 1943:66:160-71.

3. Andersson M, Carlin N, Leontein K, Lindquist U, Slettengren K. Structural studies of the O-antigenic polysaccharide of *Escherichia coli* O86, which possess blood-group B activity. Carbohydr. Res. 1989:185:211-23.

4. Anderson P. Antibody responses to *Haemophilus influenzae* type b and diphtheria toxin induced by conjugates of oligosaccharides of the type b capsule with the nontoxic protein CRM 197. Infect. Immun. 1983:39:233-8.

5. Austrian R. Some observations on the pneumococcus and on the current status of pneumococcal disease and its prevention. Rev. Infect. Dis. Suppl: 1981:S1-S17

6. Baker CJ, Kasper DL. Correlation of maternal antibody deficiency and susceptibility to neonatal group B streptococcal infection. N. Eng. J. Med. 294:753-756.

7. Batty I, Bullen JJ. The permeability of the sheep and rabbit intestinal wall to antitoxin present in the circulation. J. Path. Bact. 1961:81:447-58.

8. Beasley RP, Hwang L-Y, Steven CE, et al. Efficacy of hepatitis B immune globulin for prevention of perinatal transmission of the hepatitis B virus carrier state: Final report of a randomized double-blind, placebo-controlled trial. Hepatology. 1983:3:135-41.

9. Bellamy JEC, Ole Nielsen N. Immune-mediated emigration of neutrophils into the lumen of the small intestine. 1974:9:615-19.

10. Bellanti JA. Biologic significance of the secretory γA immunoglobulins. Pediatr. 1975:48:715-29.

11. Benenson AS. Review of experience with whole-cell and somatic antigen vaccines. Proceedings of the 12th Joint Conference of US Japan Cooperative Medical Sciences Program, Cholera Panel, Sapporo. 1976:228-42.

12. Black SB, Shinefield HR, and the Kaiser Permanente Vaccine Study Group. Pediatr. Infect. Dis. J. 1992:11:610-13.

13. Blaser MJ. Newman LS. A review of human salmonellosis: Infective dose. Rev. Infect. Dis. 1982:4:1096-106.

14. Böttiger M. Long-term immunity following vaccination with killed poliovirus vaccine in Sweden, a country with no circulating virus. Rev. Infect. Dis. 1984:6:S548-S51.

15. Bouvet JP, Bélec L, René Pirès, Pilot J. Immunoglobulin G antibodies in human vaginal secretions after parenteral vaccination. Infect. Immun. 1994:62:3957-61

16. Bruss JB, Siber G. Treatment of severe pertussis with intravenous pertussis immune globulin. Abstract ICCAAC 103761. 1993.

17. Bruton OC. Agammaglobulinemia. Pediatr. 1952:9:727-8.

18. Carlin NIA, Svenson SB, Lindberg AA. Role of monoclonal 0-antigen antibody epitope specificity and isotype in protection against experimental mouse typhoid. Microbiol. Path. 1987:2:171-183130.

19. Centers for Disease Control. General Recommendations on Immunization. MMWR. 1994:43:RR-1.

20. Centers for Disease Control. Inactivated Japanese Encephalitis Virus Vaccine. MMWR, 1993:42:RR-1.

21. Centers for Disease Control. Pertussis vaccination: Acellular pertussis vaccine for reinforcing and booster use - Supplementary ACIP Statement. MMWR. 1992:41:1-10.

22. Centers for Disease Control. Rubella Prevention. MMWR, 1981:3037-47

23. Chanock RM, Crowe JE Jr, Murphy BR, Burton DR. Human monoclonal antibody Fab fragments cloned from combinatorial libraries: Potential usefulness in prevention and.or treatment of major human viral diseases. Infect. Agents Dis.1993:2:118-31.

24. Chodriker WB, Tomasi TB Jr. Gamma globulins: quantitative relationship in human sera and non-vascular fluids. Science 1963:142:1080-81.

25. Chu CY, Schneerson R, Robbins JB, Rastogi SC. Further studies on the immunogenicity of *Haemophilus influenzae* type b and pneumococcal type 6A polysaccharide-protein conjugates. Infect. Immun. 1983:40:245-56.

26. Clemens JD, Sack DA, Chakraborty J. et al. Field trial of oral cholera vaccines in Bangladesh: Evaluation of anti-bacterial and anti-toxic breast-milk immunity in response to ingestion of the vaccines. Vaccine 1990:8:469-72.

27. Clemens JD, Sack DA, Harris JR, et al. Field trial of oral cholera vaccines in Bangladesh: results from a three-year follow-up. Lancet 1990:335:270-73.

28. Cohen D, Ashkenazi S, Green M. et al. Safety and immunogenicity of *Shigella flexneri* 2a and *Shigella sonnei* conjugate vaccines: preliminary efficacy of the *S. sonnei* conjugate in Israeli soldiers. submitted for publication. 1994.

29. Cohen D, Green MS, Block C, Slepon R, Ofek I. A prospective study on the association between serum antibodies to lipopolysaccharide and attack rate of shigellosis. J. Clin. Microbiol. 1991:29:386-9.

30. Conley AJ, Gorny MK, Kessler JA II. et al. Neutralization of pimrary human immunodeficiency virus type 1 isolates by the broadly reactive anti-V3 monoclonal antibody, 447-52D. J. Virol. 1994:68:6994-7000.

31. Douglas RM, Hansman D, Miles HB, Paton JC. Pneumococcal carriage and type-specific antibody. Failure of a 14-valent vaccine to reduce carriage in healthy children. Am. J. Dis. Child. 1986:140:1183-5.

32. DuPont HL, Levine MM, Hornick RB, Formal SB. Inoculum size in shigellosis and implications for expected mode of transmission. J. Infect. Dis. 1989:159:1126-28.

33. Eibl MM, Cairns L, Rosen FS. Safety and efficacy of a monomeric, functionally intact intravenous IgG preparation in patients with primary immunodeficiency syndromes. Clin. Imunol. Immunopathol. 1994:31:151-69.

34. Faden H, Modlin JF, Thomas ML, McBean AM, Ferdon MB, Ogra PL. Comparative evaluation of immunization with live attenuated and enhanced-potency inactivated poliovirus vaccines in childhood: Systemic and local immune responses. J. Infect. Dis. 1990:162:1291-97.

35. Ferreccio C, Prado V, Ojeda A, Cayyazo M, Abrego P, Guers L, Levine MM. Epidemiologic patterns of acute diarrhea and endemic Shigella infections in children in a poor periurban setting in Santiago, Chile. Amer. J. Epid. 1991:134:614-27.

36. Fine PEM, Clarkson J. Measles in England and Wales III: Assessing published predictions of the impact of vaccination on incidence. Int. J. Epidemiol. 1983:12:332-39.

37. Floyd TM, Higgins AR, Kader MA. Studies in shigellosis. V. The relationship of age to the incidence of Shigella infections in Egyptian children, with special reference to shigellosis in the newborn and in infants in the first six months of life. Amer. J. Trop. Med. 1956:5:119-30.

38. Fothergill LD, Wright J. Influenzal meningitis: relation of age incidence to the bactericidal power of blood against the causal organism. J. Immunol. 1993:24:273-84.

39. Fulginiti VA, Eller JJ, Donnei AW, Kempe CH. Altered reactivity to measles virus: atypical measles in children previously immunized with inactivated virus vaccines. JAMA. 1967:202:1075.

40. Gaines S, Currie JA, Tully JG. Production of incomplete Vi antibody in man by typhoid vaccine. Amer. J. Epid. 1965:81:350-5.

41. Gershon A, Steinberg SP, The National Institute of Allergy and Infectious Diseases Varicella Vaccine Collaborative Study Group. Live attenuated varicella vaccine: Protection in healthy adults compared with leukemic children. J. Infect. Dis. 1990:161:661-66.

42. Glezen WP, Lamb GA, Belden EA, Chin TDY. Quantitative relationship of preexisting homotypic antibodies to the excretion of attenuated poliovirus type 1. Am. J. Epidemiol. 1968:83:224-37.

43. Goldschneider I, Gotschlich EC, Artenstein MS. Human immunity to the meningococcus. I. The role of humoral antibodies. J. Exp. Med. 1969:129:1307-26

44. Gotschlich EC, Goldschneider I, Artenstein MS. Human immunity to the meningococcus. V. The effect of immunization with meningococcal group C polysaccharide on the carrier state. J. Exp. Med. 1969:129:1385-95.

45. Granstrom M, Olinder-Nielsen AM, Holmbad P, Marks A, Hanngren K. Specific immunoglobulin for treatment of whooping cough. Lancet. 1991:33:1230-2.

46. Gren KY, Taniguchi K, Mackow ER, Kapikian AZ. Homotypic and heterotypic epitope-specific antibody responses in adult and infant rotavirus vaccinees: implications for vaccine development. J. Infect. Dis. 1990:161:667-79.

47. Groothuis JR, Simoes EAF, Levin MJ. et al. Prophylactic Administration of Respiratory Syncytial Virus Immune Globulin to High Risk Infants and Young Children. N. Engl. J. Med. 1993:329:1524-1527.

48. Guirgis N, Schneerson R, Bax A, Egan W, Robbins JB, Shiloach J, Ørskov I, Ørskov F. *Escherichia coli* K51 and K93 capsular polysaccharides cross-reactive with Group A meningococcal polysaccharide. J. Exp. Med. 1985:162:1837-51.

49. Gupta RK, Robbins JB, Szu SC. Comparative immunogenicity of conjugates composed of *Escherichia coli* O111 O-specific polysaccharide prepared by treatment with acetic acid or hydrazine and bound to tetanus toxoid by two synthetic schemes. Infect. Immun. in press. 1995.

50. Hambleton P, Turnbull RCB. Anthrax vaccine development: a continuing story. *In* Bacterial Vaccines, Eds F.A. Liss, Inc. New York, NY 1990:105-22

51. Isacson J, Trollfors B, Taranger J, MacDowell I, Johansson J, Lagergård T, Robbins JB. Safety, immunogenicity and an open, retrospective study of efficacy of a monocomponent pertussis toxoid vaccine in infants. Pediatr. Infect. Dis. 1993:13:22-7.

52. Janeway CA, Rosen FS, Merler E, Alper CA. The gamma globulins. Little, Brown & Co., Boston. 1967.

53. Kampelbacher EH. On antigenic O-relationships between the Groups *Salmonella, Arizona, Escherichia* and *Shigella*. Antonie van Leeuwenhoek J. Micro. Serol. 1984:25:289-324.

54. Katz MA, Landesman SH, Schiffman G. A comparison of antibody concentration measured by mouse protection assay and radioimmunoassay in sera from patients at high risk of developing pneumococcal disease. Mol. Immunol. 1984:21:1061-65.

55. Konadu E, Robbins JB, Shiloach J, Bryla DA, Szu SC. Preparation, characterization and immunological properties in mice of *Escherichia coli* O157 O-specific polysaccharide-protein conjugate vaccines. Infect. Immun. 1994:62:5048-54.

56. Krugman S, Giles JP, Friedman H, Stone S. Studies on immunity to measles. J. Pediatr. 1965:66:471-88.

57. Levine MM, Ferreccio C, Black RE, Germanier R. Chilean Typhoid Committee. Large-scale field trial of Ty21a live oral typhoid vaccine in enteric-coated capsule formulation. Lancet, 1987:i:1049-52.

58. Levine MM. Immunity to cholera as evaluated in volunteers. Cholera and Related Diarrheas. 43rd Nobel Symposium. Stockholm 1978. Karger, Basel. Eds. O. Ouchterlony and J. Holmgren. 1980:195-203.

59. Levine MM, Tacket CO. Recombinant live cholera vaccines. In *Vibrio cholerae* and Cholera. Molecular to Global Perspectives. Eds. I.K. Wachsmuth, P.A. Blake, Ørjan Olsvik. American Society for Microbiology, Washington, DC. 1994:395-414

60. Lindberg AA, Haeggman S, Karlsson K, Dac Cam P, Du Trach D. The humoral antibody response to *Shigella dysenteriae* type 1 as determined by ELISA. Bull. W.H.O. 1984:62:597-606.

61. MacLeod CM, Hodges RG, Heidelberger M, Bernhard WG. Prevention of pneumococcal pneumonia by immunization with specific capsular polysaccharides. J. Exp. Med. 1945:82:445-65.

62. Mäkela PH, Herva E, Sibakov M, Henrichsen J, Luotonen J, Leinonen M, Timonen M, Koskela M, Pukander J, Gronroos P, Pontynen S, Karma P. Pneumococcal vaccine and otitis media. Lancet 1980:ii:547-51.

63. Meade BD, Kind PD, Manclark CR. Lymphocytosis-promoting factor of *Bordetella pertussis* alters mononuclear phagocyte circulation and response to inflammation. Infect. Immun. 1984:46:733-39.

64. Mosley WH. The role of immunity in cholera: A review of epidemiology and serological studies. Tex. Rep. Biol. Med. 1969:27:227-41.

65. Mosley WH, Woodward WE, Aziz KMA, Rahman ASMM, Chowdhury AKMA, Ahmed A, Feely JC. The 1968-1969 cholera-vaccine field trial in rural East Pakistan. Effectiveness of monovalent Ogawa and Inaba vaccines and a purified Inaba antigen, with comparative results of serological and animal protection tests. J. Infect. Dis. 1970:121:S1-S9.

66. Moxon R, Murphy PA. *Haemophilus influenzae* bacteremia and meningitis resulting from the survival of a single organism. Proc Natl Acad Sci USA. 1978:75:1534-6.

67. Neoh SH, Rowley D. The antigens of *Vibrio cholerae* involved in the vibriocidal action of antibody and complement. J. Infect. Dis. 1970:121:505-13.

68. Norrby E, Penttiten K. Differences in antibody to the surface components of measles after immunization with formalin-inactivated and live virus vaccines. J. Infect. Dis. 1978:138:672-80.

69. Ogra PL, Karson DT, Righthand R, MacGillivray M. Immunoglobulin response in serum and secretions after immunization with live and inactivated poliovaccine and natural infection. N. Eng. J. Med. 1968:279:883-900.

70. Ørskov I, Ørskov F, Jann B, Jann K. et al. Serology, chemistry, and genetics of O and K antigens in *Escherichia coli*. Bact. Rev. 1977:41:667-710.

71. Pappenheimer AM Jr. Diphtheria. In Bacterial Vaccines. Ed. Rene Germanier. Academic Press, NY, 1984:1-32.

72. Pappenheimer AM, Murphy JR. Studies on the molecular epidemiology of diphtheria. Lancet. 1983:2:923-25.

73. Peltola H, Mäkelä PH, Elo O, Pettay O, Renkonen OV, Sivonen A. Vaccination against meningococcal Group A disease in Finland 194-75. Scand. J. Infect. Dis. 1976:8:169-74.

74. Pierce NF, Reynolds HY. Immunity to experimental cholera. I. Protective effect of humoral IgG antitoxin demonstrated by passive immunization. J. Immunol. 1974: 113:1017-23.

75. Pittman M. Pertussis toxin: The cause of the harmful effects and prolonged immunity of whooping cough. A hypothesis. Rev. Infect. Dis. 1979:1:401-412

76. Prince GA, Horswood RK, Chanock RM. et al. Quantitative aspects of passive immunity to respiratory syncytial virus infection in infant cotton rats. J. Virol. 1985:55:517-20.

77. Provost PJ, Hilleman MR. Propogation of human hepatitis A virus in cell culture in vitro Proc Soc Exp Biol Med. 1978:160:213-21.

78. 1994 Redbook. Report of the Committee on Infectious Diseases. 1994. 23rd Edition, American Academy of Pediatrics, Rabies. 1994:383-95.

79. Redbook. Report of the Committee on Infectious Diseases. 1994. 23rd Ed, American Academy of Pediatrics, Tetanus, 1994:458-63.

80. Reynolds H, Thompson RE. Pulmonary host defenses. I. Analysis of protein and lipids in bronchial secretions and antibody responses after vaccination with *Pseudomonas aeruginosa*. J. Immunol. 1973:111:358-68.

81. Robbins JB, Chu CY, Schneerson R. Hypothesis for vaccine development: Protective immunity to enteric diseases caused by nontyphoidal *Salmonellae* and *Shigellae* may be conferred by serum IgG antibodies to the O-specific polysaccharide of their lipopolysaccharides. Clin. Infect. Dis. 1992:15:346-361

82. Robbins JB, Parke JC, Schneerson R, Whisnant JK. Quantitative measurement of "natural" and immunization-induced *Haemophilus influenzae* type b capsular polysaccharide antibodies. Pediat. Res. 1973:7:103-10.

83. Robbins JB, Pittman M, Trollfors B, Lagergård TA, Taranger J, Schneerson R. *Primum non nocere*: a pharmacologically inert pertussis toxoid alone should be the next pertussis vaccine. Pediatr. Infect. Dis. 1993:12:795-807.

84. Robbins, J.B., R. Schneerson and S.C. Szu. 1995. Persepctive: Hypothesis: Serum IgG antibody is suficient to confer protection against infectious diseases by inactivating the inoclum. J. Infect. Dis. 171: in press

85. Robbins JB, Schneerson R, Glode MP, Vann WF, Schiffer MS, Liu T-Y, Parke JC Jr. Huntley C. Cross-reactive antigens and immunity to diseases caused by encapsulated bacteria. J. All. Clin. Immunol. 1975:56:141-51.

86. Robbins JB, Schneerson R. Polysaccharide-protein conjugates: A new generation of vaccines. J. Infect. Dis. 1990:161:821-32.

87. Robbins JB. Towards a new vaccine for pertussis. In: Schlesinger, J., ed., Microbiology. Washington, DC.: American Society for Microbiology, 1994:176-83.

88. Robbins JD, Robbins JB. Re-examination of the immunopathogenic role of the capsular polysaccharide (Vi antigen) of *Salmonella typhi*. J. Infect. Dis. 1984: 47:436-99.

89. Salk D. Herd effect and virus eradication with use of killed poliovirus vaccine. Eds. W. van Henessenn. Develop. Biol. Stand. 1981:47:247-55.

90. Sato H, Sato Y. *Bordetella pertussis* infection in mice: correlation of specific antibodies against two antigen, pertussis toxin and filamentous hemagglutinin with mouse protective activity in an intracerebral or aerosol challenge system. Infect. Immun. 1984:46:415-21.

91. Sato Y, Ito A, Chiba J, Sato Y. Monoclonal antibody against pertussis toxin: Effect on toxin activity and pertussis infection. Infect. Immun. 1994:46:422-28.

92. Schneerson R, Barrera O, Sutton A, Robbins JB. Preparation, characterization and immunogenicity of *Haemophilus influenzae* type b polysaccharide-protein conjugates. J. Exp. Med. 1980:152:361-76.

93. Sellwood R, Hall G, Anger H. et al. Emigration of polymorphonuclear leucocytes in to the intestinal lumen of the neonatal piglet in response to challenge with K88-positive *Escherichia coli*. Res. Veter. Sci. 1986:40:128-35.

94. Shurin PA, Rehmus JM, Johnson CE. et al. Bacterial polysaccharide immune globulin for prophylaxis of acute otitis media in high-risk children. J. Pediatr. 1993:123:801-10.

95. Smith DH, Peter G, Ingram DL, Anderson P. Responses of children immunized with the capsular polysaccharide of *Haemophilus influenzae* type b. Pediatrics. 1975:52:637-41.

96. Springer GF, Horton RE, Forbes M. et al. Origin of anti-human blood group B agglutinins in white leghorn chicks. J. Exp. Med. 1959:110:221-44.

97. Sutter RW, PA Patriarca. Inactivated and live atttenuated poliovirus vaccines: mucosal immunity. In: Kurstak E. ed. Measles and poliomyelitis. Vaccines and immunisation. New York: Springer Verlag, 1993.

98. Syndman DR, Werner BG, Heinze-Lacey B. et al. Use of cytomegalovirus globulin to prevent cytomegalovirus disease in renal tranplant recipients. N. Eng. J. Med. 1987:317:1049-54.

99. Szu SC, Gupta RK, Robbins JB. Induction of serum vibriocidal antibodies by O-specific polysaccharide-protein conjugate vaccines for prevention of cholera. In *Vibrio cholerae* and Cholera. Molecular to Global Perspectives. Eds, Wachsmuth IK, Blake PA, Olsvik O. Washington, DC: American Society for Microbiology. 1994:381-94.

100. Szu SC, Taylor DN, Trofa AC, et al. Laboratory and preliminary clinical characterization of Vi capsular polysaccharide-protein conjugate vaccines Infect. Immun. in press. 1994.

101. Takala AK, Eskola J, Leinonen M, Kayhty H, Nissinen A, Pekkanen E, Makela PH. Reduction of oropharyngeal carriage of *Haemophilus influenzae* type b (Hib) in children immunized with an Hib conjugate vaccine. J. Infect. Dis. 1991:164:982-5

102. Taylor DN, Trofa AC, Sadoff J, Chu C, Bryla D, Shiloach J, Cohen D, Ashkenazi S, Lerman Y, Egan W, Schneerson R, Robbins JB. Synthesis, characterization, and clinical evaluation of conjugate vaccines composed of the O-specific polysaccharides of *Shigella dysenteriae* type 1, *Shigella flexneri* type 2a and *Shigella sonnei* (*Plesiomonas shigelloides*) bound to bacteria toxoids. Infect. Immun. 1994:61:3678-87.

103. Trollfors, B., J. Taranger, T. Lagergard, L. Lind, V. Sundh, G. Zackrisson, W. Blackwelder, C.U. Lowe and J. B. Robbins. 194. A double-blind, placebo-controlled trial of a monocomponent pertussis toxoid vaccine. Submitted for publication

104. Vann WF, Liu T-Y, Robbins JB. et al. *Bacillus pumilus* polysaccharide cross-reactive with meningococcal group A polysaccharide. Infect. Immun.1976:13:1654-62.

105. van Wezel AL, van Steenis G, Hannik CA, Cohen H. New approach to the production of concentrated and purified inactivated polio and rabies tissue culture vaccines. Dev. Biol. Stand. 1978:41:159-168.

106. Vialard J, LaLumiere M, Vernet T. et al. Synthesis of the membrane fusion and hemagglutinin proteins of measles virus, using a novel baculovirus vector containing the β-galactosidase gene. J Virol. 1990:64:37-50.

107. Wagner DK, Clements ML, Reimer CB, Synder M, Nelson DL, Murphy BR. Analysis of immunoglobulin G antibody responses after administration of live and inactivated influenza A vaccine indicates that nasal wash immunoglobulin G is a transudate from serum. J. Clin. Microbiol. 1987:25:559-62.

108. Waldmann TA, Strober W. Metabolism of immunoglobulins. Prog. Allergy. Karger S, Basel, 1969:13:1-110.

109. Watson DC, Robbins JB, and Szu SC, et al. Protection of mice against *Salmonella typhimurium* with an O-specific polysaccharide-protein vaccine. Infect. Immun. 1992:60:4679-86.

110. Weibel RE, Buynak EB, McLean AA, Roehm RR, Hilleman MR. Persistence of antibody in human subjects 7 to 10 years following administration of combined live attenuated measles, mumps and rubella virus vaccines. Proc. Soc. Exp. Biol. Med. 1980:165:260-3.

111. Wernet P, Breu H, Knop J, Rowley D. Antibacterial action of specific IgA and transport of IgM, IgA and IgG from serum into the small intestine. J. Infect. Dis. 1971:124:223-6.

112. Werzberger A, Mensch B, Kuter B. et al. A controlled trial of a formalin-inactivated hepatitis A vaccine in healthy children. N Eng J Med. 1993:327:453-7.

113. Wong KH, Barrera O, Sutton A. et al. Standardization and control of meningococcal vaccines, group A and group C polysaccharides. J. Biol. Stand. 1977:5:197-215.
114. World Health Organization Expert Committee on Biologic Standardization. Technical Report Series 840, 43rd Ed Geneva, Switzerland. Requirements on Vi polysaccharide for typhoid. 1993:14-32.
115. World Health Organization. Requirements for *Haemophilus* type b conjugate vaccines. WHO Technical Report Series, 1991:814.

23

THERAPEUTIC VACCINES

A Pandoric Prospect

R. E. Spier

University of Surrey
Guildford, United Kingdom GU2 5 XH

INTRODUCTION

The oxymoron "Therapeutic Vaccines" requires an explanation. The term has usage in the area of vaccines protective against cancer or autoimmune diseases; but what does it mean? Such an understanding may be derived from an elucidation of the definitions of the individual components of the expression followed by juxtaposing those expository terms to determine the sense of the oxymoronic expression.

WHICH SEEKS TO DEFINE A VACCINE

The first definition we have of a vaccine may be attributed to Edward Jenner who in 1799 used the word 'vaccine' as an adjective describing a special kind of disease, viz:

> The certainty that the having suffered the vaccine disease will prove a preservative for the infection of the smallpox.

But it was Louis Pasteur who, in 1881, in recognising the work of Jenner, generously suggested that any material that generated immunity could be considered to be a vaccine.

Vaccination: "The inoculation of an individual with any vaccine in order to induce or increase immunity". (Where the term 'immunity' derives from the Latin 'immunis,' which means exempt from a service or charge, and carries forward to the term 'immunes' or those members of the Roman army that were not required to do the fighting).

The relationship between Vaccine and Vaccination was clarified in the 1886 Oxford English Dictionary (OED) definition.

> A vaccine is 'vaccine matter used in vaccination'.

One hundred years later, the 1986 OED has a revised definition for our consideration:

> A preparation of the causative organisms or substance of a disease (or its products) that has been specially treated for use in vaccination.

Although this seems to be a modern enough definition it clearly does not take into account the situations when we want to protect against diseases such as cancer and

Novel Strategies in Design and Production of Vaccines
Edited by S. Cohen and A. Shafferman, Plenum Press, New York, 1996

autoimmune failures that are not contingent upon being infected with a causative organism. Hence we can modify this definition and come up with an expression:

A vaccine is a material that protects an organism against an infectious or non-infectious disease. (Where, for the sake of clarity, a disease is the state of an individual who is 'not at ease').

Were this to be maximally generalised, one might come up with a universal definition such as:

A vaccine is an entity used with the INTENT of *preventing* disease; a prophylactic: this is in contradistinction to a therapeutic which is an entity used with the INTENT of *curing* a disease.

This generalization brings into the vaccine net a wide variety of entities which may be construed as protecting the immune system so that the immune system can more effectively protect the person.

THE FENCE AROUND THE IMMUNE SYSTEM

It is a Jewish tradition to build a fence around the law for its protection. The provision that a Jew may not eat milk and meat at the same meal (Mishnah, Hullin 8.1) protects the more basic law given in the bible, that it is forbidden "to seethe a kid in the milk of its mother" (Exodus 23 v.19). So is it with the immune system. 'Fence Vaccines' may be seen to provide protection to the immune system in four ways: though the psyche, the stomach, the mind and through physical and chemical means (Figure 1).

Protection through Psychology

In 1988, Howard Weiner (Harvard Medical School) was able to write that the subject 'Psychoneuroimmunology....has come of age'. There is little doubt that mental stress is a predictor for bodily disease as well as being a disease of the mind. Such stress may be caused by confusion or disruption and is associated with an individual's realisation of a decrease in his/her ability to control his/her environment. To counter such disturbances different ethnic cultures have devised material objects to protect against 'evil influences'. Some consider the Phylacteries (Tefillin) as used by Jews to be one such talismanic protector (Ausubel,1964).

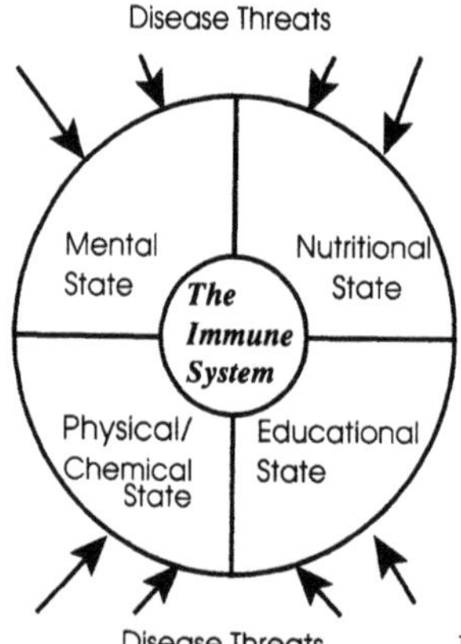

Figure 1. 'Fence Vaccines' protect the immune system.

Protection through Nutritional Status

Experiments with live type A Foot-and-Mouth disease vaccines in the late 1960s indicated that such vaccines caused disease outbreaks in cattle that were intensively stressed through lactation. (This experience heralded the end of live virus vaccines in this area). It has also been shown that the absence of Selenium in the diet predisposes individuals to infections diseases (Spinney, 1995). Notwithstanding such insults to the body, the lack of vitamins, iron, fluorine, iodine and olive oil have been held to predispose the body to particular disease states.

Educational State

Hygiene has been one of the most effective means of protecting the immune system against attack. Leora Brown (This Symposium) presents striking data showing that an effort to increase the hygienic activities of the residents of hotels in the Catskills was most effective in protecting such individuals from infection by the Hepatitis A virus. Indeed the improved sanitation and hygiene of the early 20th century has been held to have been the principle cause of the decrease in deaths due to tuberculosis; with the corollary that present increases in poverty and consequent decreases in hygiene is responsible for a resurgence of this disease.

In the strategies for the prevention of the transmission of the Human Immunodeficiency Virus (HIV), education (or propaganda) that encourages sexually active individuals to take protective measures when engaging in sexual activity has been an effective way of decreasing the rate of spread of this disease. It is not enough; but it does show how education can be included in the armamentarium of the vaccinilogist.

Physical/Chemical State

Protecting the body against invasion by microorganisms is an effective way of providing prophylaxis (Preston, 1994). The use of condoms, face masks, rubber gloves and biocontainment suites in specially designed laboratories under negative ambient pressures and fitted with cabinets and glove boxes is effective in protecting the immune system against a challenge it may fail to meet. On the other hand however there are a number of chemicals that, non-specifically, depress the immune system (cyclosporine, azathioprene, rapamycin and FK506). While others non-specifically stimulate it (superantigens of Staphylococcal enterotoxin B). Immunostimulants that are directed towards protection against a specific disease may be included in this category.

DEFINING THE THERAPEUTIC

The word therapeutic derives from the Greek 'Therapen' meaning; to minister, to treat medically. From this comes the designation of two classes of people: in Greece the Therapeutae were servants, ministers, or attendants, while in the Alexandria of Philo (born c. 10 CE) the same term delineated a Jewish sect practising their rituals at about 100 BCE. It is thought that the latter group were not progenitors of today's medical doctors but rather they were an ascetic gathering that gave up all their worldly possessions to serve, minister or attend to their god and the holy writ associated with that deity (Encyclopaedia Britannica, 1910).

Modern definitions culled from the OED have meanings such as: therapy is the branch of medicine which is concerned with the remedial (tending to relieve or redress) treatment of disease.

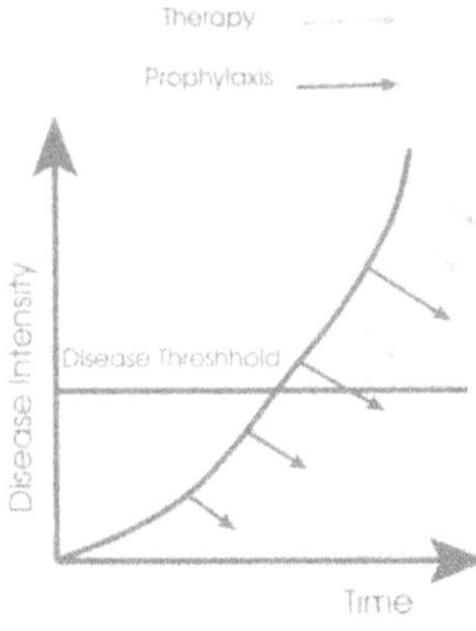

Figure 2. Therapy and prophylaxis juxtaposed.

There is little doubt that therapy involves the intent to cure starting from a situation when the patient is experiencing disease. Prophylaxis on the other hand can be applied with the intent of preventing the disease situation from worsening either before of after the recognition of being in a diseased state (Figure 2).

THE OXYMORON RESOLVED

We clearly cannot define a therapeutic vaccine as a material that prevents a disease it then heals. Nor can it be a material that heals a disease it then prevents. The term has come into existence to cover the area where we use a vaccine in those situations where once there was only the prospect of a cure and where presently we can foresee the use of agents that will prevent that disease from getting worse. As vaccines and the associated diagnostic capabilities improve to the point where vaccines can be applied before the patient reports to a physician or clinic, the term therapeutic vaccine will be dropped to be replaced by the normal expression; vaccine.

A partial listing of such therapeutic vaccines will illustrate these definitions:

- Post-exposure vaccines to infectious diseases: Rabies, Herpes, Ebola, Hepatitis B, Malaria
- Pre- or Post-exposure vaccines against diseases for which we previously only sought cures: Cancer, Diabetes, Myasthenia gravis, Atherosclerosis, Rheumatoid arthritis.
- Genetic diseases such as Cystic Fibrosis, Aminodeaminase deficiency; Pregnancy, Aging, Appearance.

A further listing of the kinds of diseases that can be approached through gene transfers are listed in Genetic Engineering News of April 15th 1994 on page 9.

THE PANDORIC PROSPECT

Pandora, the Greek Eve, has contested attributes. On the one hand the pantheon of gods gave her all the virtues; music, art, culture, beauty and hope while on the other hand she is held to be responsible for the unleashing of all the evils; plagues, gout, rheumatism, colic, envy, spite and revenge (Bulfinch,1864). Somewhere, a box (possibly belonging to the brother of Prometheus, Epimetheus) enters into the story, the opening of which floods the earth with the characteristics alluded to above. If we take Pandora to be the promulgator of both good and evil then it is clear that the prospect of therapeutic vaccines as depicted in the previous section can also be the purveyor of good and evil. We have but to consider the situation where an individual wishes to vaccinate himself/herself against some aspect of his/her appearance to realise that it is not just diseases of body that cause physical pain that are the target of the new and prospective therapeutic vaccines. Diseases of the mind that cause mental unease are just as likely to be the goals against which vaccines could be directed in the future.

To continue to make progress in this area it becomes increasingly necessary to have a clear view as to the ethics of what one is about. Ethics is the science (knowledge base) which underpins our understanding of what is right behaviour. (It is the Greek version of the Latin derived word, morals) (Spier,R.E., 1995). How then do we come to such understandings?

DETERMINANTS OF ETHICAL PRINCIPLES

Numerous authors have elucidated the different principles or schools of ethics. As yet it is not clear as to which of these principles is to be preferred in circumstances where different courses of action are predicated on the adoption of one or other of the different ethical schools. I have briefly summarised some of the main schools below;

- Utilitarianism; greatest benefit or happiness for the greatest number;
- Communitarianism; implies consensus on acceptability, often associated with democracy (which is power residing with the people);
- Casuistry; case law ethics; tradition;
- Kantian Categorical Imperative; do unto others as you would have others do unto you (also the Mosaic tradition; love your neighbour as yourself (Leviticus 19.18));
- Introspective; taking guidance from internally generated feelings (virtue);
- Theistic: the commands of a god and the associated holy writ with interpretations of such by priests;
- Biological: survive (varies as a function of time and situation).

In any particular situation, some of the approaches to ethics may concur as to how to proceed or what behaviour is to be adopted. However, there is clearly scope for disagreement by others who approach ethics from a non-consensus basis. For example; it is often argued that, as god created disease, it is inappropriate for mankind to gainsay the works of the creator by adopting such measures as therapy or prophylaxis to alleviate or prevent disease. The use of disease as a punishment by god for wrong-doing is not uncommon. It can also be argued that, as god gave mankind abilities and choice, it is incumbent upon mankind to improve the conditions for life by decreasing the incidence of disease. A third approach might be to deny the authority of gods and/or holy writ and proceed with the guidance that devolves from the acceptance of one of the other, non-theistic, schools of ethics.

Living in society we arrive at decisions about how to behave as a collective. Our elected representatives make decisions about whether or not a particular crime merits a death sentence or not. In some societies it is not lawful to not participate in elections while in others the representatives of the people determine policy with regard to the production and use of vaccines (therapeutic or otherwise). So there are circumstances when decisions are taken communally with which individuals do not agree. Under these conditions such dissenters may either swallow their pride and go along with the prevailing situation, emigrate to a society that is more in tune with their view of the way to behave or work with the other dissenting individuals to reverse the unpalatable decisions by use of the democratic process. It is generally regarded as ethically acceptable for individuals in a democratic society to have the opportunity to express their views (dissenting or consenting) via whatever communication media that society possesses. In keeping with this facility, this author holds that the use of our understandings of basic biology are not sufficiently used for the determination of the guidelines for our behaviour.

TOWARDS A BIOLOGY BASED ETHICS

Mankind made a quantum leap forward following the publication of the code of laws of Hamurabi (c.1600-1700 BCE), the Mosaic code (c.1300 BCE), the Justinian code (534 CE) and the Napoleonic code (1804). This author would contend that an equivalent step occurred following the publication of the Origin of Species by Charles Darwin on November 24th, 1859. Following the publication of this work the doctrine of the survival of the fittest as a result of the process of natural selection became a notion that was used by some nation states to determine how they conducted their internal affairs and external relationships. It led to the persecution of sectors of the workforce, the elevation of the capitalistic ethic, eugenic policies that forced individuals to become infertile and possibly even the development of concepts of master-races. But these were crude applications of Darwin's doctrines. Society is more complex and people more interdependent than would be envisaged on a simplistic application of the survival guideline. The creation in a society of a 'winners' and 'losers' situation is tantamount to the individuals in the society declaring war on one another. This is not the way modern societies can progress. Cooperation is also predicated in a survivalist ethics. Groups are often more successful at achieving their goal when the individuals within them cooperate. As communications systems advance both in terms of our abilities to transfer information as well as the movement of people to foreign countries where they can experience at first hand the products of an alternative lifestyle and ethical system, we realise that no one society or group has a monopoly on a universally acceptable ethic. This realisation makes us respectful of others and mindful that, whatever our present condition, there is room for improvement.

CONCLUSION

It is towards the objective of maintaining progress that we strive to improve our capabilities in the area of vaccines; that we develop new kinds of vaccines to take us into areas that were once monopolised by those who had but therapeutic solutions to offer. Such a transformation has ethical implications. It has been the purpose of this paper to emphasise the implications of this new condition, particularly where we need to examine our ethical principles to derive the guidelines that will enable us to handle the new prophylactic tools to our advantage. Such an examination might reconsider the teachings that could emerge from a more sophisticated and realistic appreciation of our biology. Indeed once having had our fingers burnt from a rather crude application of biological principles to human activities, it is difficult to 'turn back the clock' and go over old ground. Yet we are but living organisms, and it would be churlish to continue to neglect this avenue for enlightenment as to the elucidation of the nature of our condition and the way we should behave.

REFERENCES

Ausubel, N., 1964, The Book of Jewish Knowledge, Crown Publishers, Inc. New York 458-459

Bulfinch's Mythology, 1864, Spring Books (1967), London, 15

Encyclopaedia Britannica, 11th Edition (1910-1911) 26,793

Preston, R., 1994 The Hot Zone, Transworld Publishers, Inc.London

Spier, R.E.,1995, Science, Engineering and Ethics: Running Definitions, *Science and Engineering Ethics* 1,5-10

Spinney, L., 1995 Poor diets breed deadly viruses, New Scientist, 146,16

Weiner, H., 1988, Connecting up, *Nature* 335, 475

INDEX

Abortive infection, HIV, 85, 86
Acellular vaccines, 55–57
  combination, 127, 128
  mechanisms of protection, 173
  standardization of, 170
Acetylcholinesterase receptor (AChR), 3
N-Acetylmuramyl-D-alanyl-isoglutamine (MDP),
  2, 24, 25
Adenovirus, 87, 171
Adjuvanticity
  anti-influenza synthetic vaccines, 24–26
  Bacillus anthracis toxin mutant strains, 69–72
  dual, conjugate vaccines, 109, 110
Adjuvants
  built-in, 2
  cholera toxin and *E. coli* heat-labile enterotoxin,
    57–59
  combination vaccines, 109, 110, 130
  dimethyldioctadecyl ammonium bromide, 115–
    124
  HIV vaccines
    first-generation, 82
    peplotion, 101
  modulation of immune response, 105–111
    antibody response, 105–108
    controlled release delivery system, 106–108
    MHC classes, 109
    protein–polysaccharide conjugates, 109, 110
    T helper cells, 108, 109
  mucosal, 55–57
  polysaccharide conjugate vaccines, 137
ADP ribosylation
  cholera toxin and *E. coli* heat-labile enterotoxin,
    57
  pertussis toxin, 56
  toxoid vaccine design parameters, 61–66
AIDS vaccines: *see* HIV vaccines
Alphavirus expression systems, 31–39
  chimeras, 34, 35
  infections with cDNA clones, 34
  life cycle, 31–33
  replication and packaging-competent vectors,
    35, 36

Alphavirus expression systems (*cont.*)
  RNA replicons, 36, 37
  translational enhancer, 37, 38
  vaccine applications, 38, 41–46
Alphavirus hybrid virion vaccines, 41–46
  Salmonella as vector for Semliki Forest virus
    epitopes, 42, 43
  Sindbis virus presentation system, 42, 44–46
Aluminum adjuvants, 106, 107, 109
  combination vaccine design considerations, 130
  DDA comparison, 115–124
Amino acid copolymer (Cop-1), 2, 3
Ankara vaccinia virus, 7–11
Anthrax
  Bacillus anthracis toxin mutant strains, 69–72
  passive immunization, 172
  vaccines, 171
Antibody response
  adjuvants and, 105–111
    foot and mouth disease vaccines, 121, 123
    modulation of isotypes and subclasses, 108,
      110
    Newcastle disease vaccine, 119, 123
    rabies virus vaccines, 119, 123
    Semliki Forest virus vaccines, 117, 123
  Escherichia coli K12–*Shigella flexneri* hybrid
    vaccine, 161–163
  mechanisms of protective immunity, 172, 173
    mucosal IgG, 173
    passive, 171, 172
    serum IgG, 173
  priming with proteosomes, 25
  Pseudomonas aeruginosa exoprotein A-*Shigella*
    vaccines, 163–165
  standardization of vaccines, 170
Antigenic competition, 2
Antigenic drift, influenza virus, 50
Antigen presentation, *see also* MHC class I; MHC
    class II
  autoimmune processes, 2
  HIV, 99, 100
Antigens, synthetic, 1–4
Antitoxins, 175; *see also* Toxins/toxoids

Attenuated bacterial vaccines
  avirulent *Salmonella*, 15–20
  cholera, 74
  pertussis, 73
  Salmonella alphavirus hybrid virion vaccines,
    41–44
Attenuated virus vaccines
  alphavirus, 38, 41, 42, 44–46
  HIV, 83
  polio vaccines, 129, 171
  standardization, 170, 171
Autoimmune diseases, 2–4

Bacillus anthracis: see Anthrax
Bacillus Calmette Guerin (BCG) vaccine, 73, 74, 171
Bacterial pathogens, 171
  combination vaccines, 127–132, 128
    DTP: *see* DTP
    Shigella clinical trials, 159–165
  DNA vaccines, 51, 52
  mechanisms of protection, 173–175
  outer membrane proteins, meningococcal, 73–75
  toxins, *see* Toxins/toxoids
Bacterial polysaccharides: *see* Capsular polysaccha-
    rides; Capsular polysaccharide vaccines;
    Polysaccharide antigens
Bacterial vectors
  alphavirus vaccines, 41–44
  HBV vaccine, 16
  malaria, 17
BCG, 73, 74, 171
BHK/BRS cells, 142, 143, 145–148, 150
Bioreactors, influenza virus production, 148
Bordetella pertussis, 127, 128; *see also* DTP;
    Pertussis; Pertussis toxin; Pertussis vac-
    cines
  analysis, ELISA and flow cytometry, 153–
    157
  passive immunization, 172
  toxoid vaccine design parameters, 61–64
Botulism, 172

Canarypox vectors, 84
Cancer vaccines, 10, 11
Capsid protein: *see* Nucleocapsid proteins, virus
Capsular polysaccharides
  Gram-positive bacteria, 133–139
  mechanisms of protection, 172, 173
  *Haemophilus influenzae: see Haemophilus influ-
    enzae* type B conjugates
Capsular polysaccharide vaccines, 171
  epidemiological, clinical, and immunological
    data, 173, 174
  gram-positive organisms, 133–139
  standardization of, 170
CD1 molecules, HIV antigen presentation, 100,
    102, 103
cDNAs, alphavirus hybrids, 41–46
Cell culture, influenza virus production, 141–150

Cell-mediated immunity
  adjuvants and
    foot and mouth disease vaccines, 119–121,
      123
    Newcastle disease vaccine, 119, 120, 123
    rabies virus vaccines, 118, 119, 123, 119
    Semliki Forest virus vaccines, 117, 118, 123
  influenza virus and, 25, 26
Cellular vaccines: *see* Whole-cell bacterial vaccines
Chemical detoxification, pertussis toxin, 56
Chimeras, alphavirus, 34, 35
Chlamydia trachomatis, 75
Cholera toxin, 2
  genetic detoxification, 74
  vaccine design parameters, 62, 64–66
Cholera vaccines, 171
  attenuated and whole cell, 74
  mechanisms of protection, 174
  standardization of, 170
Clinical isolates
  HIV, first-generation vaccines, 81
  influenza virus production in cell culture, 141–
    150
Clinical trials, *Shigella* vaccines, 159–165
Combination vaccines
  development of, 127–132
    adjuvants, 130
    clinical evaluation, 130, 131
    excipients in, 129, 130
    manufacturing and regulatory issues, 131
    marketing, 131, 132
    safety, 131
  DTP: *see* DTP
  Shigella, 159–165
Competition, antigenic, 2
Complete Freund's adjuvant, 24, 107–109
  DDA comparison, 115–124
  in microsphere delivery systems, 107
  T helper cell modulation, 108, 109
Computer analysis, HIV proteins, 103
Conjugate vaccines
  dual adjuvanticity, 109, 110
  Gram-positive organisms, 133–139
  microsphere delivery systems, 107
  polysaccharide-protein, 74
  Shigella, 159–165
  standardization of, 170
Controlled release of antigens, 106–108
Cop-1, 2, 3
Corynebacterium diphtheriae: see Diphtheria;
    Diphtheria toxoid
Cross-reactivity, HIV, 96
Cytokines, 108, 110
Cytomegalovirus, 172
Cytotoxicity: *see* T cells

DDA: *see* Dimethyldioctadecyl ammonium bro-
    mide
Defective helper RNAs, 26, 27

Delivery systems, 105–111
Dendritic cells, HIV peplotion, 97–103
Diarrheal toxins, 57–59; *see also* Cholera toxin
Diet, 185
Dimethyldioctadecyl ammonium bromide (DDA),
    115–124
  foot and mouth disease virus vaccine adjuvants,
    121, 122
  Newcastle disease virus vaccine adjuvants, 121–
    123
  rabies virus vaccine adjuvants, 118, 119, 123
  Semliki Forest virus vaccine adjuvants, 116–
    118, 123
  toxicity and side effects, 122
Diphtheria, 2, 62; *see also* DTP
  mechanisms of protection, 175
  passive immunization, 171, 172
Diphtheria toxoid
  antibody response, 106, 108
  conjugate vaccine adjuvanticity, 110
  standardization of, 170
DNA vaccines, 49–52
  influenza, 49–51
  papilloma virus, 51
  tuberculosis, 51, 52
D toxoid, 128
DTP, 127, 171
  conjugate vaccine adjuvanticity, 110
  potential combination vaccines, 132

ELISA
  anthrax toxin, 70
  antibody response to toxoids, 107
  Bordetella pertussis analysis, 153–157
  capsular polysaccharide-specific antibodies, 136
  DNA vaccine assays, 50
  HIV epitope mapping, 93
Endotoxin, 74, 75; *see also* Lipopolysaccharide
Enteric pathogens
  mechanisms of protection, 174–176
  Shigella clinical trials, 159–165
  toxins, 57–59; *see also* Cholera toxin
Enterotoxinogenic *Escherichia coli*, 57–59
env, 84
Envelope, viral, *see also* Glycoproteins
  alphaviruses, 31, 33, 38
  DDA adjuvant-induced cell-mediated immune
    responses, 123
  HIV/SIV, 82, 84, 91–96
Epitope mapping, HIV, 92
Escherichia coli
  enteroinvasive, 174, 175
  enterotoxinogenic, 57–59, 61, 62
  K12–*Shigella flexneri* hybrid vaccine, 161–163,
    165
  outer membrane protein mutants, 75
Ethics, 187, 188
Excipients, in combination vaccines, 129, 130
Exoprotein A, 136, 163–165

Experimental allergic encephalomyelitis, 2, 3
Expression vectors: *see* Recombinant vaccines

Flow cytometry, *Bordetella pertussis* analysis, 153–
    157
Foot and mouth disease virus, DDA adjuvant, 121,
    122
Freund's complete adjuvant: *see* Complete Fre-
    und's adjuvant
gag, SIV, vaccinia virus vector, 9, 10
gag-pro, HIV vaccines, 84

Gene therapy, alphavirus systems, 31–39
Genetically engineered antigens: *see* Recombinant
    vaccines
Genetic toxoids, 74
  design parameters, 61–66
  pertussis toxin detoxification, 56, 57
Glycoproteins
  alphavirus envelope, 33, 34, 38
  HIV
    first-generation vaccines, 81, 82
    gp120, 80, 81, 91–96
    gp120/M77, 91–96
    gp160, 80, 100–102
Gram-positive bacteria, 133–139

Haemophilus influenzae type B conjugates, 74, 75,
    127, 128, 171
  adjuvanticity, 110
  microsphere encapsulation, 107
  standardization of, 170
Hemagglutination assays, 50, 56, 57
Hemagglutinin
  conjugate vaccine adjuvanticity, 110
  influenza virus
    alphavirus vectors, 35
    synthetic vaccines, 23–29
    vaccinia virus vectors, 8, 9
  pertussis vaccines, subunit, 73
Hepatitis A, 127
  combination vaccines, 127, 128
  mechanisms of protection, 175
  passive immunization, 172
Hepatitis B, 127
  combination vaccines, 127–129
  core antigen as carrier moiety, 15–20, 43, 44
  passive immunization, 172
Herd immunity, 174, 176
HIV vaccines
  changing paradigms, 79–88
    correlates of immunity, 87, 88
    first-generation vaccines, 80–82
    prevention of sexual transmission, 86, 87
    recovery from infection, 84–86
    sterilizing immunity, 80–83
  envelope proteins, 91–96
  peplotion, 97–103
  vaccinia virus vectors, 7, 9, 10

HLA: *see* MHC class I; MHC class II
Human immunodeficiency virus: *see* HIV
Human vaccines, adjuvants and delivery systems,
    105–111
Hybrid vaccines
    alphavirus, 41–46
    Shigella, 159–165
Hygiene, 185

Immune response
    DNA vaccine immunogenicity, 49–52
    modulation by adjuvants and delivery systems,
        105–111
Immunogenicity: *see* Antibody response; Cell-me-
        diated immunity
Immunoglobulin A, 87
Immunoglobulin G, 175; *see also* Antibody re-
        sponse
    HIV mucosal immunity, 87
    mechanisms of protective immunity, 173
Immunoglobulins
    adjuvant modulation of isotypes and subclasses,
        108, 110
    mucosal immunity, 87
Immunostimulants, 185
Inactivated bacterial vaccines, 73
Inactivated virus vaccines
    HIV, 83, 87
    mechanisms of protective immunity, 173, 175,
        176
    polio, 129
    standardization of, 171
Influenza vaccines, 171
    alphavirus vectors, 35
    DNA vaccines, 49–51
    standardization of, 170
    synthetic recombinant, 23–28
    vaccinia virus vectors, 8, 9
    virus production in cell culture, 141–150
        BHK/BRS cells, 142, 143, 145–148, 150
        MDCK cells, 142, 143, 145–148, 150
        reactor cultures, 143
        Vero cells, 142–148, 150
        virus purification, 143
Interdigitating dendritic cells, 97–103
Inulin, 108, 109
ISCOM, 101

Japanese encephalitis virus, 171

Killed whole bacterial vaccines, 73

Langerhans cells, HIV peplotion, 97–103
Latent genome, HIV, 98
Lipid moieties, HIV vaccines, 84
Lipopolysaccharide, 109
    mechanisms of protection, 172–175
    removal in OMV vaccines, 74, 75
Liposomes, 108, 109

Live virus vaccines
    alphavirus hybrid virion vaccines, 41–46
    HIV, 83
    polio, 129, 171
    vaccinia virus vectors, 7–11

MABAT, 120
Major histocompatibility complex: *see* MHC class
        I; MHC class II
Malaria vaccines, *Salmonella* expression, 15–20
Marketing, combination vaccines, 131, 132
MDCK cells, 142, 143, 145–148, 150
MDP (N-acetylmuramyl-D-alanyl-isoglutamine),
        2, 24, 25
Measles virus
    measles-mumps-rubella vaccine, 127, 129,
        171
    mechanisms of protection, 175, 176
    passive immunization, 172
    standardization of vaccines, 170
Mechanisms of action, *see* Protective immunity,
        mechanisms of
Meningococcal vaccines, 127, 171, 174
    conjugate, 74, 128
    outer membrane proteins, 73–75
    proteosomes, 25
MHC class I, 35
    adjuvant modulation, 109
    HIV antigen presentation, 99, 100
    HIV infection, 97, 98
    HIV peptides with motifs of, 102
MHC class II
    adjuvant modulation, 109
    autoimmune processes, 2–4
    BCG vaccine, 73
    HIV infection, 97
Microcarrier cultures, influenza virus production,
        148
Microspheres, 105–111
Mineral oil adjuvants, 120
Monoclonal antibodies, HIV envelope proteins, 91–
        96
Monophosphoryl Lipid A, 137
Moraxella catarrhalis, 75
Mucosal immunity
    bacterial toxins, 55–59
    cholera toxin and *E. coli* heat-labile enterotoxin,
        57–59
    HIV, prevention of sexual transmission, 86–
        88
    HIV vaccine model, 79–88
    mechanisms of, 173
    microsphere immunization, 107
    Salmonella expression systems, 19, 20
    Shigella clinical trials, 159–165
Multiple sclerosis, 2, 3
Multivalent serosubtype vaccines, 73–75
Mumps
    combination vaccines, 127–129

Mumps (*cont.*)
  passive immunization, 172
  vaccine standardization, 170
Muramyl dipeptide, 2, 24, 25
Mutagenesis, bacterial toxins, 55–57
  anthrax, 69–72
  pertussis, 56
  vaccine design parameters, 61–66
Mutant D toxin, 128
Myasthenia gravis, 3, 4
Mycobacterial infections
  BCG vaccine, 73, 74
  DNA vaccines, 51, 52
Myelin basic protein (MBP), 2, 3

Nasal immunization
  HIV, prevention of sexual transmission, 86, 87
  Salmonella expression systems, 20
nef, 83, 102
Neisseria gonorrhoeae, 75
Neisseria meningitidis, 127; *see also* Meningococcal vaccines
Newcastle disease virus, 121–123
Novasomes, 137
Nucleic acid vaccines, 49–52, 82
Nucleocapsid proteins
  alphavirus, 31, 33, 38
  influenza virus
    DNA vaccines, 49, 50
    synthetic vaccines, 23–28
    vaccinia virus vectors, 8, 9
Nutrition, 185

Oligonucleotides, influenza virus, 23–28
Optivant, 117, 118
Oral vaccines
  cholera, 74
  Escherichia coli K12–*Shigella flexneri*, 161–163, 165
  HIV, prevention of sexual transmission, 86, 87
  polio, 129
  Salmonella expression systems, 15–20
  typhoid, 74
Outer membrane proteins
  combination vaccines, 128
  meningococcal, 73–75

p195-212, 3, 4
p259-271, 3, 4
Pandora, 183–188
Papilloma virus, DNA vaccines, 51
Passive immunization
  Gram-positive bacterial infections (StaphGAM), 137–139
  mechanisms of protection, 175, 176
Passively acquired antibodies, 171, 172
Pediatric vaccinations, 128

Peptide antigens
  HIV
    antigen presentation by MHC class I molecules, 99, 100
    peplotion, 97–103
  versus polysaccharide antigens, 172, 173
Pertussis, *see also* DTP
  mechanisms of protection, 175
  passive immunization, 171, 172
Pertussis toxin
  genetic detoxification, 74
  production of *Bordetella pertussis*, 153–157
  vaccine design parameters, 61–64
Pertussis vaccines, 73
  combination, 127, 128
  killed whole-cell, 73
Plasmids, anthrax, 69
Plasmid transfer vector construction, 7
Plasmid vaccines, 49–52
Plasmodium, *Salmonella* expression systems, 15–20
PLGA microspheres, 107
Pneumococcal vaccines, 171
  conjugate, 74, 127, 128
  epidemiological, clinical, and immunological data, 173, 174
pol, 9, 10
Poliovirus
  combination vaccines, 127–129
  mechanisms of protection, 175
  mucosal delivery systems, 87
  passive immunization, 172
  standardization of vaccines, 171
Polyclonal antibodies, Gram-positive bacteria, 133–139
Poly-DL-alanine carrier, 1
Polynucleotide vaccines, 49–52
Polysaccharide antigens, 171
  conjugate vaccines, 74, 75
    dual adjuvanticity, 109, 110
    microsphere delivery systems, 107
    PRP (*Haemophilus influenzae* type B), 128
  epidemiological, clinical, and immunological data, 173, 174
  Gram-positive pathogens, 133–139
  mechanisms of protection, 172, 173
  versus protein antigens, 172, 173
  vaccine standardization, 170
  virus, *see also* Envelope, viral; Glycoproteins
Preservatives, combination vaccines, 129, 130
Primary isolates: *see* Clinical isolates
Primate models of HIV: *see* SIV
Process: *see* Production
Production
  Bordetella pertussis analysis, 153–157
  influenza virus, in cell culture, 141–150
Protective antigens
  alphavirus hybrid virion vaccines, 41–46
  anthrax toxin, 69

Protective immunity
  Bacillus anthracis toxin mutant strains, 69–72
  mechanisms of, 169–177
    attenuated versus inactivated organisms, 176
    epidemiologial, clinical, and immunological
      data, 173–175
    mucosal IgG, 173
    passively acquired antibodies, 171, 172
    polysaccharide versus protein antigens, 172, 173
    serum IgG-mediated prevention versus ther-
      apy, 173
    standardization of vaccines, 170, 171
    viral diseases, 175, 176
Protein antigens
  versus polysaccharide antigens, 172, 173
  virus nucleocapsid: *see* Nucleocapsid proteins
Protein-polysaccharide conjugates, adjuvanticity,
    109, 110
Proteosomes, influenza virus, 23–28
PRP (*Haemophilus influenzae* type B) combination
    vaccines, 128
Pseudomonas aeruginosa, 62, 74
Pseudomonas aeruginosa exoprotein A
  polysaccharide conjugate vaccines, 136
  Shigella vaccines, 163–165
Pseudovirion vaccines, HIV, 84
Public health, 185

Quality control assays, 131

Rabies virus, 171
  passive immunization, 172
  vaccines, DDA adjuvant, 118, 119, 123
Recombinant vaccines
  bacterial
    cholera toxin, 57, 64
    DNA vaccines, 49–53
    E. coli enterotoxin, 57–59
    outer membrane protein, 74, 75
    Pertussis toxin, 55, 61
    Salmonella, mucosal immunization, 15–20
    Shigella, 159–165
  viral
    alphavirus systems, 31–39, 41–46
    DNA vaccines, 49–53
    HBV, 15–20
    HIV, first-generation, 80
    influenza virus, 26–28
    vaccinia virus vectors, 8–10
Regulatory issues, combination vaccines, 131
rev, HIV, 102
Rift Valley Fever Virus, 34
RNA viruses: *see* Alphaviruses; Poliovirus; *spe-
    cific viruses*
Rotavirus, 175
Rubella vaccines, 171
  combination, 127–129
  standardization of, 170
Rubeola vaccines, 170

Salmonella typhi, 174, *see also* Typhoid; Typhoid
    vaccines
  passive immunization, 172
  standardization of vaccines, 170
Salmonella typhimurium, 175
  attenuated, alphavirus hybrid virion vaccines,
    41–44
  hepatitis core antigen expression in, 15–20
Semliki Forest virus
  adjuvants, DDA, 116–118, 123
  alphavirus expression systems, 31, 36
  hybrid virion vaccines, 41–46
Serosubtype vaccines, multivalent, 73–75
Serum IgG-mediated prevention versus therapy,
    173
Sexual transmission of HIV, prevention of, 86,
    87
Shigella
  clinical trials, 159–165
    Escherichia coli K12–*Shigella flexneri* hy-
      brid vaccine, 161–163
    Pseudomonas aeruginosa exoprotein A–
      Shigella vaccines, 163–165
  mechanisms of protection, 173–175
  structure and ADP ribosylation, 62
Simian immunodeficiency virus: *see* SIV
Sindbis virus
  alphavirus expression systems, 31–39
  hybrid virion vaccines, 41–46
Site-specific mutagenesis, toxoid vaccine design
    parameters, 61–66
SIV
  mucosal infection in primates, 87
  vaccinia virus vectors, 9, 10
SIV vaccines, 82–84
Skin HIV peplotion, 97–103
Smallpox vaccination, reactions to, 7, 8
Stabilizers, combination vaccines, 129, 130
Standardization of vaccines, 170, 171
StaphGAM, 137–139
StaphVAX, 136–139
Staphylococcus aureus, polysaccharide conjugate
    vaccines, 133–139
Stearyl tyrosine, 108, 109
Sterilizing immunity, HIV vaccines, 80–83
Stimulon, 137
Streptococci, Group B, 74
Streptococcus pneumoniae, 127, 128
Structure–function relationships, toxoid vaccine
    design parameters, 61–66
Subunit vaccines
  HIV, first-generation, 80
  pertussis, 73
Suppressed infection, HIV, 85, 86
Surface proteins, bacterial, 73–75
Syntex, 108, 109
Synthetic antigens
  influenza virus, 1–4
  outer membrane proteins, 74, 75

Synthetic vaccines, 1–4
  anti-influenza, 23–28
    built-in adjuvanticity, 24–26
    recombinant, 26–28
    synthetic peptides, 24
  Shigella, 159–165

Tailor made vaccine strains, 73–75
T cell epitopes, 24, 25, 35
T cells
  autoimmune processes, 3, 4
  CD4$^+$
    BCG vaccine, 73
    HIV infection, 97
    HIV vaccines, first-generation, 80
    vaccinia virus SIV antigen vectors, 10
  CD$^+$, HIV vaccines
    first-generation, 80
    peplotion, 97–103
  cytotoxic, 23
    HIV immunity, correlates of, 88
    HIV vaccine model, 79–88
    priming with proteosomes, 25
  helper, 24
    DNA vaccines, 49–52
    modulation by adjuvants, 108, 109
    priming with proteosomes, 25
Tetanus
  DTP: *see* DTP
  passive immunization, 171, 172
Tetanus toxoid
  antibody response, 106, 108
  conjugate vaccine adjuvanticity, 110
  microsphere administration, 107
Therapeutic vaccines, 183–188
TiterMax, 117, 118
Toxins/toxoids, 2
  anthrax, 69–72
  antibody response to toxoids, 108
  Bacillus anthracis toxin mutant strains, 69–72
  cholera, 57–59
  conjugate vaccines
    adjuvanticity, 110
    microsphere delivery systems, 107
  enterotoxinogenic *Escherichia coli*, 57–59, 61, 62
  genetic detoxification, 74
  mechanisms of protection, 174, 175
  passive immunization, 171, 172
  pertussis, 55–58
  structure–function correlations, 65, 66
  vaccine design parameters, 61–66
    cholera, 62, 64, 65
    pertussis, 61–65
Translational enhancer, alphavirus, 37, 38

T toxoid, 128
Tuberculosis
  BCG vaccine, 73, 74
  DNA vaccines, 51, 52
Tumor cell vaccines, 10, 11
Typhoid
  mechanisms of protection, 174
  passive immunization, 172
Typhoid vaccines, 171
  attenuated and whole cell, 74
  standardization of, 170

Vaccines, *see also specific pathogens and toxins*
  development of, 127–132
  standardization of, 170, 171
Vaccinia virus
  Ankara, 7–11
  HIV vaccines, second-generation, 84
Varicella virus, 127, 128, 171
  mechanisms of protection, 175
  passive immunization, 172
Vectors: *see* Recombinant vaccines
Veiled dendritic cells, 97–103
Venezuelan equine encephalitis virus, 31, 36
Vero cells, 142–148, 150
Vibrio cholerae
  mechanisms of protection, 174, 175
  standardization of vaccines, 170
  toxoid vaccine design parameters, 62, 64–66
Viral vaccines, 171
  adjuvants
    DDA, 115–124
    dimethyldioctadecyl ammonium bromide, 115–124
  alphavirus, 41–46
  combination, 127–132, 128
  DNA vaccines, 49–51
  HBV, 15–21
  HIV: *see* HIV
  influenza: *see* Influenza vaccines
  mechanisms of protective immunity, 175–176
  polio: *see* Poliovirus
  standardization of, 170, 171
Viral vectors: *see* Recombinant vaccines, viral
Virulence factors, 135, 136
vpu, HIV, 102

Whole-cell bacterial vaccines, 73, 74, 176
  Bordetella pertussis analysis, 153–157
  killed, 73
  standardization of, 170
Whole-inactivated virus: *see* Inactivated virus vaccines

GPSR Compliance
The European Union's (EU) General Product Safety Regulation (GPSR) is a set
of rules that requires consumer products to be safe and our obligations to
ensure this.

If you have any concerns about our products, you can contact us on

ProductSafety@springernature.com

In case Publisher is established outside the EU, the EU authorized
representative is:

Springer Nature Customer Service Center GmbH
Europaplatz 3
69115 Heidelberg, Germany